D0553848

# CLINICIAN'S GUIDE TO BIPOLAR DISORDER

# Related Guilford Titles

## FOR PROFESSIONALS

*Bipolar Disorder, Second Edition:*
*A Family-Focused Treatment Approach*
David J. Miklowitz

*Understanding Bipolar Disorder:*
*A Developmental Psychopathology Perspective*
Edited by David J. Miklowitz and Dante Cicchetti

## FOR GENERAL READERS

*The Bipolar Disorder Survival Guide, Second Edition:*
*What You and Your Family Need to Know*
David J. Miklowitz

*The Bipolar Teen: What You Can Do*
*to Help Your Child and Your Family*
David J. Miklowitz and Elizabeth L. George

# Clinician's Guide to
# BIPOLAR DISORDER

## Integrating Pharmacology and Psychotherapy

**David J. Miklowitz**
**Michael J. Gitlin**

THE GUILFORD PRESS
New York          London

© 2014 The Guilford Press
A Division of Guilford Publications, Inc.
72 Spring Street, New York, NY 10012
www.guilford.com

All rights reserved

Except as indicated, no part of this book may be reproduced, translated, stored in a retrieval system, or transmitted, in any form or by any means, electronic, mechanical, photocopying, microfilming, recording, or otherwise, without written permission from the publisher.

Printed in the United States of America

This book is printed on acid-free paper.

Last digit is print number:   9   8   7   6   5   4   3   2   1

LIMITED PHOTOCOPY LICENSE

These materials are intended for use only by qualified mental health professionals.

The publisher grants to individual purchasers of this book nonassignable permission to reproduce all materials for which photocopying permission is specifically granted in a footnote. This license is limited to you, the individual purchaser, for personal use or use with individual clients. This license does not grant the right to reproduce these materials for resale, redistribution, electronic display, or any other purposes (including but not limited to books, pamphlets, articles, video- or audiotapes, blogs, file-sharing sites, Internet or intranet sites, and handouts or slides for lectures, workshops, webinars, or therapy groups, whether or not a fee is charged). Permission to reproduce these materials for these and any other purposes must be obtained in writing from the Permissions Department of Guilford Publications.

The authors have checked with sources believed to be reliable in their efforts to provide information that is complete and generally in accord with the standards of practice that are accepted at the time of publication. However, in view of the possibility of human error or changes in behavioral, mental health, or medical sciences, neither the authors, nor the editors and publisher, nor any other party who has been involved in the preparation or publication of this work warrants that the information contained herein is in every respect accurate or complete, and they are not responsible for any errors or omissions or the results obtained from the use of such information. Readers are encouraged to confirm the information contained in this book with other sources.

**Library of Congress Cataloging-in-Publication Data**

Miklowitz, David Jay, 1957–
    Clinician's guide to bipolar disorder : integrating pharmacology and psychotherapy / David J. Miklowitz, Michael J. Gitlin.
        pages cm
    Includes bibliographical references and index.
    ISBN 978-1-4625-1559-2 (hardcover)
    1. Manic–depressive illness—Treatment.  2. Psychotherapy.  3. Psychopharmacology.
I. Gitlin, Michael J.   II. Title.
    RC516.M555 2014
    616.89′14—dc23
                                                                        2013045284

*To our patients—past, present, and future—*
*who have taught us at least as much*
*as we have taught them*

# About the Authors

**David J. Miklowitz, PhD,** is Professor of Psychiatry at the University of California, Los Angeles (UCLA), School of Medicine and Senior Clinical Researcher at the University of Oxford, United Kingdom. He directs the Child and Adolescent Mood Disorders Program and the Integrative Study Center in Mood Disorders at the UCLA Semel Institute. Dr. Miklowitz is a recipient of the Distinguished Investigator Award from the National Alliance for Research on Schizophrenia and Depression, the Mogens Schou Award for Research from the International Society for Bipolar Disorders, the Bipolar Mood Disorder Research Award from the Brain and Behavior Research Foundation, and the Gerald L. Klerman Senior Investigator Award from the Depressive and Bipolar Support Alliance. His numerous publications include *Bipolar Disorder, Second Edition: A Family-Focused Treatment Approach* and the bestselling self-help resource *The Bipolar Disorder Survival Guide, Second Edition: What You and Your Family Need to Know.*

**Michael J. Gitlin, MD,** is Professor of Clinical Psychiatry at the UCLA School of Medicine, where he is Director of the Adult Division in the Department of Psychiatry. He is also Director of the Mood Disorders Clinic at the UCLA Neuropsychiatric Hospital. Dr. Gitlin is the author of many scientific articles and book chapters as well as two editions of *The Psychotherapist's Guide to Psychopharmacology.* His awards include the Distinguished Educator Award from the UCLA Department of Psychiatry, the Teacher of the Year Award from *Psychiatric Times,* the Dadone Clinical Teaching Award from the Geffen School of Medicine at UCLA, and the Leonard Tow Humanism in Medicine Award from the Arnold P. Gold Foundation.

# Preface

Writing this book has been a labor of love—labor because it takes concentrated time and effort to write a book while also seeing patients, writing grants, lecturing, supervising, and serving as administrators; and love because this work reflects our combined 60-plus years of interest, knowledge, and experience in an area to which we are both passionately and deeply committed. It also reflects our strong beliefs regarding the value of integrating psychopharmacology and psychotherapy.

We have had throughout our careers wonderful mentors and colleagues who have helped us refine our thinking, ask better questions, and pursue deeper and more accurate answers. They include Dr. Michael Goldstein, who is no longer with us, as well as Drs. Kay Jamison, Connie Hammen, Lori Altshuler, Ira Lesser, Mark Frye, Ellen Frank, David Kupfer, David Axelson, Kiki Chang, Chris Schneck, and Boris Birmaher. We are indebted to our chairman, Professor Peter Whybrow, for his leadership in bipolar disorder research and scholarship for two generations. Our thanks to Melissa Baird for her cheerful competence in constructing tables and coordinating references. We are deeply grateful to our students and to Kitty Moore at The Guilford Press, who encouraged us to write this book and provided sound editorial advice.

David J. Miklowitz has been fortunate to have had wonderful graduate students, postdoctoral fellows, and psychiatric colleagues who have been central in his clinical work and research, both at UCLA and formerly at the University of Colorado. For Michael J. Gitlin, over 30 years of teaching residents at UCLA, especially in the Mood Disorders

Clinic, have been invaluable in sharpening his thinking about this fascinating and troubling disorder. Of course, we are both grateful to have met and begun working together at UCLA over 30 years ago, and for the wonderful friendship that has emerged.

Last, but not least, we would like to thank our (very patient) wives—Mary and Jeanie—and our children—Ariana, Josh, Katie, and Rebecca.

DAVID J. MIKLOWITZ, PhD
MICHAEL J. GITLIN, PhD

# Contents

# CHAPTER 1

## An Integrated Approach to Bipolar Disorder

---

When Drew consulted our mood disorders clinic, he complained of depression, anxiety and suicidal thinking. Only 35 years old, he was on his third marriage and it had followed a pattern like all the others: Relationships were exciting and lively at the beginning, full of "great sex, all night conversations, and the feeling we could be anything we wanted to be." Within 6 months after each wedding, however, Drew would grow increasingly depressed and anxious. Many explanations were offered by the various therapists Drew consulted, including seasonal depression (even though his depression had not followed the seasons), "anniversary reactions" to his father's death, and, in one case, "buyer's remorse."

Drew, who was trying to get work as an actor in the highly competitive Los Angeles entertainment industry, felt that his depressive episodes coincided with losing out on a movie role or finding out that a friend had done better than he had. He felt they had little to do with his marriages. His most recent breakup illustrated a pattern that occurred in several of his prior marriages. After losing out in a string of auditions, he grew despondent and withdrawn. His wife attempted to cheer him up by reassuring him that she loved him and that he would get back on his feet. But after enduring a year of his sullenness, irritability, disinterest in sex, and suicidal threats, she said she would leave him unless he sought help. As he described it, the pressure from his wife made things much worse because "having my arm twisted into therapy is never a good beginning." He felt that most of the individual and couple therapists he (and his spouses) had consulted over the years were "charlatans" who gave "cookie cutter advice."

Despite having had multiple evaluations with various general practitioners and psychiatrists, Drew never believed that he had received a proper diagnosis. He had seen a counselor in high school because of "the usual adolescent mood swing stuff" and a psychologist for a few sessions in college because of anxiety. In fact, he felt it was his anxiety that had led him to drop out of

1

school. Most of these clinicians had told him he had depression, and some also suggested an anxiety disorder. Attention-deficit/hyperactivity disorder (ADHD) had been put forth by others. One had suggested that he had a narcissistic personality disorder, adding that "it may work well for you in the acting business." One called him "depressed with bipolar tendencies" but did not elaborate on what that meant.

Following the advice of his third wife, a nurse, Drew met with an outpatient psychiatrist who recommended trials of various medications, including lithium (Eskalith), valproate (Depakote), quetiapine (Seroquel), and a "cocktail that mixed them all together." He did not respond well to any of these agents, and typically tried them for only a week or two, after which his depression usually worsened. Then, a new psychiatrist, convinced that his problems were all due to a "biogenic depression," had recommended magnetic resonance imaging (MRI). Although the imaging results were inconclusive, the doctor had suggested that Drew discontinue all the other agents and try escitalopram (Lexapro) and methylphenidate (Ritalin) together. She also suggested he participate in Saturday morning group support sessions, which he attended only once, describing his fellow patients as "the clown brigade." Escitalopram and methylphenidate made him feel better at first and gave him more energy, but then "I couldn't sleep, I was nervous, angry as hell . . . it made me worse." He continued to feel anxious, fearful, irritable, and fatigued, and his thoughts began to speed up. He eventually stopped escitalopram and never went back to this psychiatrist, although he continued to take methylphenidate and began "doctor shopping" to renew his prescriptions. When he consulted our clinic, he was in a depressive episode that required hospitalization and a full reevaluation of his treatment.

## OBJECTIVES OF THIS BOOK

Certainly, not all people with bipolar disorder receive the chaotic care that Drew received, but in our experience, his story is not unusual. On average, patients have 8–10 years of illness before they get the correct diagnosis, and many go even longer before finding an effective medication regimen.[1] Many report that they have never had any targeted or individualized psychotherapy related to their disorder, even if they have found therapists they liked. Some report little or no integration among the various treatments they have received; their medications have been dispensed by a general practitioner (GP) or a psychiatrist with minimal expertise in bipolar disorder, with follow-up appointments every 3 months. Their therapist, usually a practitioner in a different clinic, may have never spoken with their psychiatrist or GP, and rarely have any of the practitioners ever spoken to family members (often on purpose because they view the confidentiality of psychiatric treatment to be unassailable).

## Personalized and Integrated Treatment

*A key theme of this book is that the treatment of bipolar disorder must be individualized in an ongoing collaboration with each patient.* Our combined experience of over 60 years of working with people with bipolar disorder has convinced us that each treatment regimen, whether pharmacological or psychosocial, must involve careful planning to fit the needs of the individual. Moreover, it is critical to have a dialogue with the patient about the factors in the immediate milieu that play a role in the mood swings.

For most patients, a healthy balance of pharmacotherapy and psychotherapy are developed as an integrated and individualized plan. As shown repeatedly in the research literature, the integration of targeted forms of psychotherapy with pharmacotherapy enhances outcomes in functional as well as symptomatic domains.[2] To implement personalized treatment, there must be a number of factors in place: (1) an ongoing dialogue about treatment goals between the clinician and the patient; (2) ongoing communication between the physician and therapist (assuming that the patient is receiving both medication and psychotherapy and that the two clinicians are separate individuals), with each provider facilitating the goals of the other's treatment; and (3) flexibility over time, with the acknowledgment that the patient's needs will change over the course of treatment.

In individualizing pharmacological interventions, many factors need to be considered. A patient's history with certain medications (positive or negative), plus his lifestyle, economic resources, and support network, almost always influence what treatments are prescribed and when. Thus, a patient involved in a stressful relationship will often need a different medication regimen (or different dosages) than a patient who has a supportive partner. A cognitively disabled patient with a complex medication regimen will surely need support from family members to comply with the prescribed treatment. Ideally, Drew's psychiatrist would have designed an approach not only to treat his bipolar disorder, which was clearly the appropriate diagnosis, but one that also considered his dislike of medications and general mistrust of psychiatry, and the relationship problems and other situational factors contributing to his course of illness. Given his interest in an acting career, it might have meant avoiding medications that cause weight gain, even though some of them (e.g., quetiapine) would probably stabilize his mood. And it certainly would have included establishing a strong therapeutic alliance to encourage his collaboration in his own treatment.

In terms of the type of psychotherapy to offer, this, too, will vary depending on the patient's circumstances—his age, the degree to which current family or spousal relationships are problematic, recent events (e.g., loss experiences or work problems), and the patient's working knowledge of how to cope with bipolar disorder. The type and intensity of therapy may also change over time as a function of changing illness states or emergent life events, during periods in which medications are changing, or when the patient has discontinued all medications.

Why place so much emphasis on psychotherapy? As Drew's story illustrates, the functional consequences of bipolar illness are as important as the frequency or severity of symptoms. Bipolar disorder has wide-ranging effects on a patient's school, work, social, or family life, even when the patient is on an optimal medication regimen. Many patients remain functionally impaired even when only minimally symptomatic.[3] Despite the difficulties inherent in measurement of functioning, clinicians must be attuned to the specific effects of the illness on the patient's quality of life and, furthermore, to the factors that may contribute to poor functioning, including unremitting depressive symptoms, cognitive impairment, loss of social supports, or adverse reactions to medications.

### Treatment as a Moving Target

The treatment of bipolar disorder is a moving target and needs to be continually reassessed and revised as the patient's symptoms and life circumstances change. Yet many patients with bipolar disorder say that they have been repeatedly given the same treatments in the ill-conceived hope that eventually they will respond. If their practitioner has changed any aspect of treatment, it has generally been to increase the dosage of a given medication or substitute another in the same class. Likewise, psychotherapists have been known to stick to the same treatment well after it is clear that the patient is stalled. *A second major theme in this book is the need to continually reevaluate a patient's situation—his symptoms, level of improvement, and functional capacity—such that treatment plans can be adjusted accordingly.* Sometimes the best course of action is to stop a treatment rather than introduce a new one; in other cases, it may involve using novel pharmacological agents or introducing behavioral plans such as sleep–wake cycle regulation.

## The Role of the Family

When we asked Drew to tell us more about his experiences with psychotherapy, he grimaced. He had found insight-oriented individual therapy to be somewhat helpful, but he stopped after 6 weeks, saying "I got what I could out of the lady." He explained that his marital treatments were focused only on "things we could do to be nicer to each other." He felt particularly humiliated by an in-session exercise in which he was asked to rub his wife's back for 3 minutes whenever she said something that made him feel more confident about his acting career.

Drew's third wife, a nurse, had significant medical knowledge and was the first to suggest that he might respond to mood stabilizers. She encouraged him to put his work away and be in bed by midnight. Yet when Drew worsened (writing lengthy letters of introduction to movie directors, then trying to reach them well into the night) and she tried to contact his psychiatrist, the doctor never returned her calls. When Drew asked the psychiatrist about this, she explained that Drew had never given her permission to talk with his wife. Eventually, the psychiatrist invited Drew's wife in for a consult, but insisted that Drew not be present, to allow his wife to talk freely. Drew felt alienated by this encounter, which contributed to his decision to quit taking his medications.

In addition to the "one-size-fits-all" quality of his prior treatment experiences, none of Drew's treatment had involved *psychoeducation*. None of his clinicians had discussed the possibility that he had bipolar disorder, or explored the genesis of his depression or its effects on his relationships. Of course, milder cases of bipolar disorder can be easily missed by even the most experienced clinicians. Often, depression dominates the clinical picture to the extent that periods of hypomania or subthreshold mixed symptom states are missed.

In our view, the clinician should view the bipolar patient's interpersonal problems within the context of the symptoms of the disorder. For example, knowing that a patient tends to behave aggressively and be self-absorbed when hypomanic may help us to understand why he has recently lost his job, even though he might see and explain things quite differently. Marital or relational conflicts may have different implications if they only emerge during depressive episodes and resolve during periods of remission.

This brings us to the third theme of this book: *Family members are integral members of the treatment team*. They provide information critical to making the initial diagnosis. Moreover, they are often the first to notice changes in the patient's mood or behavior, and can therefore help prevent worsening of manic or depressive symptoms. They can offer immeasurable help in maintaining the patient's consistency with the treatment regimen. For example, they can help to ensure the bipolar person maintains regular daily routines and sleep–wake cycles. They may describe instances of medication nonadherence that the patient has either forgotten or thinks are insignificant.

Family members are often quite willing to give input into their relative's treatment, and are often bewildered by mental health professionals' seeming lack of interest. Throughout this book, we provide examples of how best to engage family members, so that they become allies in the treatment; how and when to set limits with them; and ways to make their involvement both palatable and helpful to patients.

## HOW IS THIS BOOK DIFFERENT FROM ANY OTHER BIPOLAR BOOK?

Books on bipolar disorder have proliferated. Amazon.com lists over 100 books on the disorder, including first-person accounts; self-care books for patients, parents, or spouses; books about bipolar children or teens; managing bipolar disorder during pregnancy; and a host of "how-to" books for clinicians. Some of these books are clearly designed for psychopharmacologists, and others equally clearly are for psychotherapists. What has been missing is a clinically useful integration of pharmacology and psychotherapy as the foundation for treatment, including a realistic appraisal of the complexities of these interventions and what to do in specific situations.

What you do find in these books, for example, are discussions of medications, set out one by one. There is a chapter on lithium, one on valproate or carbamazepine, another on lamotrigine, one on antipsychotics, and one on "novel agents." These books usually survey the clinical trial literature on acute efficacy (e.g., how many studies have shown that the drug, when used as a monotherapy, does better than placebo in stabilizing a manic or depressive episode). We realize the importance of such reviews to an academic audience, but practicing clinicians may not find them useful. Although at times psychiatrists may have to decide among medications to treat patients' acute episodes, more often they seek information on what to do in very specific clinical situations. For example, they want to know how to consider the treatment options for bipolar I depression versus bipolar II depression—when to introduce changes, and how to make adjustments correctly. What these books miss, then, is helping clinicians resolve critically important treatment questions:

What combination of medications should a clinician choose for a particular patient in an acute episode?

In what order should they be given and at what starting dosage?

How does the clinician adjust this regimen if symptoms worsen, or if the patient switches into the opposite polarity?

What is the protocol when weaning patients off certain agents as they recover?

Clinicians often need to weigh cost–benefit ratios between side effects and efficacy at different points in the illness. They may want to know more about ways to prevent recurrence in a patient with subsyndromal symptoms than about how to stabilize an acute manic episode. In this book, our goal is to provide much-needed advice on how to make treatment decisions at different change points in the illness, based as much as possible on the available literature—what the science tells us and what it does not—and on our own experiences from treating numerous patients.

Most existing books on bipolar disorder address psychotherapy in a single chapter in which different treatment models (interpersonal therapy, family therapy, cognitive-behavioral therapy, or group psychoeducation) and their supporting evidence are reviewed. Although it can be useful to compare and contrast the models now in use, there are few studies that directly test these methods against each other or try to match patients to treatments. Other books focus on only one psychotherapy method and take the reader, chapter by chapter, through that type of therapy.

Most clinicians do not have the time or the resources to obtain extensive training in manual-based psychotherapies. Moreover, in our experience, clinicians want training in *strategies* as opposed to lockstep manualized treatments. These strategies cut across psychotherapeutic (i.e., psychodynamic, cognitive-behavioral, or interpersonal) models. For example, they seek ways to educate patients and family members about bipolar disorder; to help patients identify the early warning signs of recurrence and coach them on what to do when these appear; to assist them in coping with stressors that elicit symptoms; to clarify or challenge the patient's thinking about medications; or to counsel the patient about substance abuse. Indeed, adapting these principles of evidence-based psychotherapy and putting them into treatment individualized to the patient is both feasible for the clinician and beneficial to patients. Learning about these strategies involves borrowing from the literature on specific psychotherapies and focusing on common elements. In this book, we emphasize common and effective psychotherapy strategies and how to time them to address the challenges of different stages of illness.

Finally, most of the existing books do not consider the heterogeneity of illness presentations with which clinicians in community mental health settings deal daily. Many clinicians do not see patients in an acute manic state. Most patients seek treatment because of subthreshold depressive or mixed states, or because they are functioning at a low level even though their symptoms do not appear to be severe. Some patients are chronically hypomanic, with occasional periods of depression, or they straddle the line between bipolar disorder and borderline personality disorder. Others may follow a bipolar illness course, but their real problems have more to do with anxiety.

In this book, we provide numerous cases of patients with a wide variety of clinical presentations. These examples illustrate the complexity of the illness, as well as the principles to follow when deciding what to do and when to do it. We offer ways to think about complex or highly comorbid patients from a longitudinal perspective, with changing treatment targets. There are suggestions on how to prioritize pressing concerns (e.g., suicidality) that may take precedence over other mood symptoms, and how to revise these priorities as the patient improves. It is our hope in presenting these examples that clinicians will be able to generalize the recommended approaches to the majority of patients in their practices.

We base our recommendations for clinical diagnosis and treatment on research evidence whenever possible. However, we have opted to use representative references on a given topic rather than an exhaustive list of references, or extensive comparisons of studies that went about addressing the same question differently. The reader who is well acquainted with the bipolar literature may at times wonder why we cite one study instead of another. Although we acknowledge the limitations inherent in noncomprehensive reviews, we believe that our approach improves accessibility and readability while maintaining our dedication to evidence-based practice. When appropriate, we refer the reader to comprehensive reviews of the literature on specific topics.

Given that we are writing this book for practicing psychotherapists *and* psychopharmacologists, we realize that readers will differ in the level of detail and amount of information they want or need. Psychopharmacologists may focus more on the details of constructing a pharmacological treatment plan for acute mania or hypomania, while psychotherapists may want more detail about the psychotherapeutic strategies during maintenance treatment. Yet given our belief that treatment needs to be well integrated, we believe it would be helpful to peruse the entire volume.

Additionally, we assume that readers will differ in their familiarity with some of the technical language used, especially with regard to medication names and side effects. In general, whenever we introduce a medication in a chapter, we use its generic name, with its more commonly known trade name in parentheses, as in "fluoxetine (Prozac)." Thereafter, the medication is referred to by its generic name only. If that same medication is referred to in another chapter, both names are again provided. Appendix B is a table that provides both generic and trade/proprietary names for easy reference. It is a comprehensive list of all medications relevant to the treatment of bipolar disorder.

Similarly, some side-effect names—such as dry mouth—are self-explanatory. Others, such as agranulocytosis—when the bone marrow stops making white blood cells—require explanation and are provided for those readers unfamiliar with these terms.

A word about gender terminology: We refer to the patient as "he" in some places and as "she" in others. We realize this can be confusing, but we find referring to each patient as "he or she" is awkward. We at times refer to the treating clinician as "the psychiatrist" and at other times as "the therapist" or "the clinician," recognizing that patients with bipolar disorder are treated by health care professionals of all trades and degree status. All of the case studies have been disguised so that individuals cannot be identified, but the reader can be assured that the cases are all based on real-life situations we have faced in our practices.

## STRUCTURE OF THE BOOK

This book is organized by the illness phases in which clinicians typically encounter patients with bipolar disorder, with both pharmacological and psychosocial advice to consider at every phase. Chapter 2 describes the basics of bipolar disorder: how manic and hypomanic episodes differ and the significance for treatment of diagnosing bipolar I disorder, bipolar II disorder, or subthreshold bipolar disorder; how bipolar disorder is distinguished in DSM-5 from "near-neighbor" disorders; and the significance of the duration of episodes. We explore the controversies currently being debated among clinicians and researchers, including issues such as whether a major depression with only one or two manic symptoms should be considered a part of the bipolar spectrum and the distinctions between bipolar disorder and borderline personality disorder. Chapter 2 covers the most recent research on the phenomenology of bipolar disorder, and new ideas on how to approach the more diagnostically ambiguous cases in practice.

Chapter 3 offers recommendations for conducting intake evaluations. The psychiatrist, psychologist, or social worker undertaking the evaluation—whether this occurs on an inpatient or outpatient basis—should be aware of biological, genetic, and environmental factors that may be relevant to the patient's diagnostic presentation. We are trying to help clinicians avoid the situation Drew faced in never receiving a full diagnostic evaluation, or if he did, never getting the results.

In discussing the initial encounter and history taking, suggestions are offered on how to ask certain questions and probe further when a clinician is not getting her questions answered. We emphasize obtaining information from key relatives or other "collaterals" whenever possible, and offer strategies as to how to address the patient's concerns about the involvement of parents or spouses.

Chapters 4 and 5 describe modern pharmacological approaches to treating acute mania and acute depression, respectively. Acute episodes present challenges for planning both pharmacological and psychosocial interventions, although most of the research literature deals only with pharmacotherapy. The careful balancing act of finding the most effective but tolerable dosage requires some trial and error, yet following a basic algorithm—with opt-in and opt-out decisions along the way—can stabilize the episode and set the stage for maintenance treatment. The strategies will be different when the patient is acutely manic, mixed or depressed, psychotic, cognitively impaired, or younger versus older, but there are common themes as well.

Chapter 6 discusses pharmacological treatment during the maintenance phase, during which medication regimens may be simplified. Here, the challenge becomes one of controlling subsyndromal symptoms to reduce the likelihood of relapse, and trying to enhance the patient's return to functioning in the community. One of us (M. J. G.) has shown that even minor subsyndromal depressive symptoms (scores as low as 6 on the Beck Depression Inventory) can be associated with functional impairment in the maintenance phases after a bipolar depressive episode.[3]

Psychotherapy can be effectively introduced during acute episodes. The strategies may be very simple, such as offering emotional support to the patient and family, encouraging practical strategies such as the monitoring of mood states, or explaining the importance of consistency with medications. In fact, the strong therapeutic alliance that is often built during the most extreme phases of illness sets the stage for more intensive treatment during the maintenance phases. Chapter 7 addresses the challenges of maintenance treatment from the psychosocial viewpoint. We emphasize psychosocial *strategies* rather than particular manualized treatments. The approaches include educating the patient (and family, if available) about bipolar disorder, social and circadian rhythm tracking, behavioral activation, and relapse prevention planning. Family caregivers play a key role during maintenance treatment in helping to track residual symptoms and identifying prodromal periods (i.e., the beginning of new episodes) or other change points. During Drew's maintenance treatment, he and his wife agreed to collaborate in identifying daily changes in his irritability and activity levels (his position: "I'll do it if you'll also do it on yourself").

The medically nonadherent patient presents special challenges (Chapter 8), but clinicians can enhance the outcome of pharmacological treatment by exploring the issues that get in the way of adherence. Often, nonadherence can simply be traced to the side effects of a particular medication. In other cases, nonadherence is associated with psychological conflicts of the individual (e.g., equating medications with a loss of independence), cognitive limitations (e.g., forgetting pills), or family factors (e.g., caregivers who constantly remind the patient that he is ill or insist on evidence of medication consistency). Drew was in constant conflict over his medications, which to some degree derived from their side effects (e.g., weight gain on quetiapine) or their meaning (i.e., feeling like a child) within his marital relationships. Chapter 8 includes many examples of how to talk to patients about nonadherence and to normalize it, and how to avoid setting oneself up as an authority figure who must be obeyed. Exploring the patient's long-term values or goals—and how medications do and do not fit with those goals—can be quite powerful, especially in the aftermath of an episode.

The unique issues faced by women during pregnancy and the postpartum period are covered in Chapter 9. Certain medications pose dangers to the developing fetus, but these dangers must be balanced against the risks of untreated bipolar disorder during pregnancy. Psychosocial interventions such as mindfulness-based cognitive therapy can enhance the patient's resilience during and following pregnancy. Current guidelines for the pharmacological treatment of postpartum bipolar depression, including the risks of breastfeeding when on lithium or other agents, are reviewed in this chapter.

In Chapter 10, on suicide prevention, we highlight the importance of an integrated, team approach to illness management. There are few data to guide the treatment of suicidality among bipolar patients, even regarding the oft-repeated recommendation to add lithium to every regimen. Safety must be maximized during the postdepressive-illness phases, when many patients are still at risk despite their denial of suicidal intention. Including family members in suicide prevention planning is crucial because of the loss of insight among patients during acute episodes. Communicating closely with family members to enhance support can be protective during these high-risk intervals.

Finally, in Chapter 11—a "special topics" chapter—we discuss comorbid disorders such as ADHD, anxiety disorders, substance or alcohol abuse, personality disorders, or general medical illnesses, all of which frequently co-occur with bipolar disorder. Sometimes, the solutions to treating these complex combinations of disorders are straightforward (e.g., avoiding divalproex [Depakote] with patients who have hepatic problems). In other cases, they require weighing the benefits and costs of adjunctive treatments, such as when a patient has significant anxiety but has been destabilized by selective serotonin reuptake inhibitors (SSRIs) in the past. The dilemmas faced by clinicians when treating patients who have bipolar disorder and borderline personality disorder—such as when to rely on pharmacotherapy to stabilize mood and when to introduce dialectical behavior therapy or other psychosocial strategies—are discussed in this chapter.

In Chapter 11 we also discuss a related special topic: how to implement "split treatment" effectively when pharmacotherapy and psychotherapy are provided by different providers. There are ways to make shared treatment plans effective even when both practitioners are extraordinarily busy or do not fully comprehend each other's approach. Simple principles, such as optimal (rather than frequent) communication, mutual respect for another's area of expertise, and consistent messages to patients about the importance of both approaches, can make split treatment work quite effectively in practice.

In all, it is our hope that this book will help the clinician view the treatment of bipolar disorder in a fresh and new way: one that integrates individualized approaches to pharmacotherapy and psychotherapy, considers treatment as a moving target, offers flexibility when treating nonadherent patients or those with complex clinical presentations, and involves family members as important allies throughout treatment. But first, let us consider what we mean by bipolar disorder.

# CHAPTER 2

# Bipolar Disorder
## *The Basics*

On the surface, the diagnosis of bipolar disorder should be rather straightforward: It is a disorder characterized by highs and lows (or manias and depressions) and can therefore be easily distinguished from unipolar depression (major depressive disorder in DSM-5) by the presence of manic or hypomanic episodes, and from other disorders by its characteristic clear cycling. Certainly, in many cases, the diagnosis is just that simple. Yet, in many other cases, even knowledgeable clinicians disagree as to when a patient has bipolar disorder rather than another mood disorder. In this chapter, we define the classic presentations of bipolar disorder, describe the equally classic subtypes of the disorder, and focus on the diagnostic confusions and controversies in the area. We also review the genetics and natural history of bipolar disorder and consider the functional consequences of illness episodes and the role of life events in the course of the illness.

## CORE SYMPTOMS OF BIPOLAR DISORDER

### *Mania/Hypomania*

The hallmark features of classic mania are clear and well described in DSM-5. A *manic episode* is characterized by an abnormality of mood that is either euphoric, expansive, and elevated or irritable plus increased energy (a new core criterion in DSM-5), along with a group of "B" signs and symptoms, such as inflated self-esteem or grandiosity, decreased need for sleep, pressure of speech or being more talkative than usual, flight of ideas or racing thoughts, distractibility, an increase in goal-directed behavior, psychomotor agitation, or poor judgment

13

and impulsive decision making, resulting in unwise and/or dangerous behavior.[1] These destructive behaviors occur most often in the areas of spending money, sexual activity, and inappropriate interpersonal behavior. Manic symptoms need to be present for at least 1 week (with duration being irrelevant if the person is hospitalized or requires emergency treatment), although the average length of an untreated manic episode is 3 months.[2] Over half of manic episodes are also characterized by psychotic symptoms such as delusions and hallucinations, with the psychotic themes typically but not invariably related to manic themes of grandiosity or specialness.[3]

Of note, the sleep disturbance consistent with mania is not insomnia but rather a decreased *need* for sleep—the individual may sleep only a few hours per night but perceives that as a sufficient amount and, in fact, has excessive energy during the day. This contrasts with *nonspecific insomnia,* seen in an endless variety of psychiatric disorders, in which sleep is disrupted or lessened and the individual sleeps fewer hours than normal but feels appropriately fatigued the next day. The failure to distinguish decreased need for sleep from insomnia is one source of unreliability among clinicians making the diagnosis.

The classic grandiose, expansive, euphoric mood state is not always present in mania. In 70% of episodes, mood is characterized by irritability rather than euphoria, although both may be present.[3] When the mood is dominated by irritability, with little euphoria, it is usually more difficult to make an accurate diagnosis of mania.

A mild manic episode is called *hypomania.* The symptoms of hypomania are the same as those of mania, with a shorter—and rather arbitrary—minimum time threshold (according to DSM-5) of 4 days. The core distinction between mania and hypomania is the extent of functional impairment caused by the episode. Mania is a destructive state that causes significant impairment in the areas of work and/or social relationships. For example, if the episode causes the patient to be fired, to hurt a loved one or damage a relationship, or to spend significant and damaging amounts of money unwisely, the individual is manic. Similarly, patients who are psychotic or hospitalized during a highly active state are manic, not hypomanic. Thus, there can never be a hospital admitting diagnosis of hypomania; if the episode is severe enough to require hospitalization, it is mania, not hypomania. Conversely, in a hypomanic episode, a relationship may be strained but not seriously damaged or the patient may spend more money than usual but not enough to threaten solvency. This distinction between hypomania and mania involves value judgments, especially since the intensity of the patient's episode expresses itself on a continuum.

Barry, a 47-year-old man, was creative director of a nonprofit organization. He had a long history of mood swings. On intake into our clinic, he described a month-long period in which he slept only 5 hours per night—2 hours less than normal—but experienced more energy than usual during the day. He also said that he had generated an unusual number of new ideas, some of which were viable. He found himself shopping more online but did not go overboard, only spending $500, which was affordable to him. During this period, he was more flirtatious with coworkers, which was noticeable but not at the level of being offensive or causing disruption. With his wife, he became more sexual than usual, but she appreciated his renewed activity. Given similar episodes in the past, Barry recognized this as a period of hypomania and called his psychiatrist to ask about a possible change in his medication regimen.

With hypomania, the symptoms may be mild, and some symptoms may have positive consequences, such as increased sexual interest, heightened creativity, or increased productivity. The episode may not be recognized by the bipolar individual or by family members or friends as a significant departure from normal behavior. In contrast, it would be clear to any observer that a patient with mania—who may be psychotic, with behavior that is dangerous and debilitating—is psychiatrically ill. Therefore, in making a diagnosis of bipolar disorder—and especially in diagnosing hypomania—obtaining collateral information from a significant other is somewhere between helpful and mandatory.

Some bipolar individuals minimize hypomanic symptoms for the usual reasons, one of which is the desire to not be seen as psychiatrically ill. Other individuals simply do not recognize hypomanic symptoms because they are so ego-syntonic (i.e., consistent with their self-concept). Of course, in many hypomanias, the individual may feel so good—often better than at any other time in his life—that he may be exceedingly reluctant to give it up.

Sam asked for a diagnostic evaluation/second opinion. Sam had already seen another clinician, who felt that he indeed had bipolar disorder, but Sam felt that the psychiatrist did not understand him, and he refused to return for treatment. His mother, with whom Sam had a conflicted relationship, was clearly bipolar. He told the interviewing clinician that his wife insisted that he had mood swings and needed to be evaluated and treated. Over two sessions with the new clinician, Sam described times in which he was clearly depressed and other times when he seemed slightly more energetic. Yet he was rather vague about other, associated symptoms (e.g., decreased need for sleep, alterations in sexuality or spending money). The clinician asked to meet with Sam and his wife; Sam initially declined the request but eventually reluctantly acquiesced. Sam's wife described an absolutely clear pattern of recurrent hypomanic episodes, with equally clear changes in sexual behavior, energy, and his relationships with others. When asked about the disparity between the descriptions put forth by himself and his wife, Sam acknowledged that these internal shifts felt so good that he did not want them to be "medicated away." Additionally, he expressed his resentment at being identified with his mother's psychiatric disorder.

---

## Depression

Depressive episodes associated with bipolar disorder share the same diagnostic criteria and, in general, are characterized by the same symptoms as nonbipolar depression. Thus, a mood component—either depressive mood or apathy—is a required "A" symptom along with a group of "B" symptoms, such as changes in sleep (either insomnia or hypersomnia); appetite/weight changes (either diminished appetite and weight loss or hyperphagia and weight gain); fatigue, psychomotor retardation or agitation; feelings of worthlessness or guilt; diminished concentration; and morbid thoughts, including suicidal ideation, intent, or plans. Some depressions, like some manias, may be associated with delusions or hallucinations. Psychotic symptoms are more common in manias (over 60%) compared to bipolar depressions (30%).[3] Delusions are more common than hallucinations.

As with nonbipolar depression, concerns about suicide are paramount in evaluating and treating bipolar depression. Approximately 50% of all suicides in our society—the largest subgroup—are associated with a depressive disorder.[4] Overall, rates of suicide for bipolar depression versus unipolar depression are crudely comparable and at least 10 times higher than the general population risk.[5]

Not surprisingly, within bipolar disorder, the vast majority of suicides occur during the depressed phase, with a smaller number of suicides occurring during a manic episode with mixed–irritable–dysphoric features. Suicides rarely occur during euphoric manias, although fatalities do happen due to impulsivity (e.g., reckless driving), bad judgment (e.g., getting involved with dangerous people), or psychotic behavior. Because concerns about suicide are so central in mood disorders, we focus in Chapter 10 on dealing with suicidality.

Some symptoms occur more frequently in bipolar than in unipolar depression. Relative to unipolar depression, bipolar depression is more likely to be associated with hypersomnia, hyperphagia–weight gain, psychomotor retardation, and psychotic symptoms, and less likely to be associated with anxiety and somatic complaints.[6] However, no single symptom or even group of symptoms reliably distinguishes bipolar from unipolar depression.

## CLASSIFICATION OF BIPOLAR SUBTYPES

### *Bipolar I and Bipolar II Disorder*

Bipolar I disorder is characterized by at least one full manic episode. In bipolar II disorder, all upswings are hypomanic, not manic. Thus, bipolar II disorder can evolve into bipolar I, but bipolar I disorder can never evolve into bipolar II disorder. Once a pattern of recurrent hypomanic episodes is established, the individual is likely to remain in the bipolar II disorder category: Only 15% of those with three or more hypomanic episodes will later evolve into having bipolar I disorder.[7] Thus, for most individuals, bipolar II disorder is a stable diagnosis.

A mixed state, or *mixed mania*, describes an episode with simultaneous manic or hypomanic and depressive symptoms. DSM-5 considers mixed features as a "specifier," which means that it is not a separate type of episode but is given as an added descriptor to a manic or hypomanic episode. In DSM-5, a mixed state is diagnosed when the full criteria of a manic or hypomanic episode are met and three depressive symptoms from the major depression criteria (excluding appetite or concentration changes) coexist. These modifications are consistent with how most clinicians use the term *mixed*, describing a manic (or hypomanic) episode with some depressive symptoms.

Because individuals with mixed features usually do not exhibit the euphoria and grandiosity seen in classic mania, these episodes can be misdiagnosed as agitated depressions. In mixed manias, the manic symptoms are the central features defining the mood state, although the patient may complain more about depressive symptoms. Thus, mixed manias/hypomanias should be conceptualized and treated in the same way as manic/hypomanic episodes, not as depressive episodes (see Chapter 4).

### *Rapid Cycling*

Rapid-cycling bipolar I or bipolar II disorder, seen in 15–35% of bipolar individuals, describes a subtype characterized by more frequent episodes than usual.[8] In DSM-5, *rapid-cycling bipolar disorder* is a specifier and is defined as a bipolar disorder with four or more episodes of full time duration—mania for 1 week (if not interrupted by intervention), hypomania for 4 days, or depression for 2 weeks or more—within a 12-month time period. (See Chapter 6 for details on the treatment of rapid-cycling bipolar disorder.)

Classic rapid cycling, equally common in bipolar I and bipolar II individuals, may be seen in the beginning or may emerge later in the course of the disorder, after many years and many episodes. For some of these later-onset rapid cyclers, the chronic use of antidepressants may have accelerated the cycling and can be considered to have "caused" the rapid cycling. For others, however, the later onset of rapid cycling simply expresses the natural course of bipolar disorder.[9]

Unfortunately, the term *rapid cycling* has also increasingly been used to describe other forms of rapid mood alterations. One such form is four or more episodes within a 1-month time frame. Clearly, this time frame cannot encompass episodes meeting full time criteria and is often called "ultrarapid" cycling. Even more problematic has been the use of the term *rapid cycling* to describe individuals with mood swings that shift within hours, often many times over the course of a day. This within-day cycling is usually described as "ultradian" (recurring within a 24-hour period) cycling.

There are three problems with these different uses of the term *rapid cycling*. First, communication between professionals suffers when one term refers to multiple, distinct psychiatric/psychological entities. Second, the meaning of *rapid cycling*—that it is a subtype of bipolar disorder less responsive to lithium (and probably to other mood stabilizers)—refers to the classic, original definition of the term only. Third, ultradian cycling is also a clinical feature of nonbipolar psychiatric disorders. Those with borderline personality disorder without bipolar disorder often exhibit within-day mood shifts, usually in response to environmental factors. Similarly, those individuals with drug-related syndromes—either acute intoxication or withdrawal—often have within-day mood swings. Conflating all of these varied forms of psychopathology by the term *rapid cycling* creates problems both with diagnosis and communication between professionals.

Rapid cycling may be chronic or transient. For some bipolar individuals, it is simply a "bad patch" in which they experience greater than normal mood instability and more episodes per unit time. Later, they settle into a less rapidly cycling phase of the disorder. In fact, when followed for the next 5 years, the vast majority of those with rapid cycling do *not* continue to cycle rapidly.[9]

---

Harriet had bipolar II disorder. With a combination of medication and psychotherapy, her disorder was kept in reasonable control, with one mild hypomania and two relatively brief (1 month) depressions occurring over the last 5 years. Following a series of stressful events, she had gone through a 1-month hypomania, followed by a 3-month depression. After stabilizing and doing relatively well (but feeling fragile) for 6 months, she had another biphasic mood swing with another hypomania, followed by another depression. At that point, Harriet became worried that her previously quiescent mood disorder was now spiraling out of control, leading to concern that she would lose important aspects of her life, mainly her job and her long-term romantic relationship. Despite ongoing collaborative work with her psychiatrist and her therapist, she had a third depression (and fifth episode overall) 4 months after the previous episode. After this cycle, she became euthymic. Harriet remained well for the next few years, with no further recurrences but not without fall-out. The period of rapid cycling oversensitized Harriet, and she became far more vigilant and less secure about her moods after that time period.

## Cyclothymia

Rarely diagnosed in clinical settings but seen more frequently in epidemiological samples, the DSM-5 definition of *cyclothymia* describes a chronic—at least 2 years—low amplitude, frequent cycling bipolar variant. The mood swings of individuals with cyclothymia occur most of the time (in the DSM-5 definition, no more than 2 consecutive months have been symptom-free within a 2-year period) and never exhibit the number of symptoms or the length of time consistent with a hypomanic/manic episode or a depression.

## Bipolar Spectrum Disorders

In DSM-5, bipolar I and bipolar II disorder are clearly delineated from each other by the intensity of the upswings. Yet, as in virtually all of psychopathology, mood swings occur on a continuum; they are dimensional, not categorical. Thus, even the distinction between hypomania and mania is a bit arbitrary. For some patients, the level of functional impairment could make one reasonable clinician call an episode mania, whereas another would describe it as hypomania (giving rise to the whimsical diagnosis of bipolar disorder 1.5 for those cases on the border between the two). In recent years, there has been increasing thought and attention to extending the dimensional nature of mood swings to include individuals who have a disorder characterized by mood swings that do not fit clearly into any of the classic subtypes (bipolar I, bipolar II, cyclothymia) described in DSM-5, where they are lumped into the "wastebasket" term *other specified bipolar and related disorders* (in DSM-IV, the term was *bipolar disorder not otherwise specified [NOS]*) but, colloquially, they are referred to as bipolar spectrum disorders. Clinicians who use this term assume that these disorders are indeed variants of bipolar disorder and typically treat these patients pharmacologically as if they had classical bipolar disorder, a reasonable assumption but one based on essentially no studies at all.

One of the most controversial definitional questions in the bipolar spectrum area is that of pharmacologically induced mania/hypomania: How does one think about patients who suffer from depressions but whose only hypomanias (or manias) occur in association with antidepressant medications? In DSM-5, manic or hypomanic episodes that emerge during antidepressant treatment are considered bipolar disorder only if a full manic/hypomanic syndrome (not just irritability or agitation) persists beyond the physiological effects of the treatment. For instance, if a depressed patient given an antidepressant becomes hypomanic and these symptoms persist for more than 1 week after discontinuing the antidepressant, the diagnosis should now be bipolar II disorder. If the hypomanic symptoms resolve within a few days of stopping the antidepressant, the diagnosis of major depression remains. Even these broad definitions, however, mask a host of clinically relevant questions: Does it matter how long the patient has been taking the antidepressant when the hypomania/mania occurs? Does one think differently if the answer is 3 weeks versus 1 year? (One could certainly argue that there is a higher likelihood of a causal link between the antidepressant and the emergent mania in the former than the latter time frame.) What if the patient is prescribed an antimanic agent at the same time as the antidepressant is withdrawn and the patient's hypomanic symptoms resolve, such that it would be impossible to know what caused the improvement? Should that patient be rediagnosed as bipolar?

Until we know more, common sense usually dictates the answers in these scenarios. For example, most experts use a 2- or 3-month cutoff to define the time frame after an antidepressant is started or increased to consider it causally related to an emergent hypomania. Episodes much later on, such as 1 year, are more likely to be the result of the natural history of the disorder.

As is common with atypical variations on a classic theme, there are no accepted subtypes of bipolar spectrum disorder, with multiple authors, as well as DSM-5, defining their own set of unique subtypes. Table 2.1 presents the commonly suggested variants of bipolar disorder. Some of these clinical subtypes differ from the classic forms by some difference in symptom description—length of episode, number of symptoms, or core symptoms. For example, there was much discussion for the DSM-5 as to whether the time criteria for hypomania should be shortened from 4 days to 2 days, given the evidence that some patients with clear bipolar I or II disorder describe brief (less than 4 day) episodes. If a patient has *only* 1 to 3 day episodes, does the diagnosis of bipolar disorder apply? (DSM-5 classifies these short hypomanias plus

**TABLE 2.1.** **Bipolar Variants and Clinical Features Suggested to Be Associated with Bipolar Spectrum Disorders**

Bipolar variants

- Hypomanias of less than 4 days' duration[a]
- Hypomanic episode without mood symptoms but with hyperactivity
- Pharmacological manias/hypomanias[a]

Suggested clinical features of bipolar spectrum disorders

- Major depression with bipolar family history
- Mixed depressive syndromes[a]
- Early age of onset of depression
- Highly recurrent depressions
- Psychotic depression
- Atypical depressive features
- Treatment-resistant depressions
- Recurrent antidepressant tolerance

[a]Described in DSM-5.

depressions in the "other specified bipolar and related disorders" section.) Should mood stabilizers be the pharmacotherapy of choice for these individuals? Similarly, how do we think about individuals whose core symptom is that of increased energy but without (as is required in DSM-5) a mood alteration such as euphoria or irritability?

Other than variations in bipolar symptom definitions, some clinical researchers suggest that certain features (presented in Table 2.1) within clearly nonbipolar symptom patterns should be considered as consistent with bipolar spectrum disorders, despite a lack of any formal manic/hypomanic symptoms. Thus, early onset of a mood disorder, seasonal variation of symptoms, a family history of bipolar disorder, atypical features (e.g., hyperphagia and hypersomnia), psychotic features during depressions (which are more common in bipolar depression than in unipolar depression), more recurrent depressive episodes (more than three), antidepressant treatment failures, antidepressant tolerance (in which the depressed patient seems to respond acutely to an antidepressant but the positive effects "wear off," resulting in the recurrent failure of maintenance treatment), have all been suggested as being consistent with bipolar spectrum disorders.[10] DSM-5 does not consider any of these as evidence of bipolar disorder due to insufficient research.

Implied in some of these clinical descriptors is the assumption that some patients can be in the bipolar spectrum without ever having any hypomanic periods or even hypomanic symptoms. The working hypothesis—for which there is little evidence in either direction—is that patients can have some genes associated with bipolar disorder but simply not express the manic part of the disorder, as if they have bipolar disorder without the highs!

Finally, mixed depression is included as a course specifier in the "depressive disorders" section in DSM-5, not the "bipolar disorders" section. As an analogue of mixed mania, in which patients present with a manic syndrome plus a few depressive symptoms, mixed depression describes a depressive syndrome plus a few manic symptoms such as irritability, psychomotor agitation, racing thoughts, increased energy, and grandiosity or elevated mood. The results of some studies have suggested that, compared to those without mixed features, depressed patients who exhibit mixed symptoms have a greater family history of bipolar disorder, a younger age of onset, a greater likelihood of antidepressant-induced manic switches, and more manic symptoms at follow-up.[11] As noted earlier, however, no study has systematically examined whether people with manic symptoms within a depression should be treated any differently than those without these symptoms.

## DIFFERENTIAL DIAGNOSIS OF BIPOLAR DISORDER

A list of psychiatric disorders that may share at least *some* clinical features with bipolar disorder would be rather long. Most would be psychiatric or medical disorders associated with depression. Yet there are a few of these disorders, listed in Table 2.2, that should be specifically ruled out when making a diagnosis of bipolar disorder or mania/hypomania. Additionally, it is vital to remember that some of these disorders— borderline personality disorder, attention deficit disorder, drug abuse

**TABLE 2.2. Differential Diagnosis of Bipolar Disorder**

Other psychiatric disorders

- Major depression
- Substance-induced mood disorders (especially stimulant abuse)
- Borderline personality disorder (especially for bipolar II)
- Schizoaffective disorder
- ADHD (especially for bipolar II)

Other medical disorders

- Hyperthyroidism
- Corticosteroid-induced mania/hypomania

syndromes—are commonly seen in conjunction with bipolar disorder. In these cases, the question should be whether the patient has one or the other of these disorders, or both. For other disorders, including major depression, schizoaffective disorder, and substance-induced mood disorder, individuals cannot have comorbid bipolar disorder.

## Major Depressive Disorder

At first glance, distinguishing bipolar disorder from major depression should be rather simple: Individuals who have manic or hypomanic periods are bipolar, and if they experience only depressive episodes, they have major depression (unipolar depression). The reality, of course, is that making this distinction can be quite difficult in practice. Many depressed patients have clear histories of bipolar I or II disorder but are treated for major depression only.[12] The two most likely reasons for misdiagnosis are (1) incomplete information gathered during the clinical history, as a result of the patient's limited insight into mania/hypomania, often compounded by state-dependent memories of manic or hypomanic episodes, the ego-syntonic nature of mild hypomania, and lack of recognition of the relationship of manic to depressive episodes; and (2) not including significant others during the diagnostic evaluation (as exemplified by the case of Sam, presented earlier in this chapter).

Many patients who are ultimately (and correctly) diagnosed as bipolar have had one or more depressive episodes before developing their first hypomanic or manic episode. Thus, inquiring about the patient's history of depression should help establish the diagnosis. Likewise, any patient who presents with depressive symptoms should always be asked about a history of manic or hypomanic symptoms. (Chapter 3 provides substantial detail on ways to probe for manic/hypomanic symptoms.)

## Substance-Induced Mood Disorder

A host of medications is associated with the emergence of manic/hypomanic systems. The most common of these are corticosteroids, such as prednisone, used to treat an endless variety of inflammatory and autoimmune disorders, which can also cause depression, or L-dopa (typically marketed as Sinemet), used to treat Parkinson's disease.

Among street drugs, stimulants such as cocaine or methamphetamine (speed) can induce a state that is clinically indistinguishable from mania. Of course, patients with substance abuse frequently minimize or outright lie about their use of illicit drugs. They may give a history that seems entirely consistent with episodes of what sounds like hypomanic episodes, leaving out the use of stimulants in association with these energized times. As discussed more in Chapter 3, evidence from dual-diagnosis clinics suggests that a number of individuals with a history of substance abuse who present with a prior diagnosis of bipolar disorder do not have a primary mood disorder when systematically evaluated with a structured interview. Structured interviews involve more systematic attempts to distinguish between substance-induced symptoms and endogenous symptoms.

The best method to distinguish between medication- or substance-induced and "real" bipolar symptoms is to take a careful history—both medical and psychiatric—with collateral information (discussed in more detail in Chapter 3). Obtaining a urine toxicology screening test to clarify current drug use is usually quite informative, although the patient may refuse such testing.

### Schizoaffective Disorder

Patients with mood symptoms, as well as psychotic symptoms, may present a specific diagnostic challenge because a number of separate diagnoses share a core set of symptoms. As examples, it is clear that a substantial subset of patients with schizophrenia have depressive symptoms *and* a substantial subset of patients with bipolar disorder have prominent psychotic symptoms. *Schizoaffective disorder* describes an illness halfway between schizophrenia and a mood disorder with psychotic symptoms. In DSM-5, schizoaffective disorder is defined by one or more full mood episodes with psychotic symptoms or negative symptoms but, additionally, by psychotic symptoms for 2 weeks or more in the absence of a mood episode. A new criterion of schizoaffective disorder in DSM-5 is the requirement that the mood symptoms/episodes must be present for the majority of the total duration of illness. Therefore, a patient who has mood episodes but is psychotic most of the time (i.e., more than 70%) without mood symptoms has DSM-5 schizophrenia, not schizoaffective disorder.

Schizoaffective disorder may also be subdivided into schizoaffective disorder, bipolar subtype or schizoaffective disorder, depressive subtype. Some, but not all studies, suggest that on the basis of family history, prognosis, and other features, schizoaffective disorder, bipolar subtype, is closer to bipolar disorder, with prominent psychotic features, whereas schizoaffective disorder, depressive subtype, represents a mixture of schizophrenia with prominent depressive features.[13,14] It must be acknowledged, however, that schizoaffective disorder is an unstable diagnosis, in that less than 50% of those with the disorder continue to have that diagnosis at long-term follow-up.[15] The majority of the individuals whose diagnoses shifted were later diagnosed as having either bipolar disorder or schizophrenia.

---

Bill, 24 years old, has had his third psychotic mania. Each of the two prior episodes had required hospitalization for hyperactivity and psychotic thinking and behavior (e.g., he would drive late at night on the left side of canyon roads, sure that he would "always know" when a car might emerge from the opposite direction). During this third episode, he was treated with valproate (Depakote) and quetiapine (Seroquel). Over 3 weeks, his hyperactivity diminished markedly and his sleep increased to 6 hours nightly. After discharge from the hospital, however, he continued to have delusions that he knew what would happen before the event. He also thought people were looking at him as he walked on the street, understanding that he was special in both positive and negative ways. These psychotic symptoms continued for 2 months despite Bill's taking his medication regularly. By the fourth month, the delusions receded, and they were gone by the fifth month after hospitalization.

---

On the one hand, there is the inherent desire to make the right diagnosis (in this circumstance, to distinguish between bipolar disorder with psychotic features and schizoaffective disorder). On the other hand, it is unclear that a more accurate diagnosis according to a diagnostic system such as DSM-5 will lead to better treatment. A bipolar patient with prominent psychotic symptoms will typically be treated with a mood stabilizer plus an antipsychotic. Most clinicians would treat schizoaffective disorder, bipolar subtype, with the same combination of medications.

### Borderline Personality Disorder

Distinguishing between bipolar II disorder and borderline personality disorder is among the most difficult and important diagnostic challenges. Both disorders are characterized at times by intense affect, affective lability, irritability, and impulsivity. Additionally, patients may have both disorders, making accurate diagnoses even more difficult. Yet a number of differences, listed in Table 2.3, may help to clarify the diagnoses. Of paramount importance, the mood swings of borderline personality disorder are far more rapid than those of bipolar disorder, with mood shifts seen within hours in the personality disorder. Although, as noted earlier, ultradian cycling may be seen in bipolar disorder, mood swings associated with a primary mood disorder tend to last longer—days to weeks to months.

**TABLE 2.3. Distinctions between Bipolar Disorder and Borderline Personality Disorder**

| Bipolar disorder | Borderline personality disorder |
|---|---|
| Mood swings are usually measured in days/weeks/months. | Mood swings are usually measured in hours to days. |
| Mood swings are frequently not triggered by life events. | Mood swings are usually triggered by life events, especially narcissistic slights. |
| There is a family history of bipolar depression and major depression. | There is a family history of drug abuse, impulsivity, and depression. |
| Manic/hypomanic episodes are characterized by classic symptoms. | Mood swings are rarely characterized by decreased sleep, increased energy, elation, or grandiosity. |

Compared to those of bipolar disorder, the mood swings of borderline personality disorder tend to be more responsive to environmental triggers. Classic manic symptoms such as psychomotor activation associated with euphoric mood and decreased *need* for sleep are not typically seen in borderline patients. In contrast, insomnia is unhelpful diagnostically. In bipolar disorder, impulsivity and irritability are episodic, seen specifically during hypomanic episodes and typically disappearing when the hypomanic episode ends, in contrast to the chronicity of these traits in borderline personalities.

An increase in spending money may be a difficult behavior to interpret because it can occur in both disorders. However, in bipolar disorder, extravagant money spending, as with impulsivity, is typically seen only during manias/hypomanias and is therefore episodic, present for weeks or months, then absent for long periods of time. After a hypomanic or manic episode resolves, the individual finds the recent extravagant purchases ego-dystonic, feels remorse, and attempts to return some or all of the items. In contrast, increased money spending in borderline patients typically represents a narcissistic self-soothing behavior, is more sporadic, and often follows a perceived slight from another person. Borderline patients may later regret the financial problems caused by the extravagance, but they justify the purchases and generally do not try to return the items bought.

One would expect to see far more bipolar disorder in the families of bipolar patients compared to those with borderline personality disorder. In the latter, drug–alcohol abuse, impulsive character traits, and depression are typical.[16] However, because bipolar patients themselves as well as their first- or second-degree relatives frequently have comorbid drug–alcohol abuse, family histories are only sometimes useful in making the proper diagnosis.

---

Barbara, age 28, came for treatment with the diagnosis of rapid-cycling bipolar disorder. She described a tumultuous childhood with an alcoholic, volatile father and a chaotic, narcissistic mother. There was an extensive family history of drug abuse. From the time she was a teenager, Barbara perceived herself as *moody*, a term her friends and family would agree was accurate. Her moods often shifted multiple times over the course of the day, almost always (but not always) in response to interactions that affected her self-esteem. She developed intense relationships that always exploded due to some miscommunication or interpersonal slight. She would then become more depressed, cut herself, increase her drug use, and buy more clothes. During the brief good times in a romantic relationship, Barbara was ecstatic and said she experienced the best "highs" of her life. During these periods, she behaved arrogantly toward others. Despite the mood swings, she still regularly slept 8 hours a night. A previous clinician had diagnosed her with rapid-cycling bipolar II disorder. A trial of lithium made her feel a bit calmer and duller but did little to change her mood swings. Her diagnosis was eventually changed to borderline personality disorder.

---

### Attention-Deficit/Hyperactivity Disorder

ADHD shares traits of impulsivity, distractibility, irritability, and aggressiveness with mania/hypomania. Additionally, as with borderline personality disorder, the two disorders can coexist. There is also evidence that children who later emerge as bipolar have high rates of attentional difficulties, implying that, for this subgroup, the ADHD is an early expression of the bipolar disorder. In adults, however, a number of differences should make the diagnostic distinction clearer. First, ADHD is a developmental disorder: It always arises in childhood (whether it is diagnosed then or not), whereas bipolar disorder typically emerges later, in adolescence or early adulthood. Second, the cognitive symptoms of ADHD are chronic, whereas the distractibility of hypomania or mania is confined to the episodes. (Making this distinction more difficult, however, is the consistent evidence that a subset of bipolar adults have cognitive deficits during their euthymic periods that cannot easily be attributed to medication side effects.[17]) Of note, these cognitive deficits do not necessarily resemble classic ADHD. Third, whereas the impulsivity of ADHD is usually chronic, impulsivity in bipolar disorder is seen only episodically during hypomanic or manic episodes.

Harold, now 24 years old, has always been a high-energy guy. During elementary school, he was always the jokester, often disrupting the classroom. He was not interested in studying but received at least average grades due to his innate intelligence. His high-energy style continued throughout high school and college, where he was an average student. He slept erratically and if excited by a project (typically related to video games) could stay up all night. Much to his own annoyance, Harold regularly misplaced his keys and wallet. Much to the annoyance of others, he was chronically late. He had a temper and was frequently irritable. He had never been clinically depressed.

Harold's route to psychiatric treatment was somewhat circuitous. A new girlfriend whose father was bipolar told Harold that she thought he, too, was bipolar and insisted that he be evaluated for it. He acquiesced, and his first psychiatrist suggested trials of lithium and valproate. Both medications proved to be unhelpful and caused intolerable side effects. Eventually, Harold was correctly diagnosed with ADHD and responded well to a psychostimulant (methylphenidate [Concerta]).

## GENETICS OF BIPOLAR DISORDER

Without a doubt, bipolar disorder runs in families. Equally true, *most* of the familial risk is genetic, not environmental. The major methods of determining familial and genetic risk are as follows:

1. Careful family history studies, in which the relatives of those with bipolar disorder are compared with relatives of patients with other disorders or normal controls, and in which the relatives are interviewed without knowledge of the proband's diagnosis (or lack thereof). Family studies can demonstrate whether bipolar disorder is familial and whether other disorders are also seen in family pedigrees, but they cannot distinguish between genetic and environmental factors since families typically share both genes and environments.
2. Twin studies in which the comparisons are between monozygotic and dizygotic twins. The former are genetically identical, whereas the latter share 50% of their genes. Higher concordance rates—the likelihood of the co-twin having the same disorder—in monozygotic versus dizygotic twins would suggest stronger heritability.
3. Adoption studies in which adoptees share genetic risks with biological parents but share environments with their adoptive families. One can compare whether the adoptees' risk for the disorder more resembles that of the genetic versus adoptive parents.

Family studies demonstrate the clear familial nature of the disorder. Overall, the relative risk for bipolar disorder in first-degree relatives of bipolar individuals is 10.7 times that seen in the general population.[3] In the families of individuals with bipolar I disorder, there is an increased risk for both bipolar I and bipolar II disorder. In the families of bipolar II individuals, one sees a substantial risk for other bipolar II disorders and a lesser (albeit increased) risk for bipolar I disorder, indicating that these two subtypes of bipolar disorder may breed true.[18] Of note, there is a strong increased risk for major depression in the families of both bipolar I and bipolar II individuals. In fact, in the families of bipolar individuals, there is a higher risk for major depressive disorder than for bipolar disorder.

Twin concordance rates for monozygotic twins range mostly between .75 and .80.[19,20] Heritability estimates in twin studies (where complete genetic heritability would be 1.0) range from .71 to .87, indicating that the substantial majority of the familial risk is genetic.[20] One of the best studies found equal concordance rates among twin pairs with bipolar I disorder and twin pairs with bipolar II disorder.[19] The results of the few adoption studies also suggest the strongly genetic nature of bipolar disorder.[21]

Clinically, the importance of these findings is that in the family trees of bipolar individuals, one is very likely to see other members with mood disorders, both bipolar disorder and major depression. Often, patients feel less stigmatized when they learn that the disorder runs in their family, particularly if they have been led to believe that their symptoms are a product of poor impulse control or lack of effort. However, knowledge of one's family history of mood disorder can also lead to rejection of the bipolar person by other family members, particularly among offspring who do not want to believe that their personal problems are an emerging sign of mania or depression. In Chapter 7, we discuss psychoeducational approaches to bipolar disorder that involve family members.

## NATURAL HISTORY OF BIPOLAR DISORDER

Constructing a thoughtful, coherent treatment plan requires knowledge of the natural history of the disorder being treated. The mean age of onset of bipolar disorder, regardless of whether it is recognized, accurately diagnosed, or treated, is the late teens or early 20s. Thus, teenage bipolar disorder is far from unusual.[22] A substantial subset of bipolar individuals are still deeply involved with their families of origin at the time of the first episode. Therefore, optimal strategies to involve the family at these times become imperative (see Chapters 7 and 8). Those individuals with early onset (in the teenage years) of bipolar disorder tend to have a somewhat poorer course of illness, with increased rates of psychosis, rapid cycling, and comorbid substance abuse.[22] The risk for bipolar disorder does not differ by gender.[23]

A smaller subset of bipolar patients have first episodes later in life, from age 50 on. This subgroup is less likely to have a strong family history of the disorder and is associated with higher rates of neurological abnormalities.[24] Nonetheless, some individuals with later-onset bipolar disorder have no evidence of neurological problems and simply have a later onset of the classic symptoms.

The first episode of bipolar disorder is mania in half of the cases and depression in the other half. Thus, a number of individuals with a first episode of depression go on to become bipolar later on. Since bipolar disorder tends to emerge at a somewhat younger age than unipolar depression, after the first depressive episode teenagers or young adults are at higher risk for a later manic or hypomanic episode than those with a first episode of depression in their 30s or 40s.

The natural course of bipolar disorder (without treatment) is characterized by recurrent episodes. Studies from the 19th century until the last 30 years described a significant proportion of bipolar individuals with only one episode in a lifetime. This is partly explainable by the varying nature of the definition of an episode. In earlier times, an episode was defined by a hospitalization, in contrast to our current method of using signs and symptoms (in the manner of DSM criteria). Nowadays, when a patient has an episode of mania followed by an episode of depression, we describe that individual as having had two episodes. In contrast, in Kraepelin's time (late 19th, early 20th century), an individual who entered the hospital at age 18, was in the hospital for 20 years with continuous cycling, and had 30 or more discrete manias and depressions would be described as having had one episode, since there was only one hospitalization! More recent studies demonstrate that 85–95% of bipolar individuals have a recurrence over follow-up times ranging from 5 to 30 years.[3] Thus, even though a small subset of bipolar individuals has only one episode in a lifetime, the vast majority have recurrent episodes. Because of this reality, treatment strategies must include anticipation of and preparation for future episodes.

Beyond the dominant tendency for recurrence in bipolar disorder, there is the question of cycle frequency; that is, do bipolar individuals have a set and predictable amount of time between episodes or do the episodes vary over time, becoming either more or less frequent? About

20 years ago, there was considerable interest in the theory of "kindling," in which episodes were thought to occur more and more frequently as the disease progressed, with one episode begetting another.[25,26] This theory has not been shown to fit the course patterns of the majority of patients, however.[27]

A good generalization is that for approximately 50% of bipolar individuals, the clock "speeds up" for at least the first three episodes, in that the length of time between episodes gets progressively shorter. For the other 50% of bipolar individuals, the time between episodes tends not to vary greatly, beginning with the first episode. However, even among those whose episodes initially occur in this accelerating course, this pattern tends to disappear after the third episode.[28] Overall, bipolar disorder is associated with incredible variability, with some patients having more than 100 episodes over a lifetime and others having only a few.

Another important question about the natural course of bipolar disorder is the relative frequency of manic versus depressive episodes. To summarize a number of modern studies, if one examines groups of bipolar individuals who are in naturalistic treatment (taking medications as decided by their individual doctors and not according to some predetermined treatment protocol), the number of depressive vs. manic/hypomanic episodes is approximately 3:1.[29,30] Thus, even though mania is the defining characteristic of bipolar disorder, depression is the dominant pole. Some, but not all studies, have additionally found that in bipolar II individuals, depression is even more dominant, with one long-term study showing a 37:1 ratio of depressive to hypomanic weeks over an average follow-up of more than 13 years![31]

It would be unethical to withhold maintenance treatments for long periods of time to examine the natural history of untreated bipolar disorder. Therefore, over the last few decades, studies have concentrated on the "natural history of treated bipolar disorder"—what the course of the disorder looks like when patients are treated by a variety of mental health professionals. Some of these patients are treated with aggressive pharmacotherapy, whereas others are not; some are in psychotherapy, but most are not. Some patients stop their treatment against medical advice, whereas others continue. These studies provide a snapshot of bipolar disorder as it looks in the community. Surprisingly, these studies present the picture of bipolar disorder as a much more recurrent disorder, even with treatment, than would have been anticipated. Typical episode relapse rates over 1–2 years in these *treated* groups are 40–60%, whereas 4- to 5-year relapse rates are 60–85%.[27,29]

Additionally, the classic notion that bipolar disorder is characterized by discrete episodes between which patients are asymptomatic also seems to be mythical. As an example, in one long-term follow-up in which patients tracked symptoms on an ongoing basis over more than 10 years, bipolar I individuals were symptomatic (to some degree) for 47% of weeks, whereas bipolar II individuals were symptomatic for 54% of weeks.[30,31] In the same study, bipolar patients were mildly symptomatic (i.e., subsyndromal) for a longer duration than the time they spent in full-blown episodes.

Thus, bipolar disorder should probably be thought of as a highly recurrent disorder even while it is being treated. Bipolar individuals are symptomatic for a substantial proportion of the time and spend more time being mildly symptomatic than in full-blown episodes. The implications of these findings should be obvious: We need to marshal as many therapeutic resources—medications, psychotherapy, environmental changes—as we can to ameliorate the rather stormy course of this disorder.

## STRESS AND THE COURSE OF BIPOLAR DISORDER

Despite the clear genetic nature of the underlying vulnerability for bipolar disorder, it is equally clear that environmental variables, such as stressors and life events, are common triggers for bipolar episodes, both manias/hypomanias and depressions. It is easy for individuals with the disorder and for clinicians to look retrospectively and always find a trigger; when events such as a mood episode occur, people naturally look at their lives and find *some* reason why the episode occurred at this particular time. Studies with prospective ratings of life events, in which the recognition of life events or stressors is established before an episode begins, demonstrate that life stressors are indeed more common before mood episodes than at other times in individuals' lives.[32] Of course, some events are inherently stressful for everyone—death or illness of a loved one, divorce, financial difficulties. For other life events, the importance of the event depends on the individual and his specific sensitivities and vulnerabilities. Whereas some events are independent of the person's behavior (e.g., natural disasters, layoffs at a plant), others may be highly dependent on the behavior of the person (e.g., a car accident associated with reckless driving). It appears that patients with bipolar disorder are more likely to have episodes after behavior-dependent events than after independent events when compared to those with major depression.[33]

It should also be recognized that bipolar patients may be "stress generators": Impulsivity and poor judgment may result in behaviors that create stressors, which then trigger a full episode.[34] Thus, a common scenario to consider is a bipolar individual who becomes hypomanic, then engages in unwise behavior (e.g., telling off the boss) that creates a stressful event (e.g., getting fired), which then triggers a full-blown mania.

Another, more biological form of stress is sleep deprivation, which is not always caused by mania/hypomania. Studying all night or taking a "red eye" flight are classic examples. Sleep deprivation is a well-established trigger for manic/hypomanic episodes but not depression.[35]

Stress can come in other forms as well, such as when family relationships are highly conflicted or marriages are in jeopardy. Patients who live in households where one or more family members (parents, spouses) are high in "expressed emotion" (highly critical, hostile, or overprotective/enmeshed relationships with the patient) are as much as five to six times more likely to have recurrences in the 9 months following a hospital discharge than those who have more benign family relationships.[36-38] Methods for treating families, as well as patients, in the aftermath of episodes are covered in Chapter 7.

Clinically, the implications of the relationship between life events (either independent or self-generated), family stressors, and bipolar mood episodes are clear. For optimal treatment of the disorder, attention must be paid to stresses in the bipolar individual's life and how she copes with these stresses. We can and must work with our patients and their families to enhance coping skills, especially when dealing with stressors that may evoke symptoms. Teaching coping strategies may result in a diminished stress response and help to avert mood episodes. In Chapter 7, ways to enhance coping and manage sleep–wake cycles—at individual and familial levels—are explored in detail.

## FUNCTIONAL OUTCOMES OF PATIENTS WITH BIPOLAR DISORDER

As reviewed earlier, most longitudinal studies of bipolar disorder define outcome in terms of episodes: How many? How frequently? Another, much less frequently used method of measuring outcome is to assess function using the criteria we all tend to use when we observe our own lives, those of our children or our friends. As must be obvious, one reason why most studies have measured episodes instead of functioning is that it is much easier. Counting symptoms and episodes can be done simply: We have predefined criteria for measuring episodes. Measuring functional outcome is more difficult, and there are many fewer established methods of measurement. Nonetheless, one might legitimately argue that functional outcome is more important, at least from the point of view of patients and their families. For most families, it is less important to describe the individual as having had three episodes in 5 years than to describe him as working a full-time job but still having some difficulties in relationships.

No single functional rating scale has achieved universal acceptance, in contrast to the accepted depression and mania rating scales (discussed in Chapter 3). Most functional scales assess at least two domains—role function and social function—with many also assessing other areas, such as recreation and quality of life. Role functioning includes work, school, or time spent as a homemaker to allow comparison of the diversity of roles, if only in a crude way. Social functioning may include romantic relationships, interactions with family members, and/or friendships. Quality-of-life measures attempt to describe the general sense individuals have of their lives (i.e., do they feel satisfied or fulfilled?). Thus, quality of life is more subjective than either symptom-based measurement or role–social functioning measurements that compare individuals to an expected standard.

For the last 100 or more years, bipolar disorder has always been considered the "good-prognosis" disorder, at least in comparison to schizophrenia. Earlier studies distinguished what was perceived as the inexorably downhill course of schizophrenia (consistent with its 19th- and early 20th-century name of "dementia praecox") versus the tendency of bipolar disorder (called manic–depressive insanity) to show discrete episodes of manias and depressions but with full recovery from each episode and, therefore, a much better long-term prognosis. This generalization is crudely accurate: Bipolar disorder has a better long-term prognosis than does schizophrenia. However, as we discussed earlier in this chapter, bipolar disorder is a far more virulent disorder than the earlier caricature would suggest. Compared to those with no major psychiatric disorders, bipolar individuals have marked, long-term functional impairment.[39] These impairments can be seen in all areas of functioning, including work, family interactions, self-reported quality of life, and social relationships.

In the short term, patients who have completely recovered from their mood episodes often experience functional impairment.[40,41] Thus, one often sees a bipolar individual who has symptomatically recovered from either a recent mania/hypomania or a depression, but who, months later, has still not returned to school full time or cannot work at the same level compared to pre-episode standards.

Jared was a 19-year-old sophomore in college when he had his first manic episode, characterized by accelerating amounts of energy, increased talking and generation of ideas, some hypersexuality, and delusions of extraordinary creativity, among other classic symptoms. He was hospitalized for a week and a half and responded well to valproate plus an antipsychotic agent. After hospital discharge, he was still somewhat manic, but his activation diminished over the next month. Two months after he left the hospital, Jared showed no manic symptoms, yet he felt he could not return to college full time. He denied being significantly depressed but was clearly less confident than usual. He could not describe why he did not want to resume normal college life but kept insisting that he was just not ready yet.

Even though they have the same levels of education as persons in the general population, patients with bipolar disorder do not achieve comparable levels of socioeconomic status.[42] Over the longer term, bipolar patients show consistently higher levels of unemployment and work absence compared to the population at large. Interpersonally, compared to control or other psychiatric populations, bipolar individuals show higher rates of separation, divorce, and relationship distress.[43,44] Family members of bipolar individuals clearly show distress related to caregiver roles.[45] Chapters 7 (on psychosocial interventions) and 8 (on medication adherence) both address the treatment of bipolar disorder within a family context.

## What Are the Causes of Functional Impairment?

From the point of view of clinicians, patients, and families, the important question is to understand what factors contribute most to the functional impairment of bipolar individuals. If we know what is causing the impairment, then we can construct treatment strategies—both psychological and pharmacological—to ameliorate these factors. First, it is obvious and true that a greater number of mood episodes correlates with greater functional impairment. Additionally, and maybe counterintuitively, depressions contribute more to long-term functional impairment than do manias.[46] In fact, *subsyndromal depressive symptoms*—depressive symptoms that are not severe enough to be described as a major depression—seem to play a major role in long-term functional disruption.[47] As noted earlier, depression is the dominant pole of bipolar disorder. Thus, much more attention needs to be paid to the recognition and treatment of depressive symptoms, even when they are relatively mild. Treatment of bipolar depression during the acute and maintenance phases is discussed in Chapters 5 and 6.

Second, cognitive impairment in bipolar individuals may also play a role in functional impairment, presumably more in work than in social functioning. A number of studies have demonstrated that a subgroup of bipolar individuals show clear deficits in cognitive function that are not easily explained by medication factors (e.g., sedation or cognitive dulling).[48] Results of other studies have suggested that, as with overall functional outcome, the cumulative effects of depressions, such as number of depressive episodes or number of months depressed over a lifetime, correlate with the extent of cognitive impairment.[49]

## SUMMARY

This chapter has provided an overview of the symptomatic and functional course of bipolar disorder, and risk factors for recurrences and functional impairment. As clinicians, we need to be vigilant in addressing any and all factors associated with a poorer long-term course of our patients' illnesses. Knowledge of how this material applies to specific life situations can be of immeasurable help to the clinician in assisting patients and families during the most difficult periods of illness. For example, younger patients and their families may not be aware of the highly recurrent course of the disorder, and may expect that after a major episode life should resume as before. Patients are often frustrated that they have not regained their prior level of functioning despite following treatment plans to the letter, and want to stop their medications. Some are reassured by knowing that the 6- to 9-month period after an acute episode is the most difficult for patients and families, that it is a period of convalescence during which even the patient's most established abilities are challenged. With this reassurance, they may agree to wait until they have achieved full recovery before deciding to stop their medications.

Unresolved depressive symptoms sometimes inhibit recovery, even though patients are not always aware of them. Furthermore, life events and conflict in one's family, romantic, or work life can affect the patient's level of functioning. All of these course of illness features suggest the importance of carefully planned pharmacotherapy (Chapters 4–6), integrated psychosocial interventions (Chapter 7), and psycho-education to address nonadherence (Chapter 8).

Central to the assumptions in these chapters is that the clinician has been able to take a detailed history and make a proper assessment of the primary and comorbid diagnoses. We discuss the intake interview in the next chapter.

# ─── CHAPTER 3 ───

# The Intake Evaluation

As we discussed in Chapter 2, diagnosing bipolar disorder involves characterizing the patient's current symptoms of mania, hypomania, depression, or mixed disorder, with a focus on the duration and severity of the current episode. Beyond these immediate concerns, a good diagnostic evaluation includes examining the past history of the disorder: whether depression, mania, or psychosis has dominated the clinical picture; whether any past episodes have been associated with substance abuse; the potential role of antidepressants in prior cycles; and evidence of comorbid disorders (e.g., ADHD). The intake evaluation may help the clinician determine whether the patient's prior course of illness resembles that of most bipolar patients: highly recurrent; depression for a substantial proportion of time (as much as 1 of every 2 weeks of the patient's life); and mildly to moderately symptomatic (with functional impairment) between episodes. The evaluation may also point to risk factors (e.g., drug abuse) or protective factors (e.g., supportive family relationships) that may alter the course of the disorder.

A thorough intake evaluation involves understanding the degree to which the patient's current and past mood episodes have affected and been affected by work, family, and social factors. To do so, one needs to evaluate the *psychosocial context* of the illness. The clinician may recognize not only that life events (e.g., new relationships) have played a substantial role in the onset of manic episodes, but also that the patient's symptoms have generated stressful circumstances (e.g., becoming overly enmeshed in a new relationship) that in turn have led to more severe symptoms.

Different clinical settings dictate different time frames for a diagnostic evaluation. For instance, many managed care contracts only reimburse for an hour of diagnostic evaluation. In other settings, a clinician may be able to spend a few full sessions doing a thorough evaluation.

In either case, efficient methods of collecting diagnostic data can save a lot of time later. The information in this chapter is intended to complement the differential diagnostic information described in Chapter 2. Here, however, we focus on (1) the efficient evaluation of current and past symptoms; (2) interview questions that help determine the diagnosis, rule out competing diagnoses, and determine the presence–absence of comorbid disorders; and (3) evaluation of the psychosocial context. We will make recommendations for how to collect a lot of information quickly, including the role of paper-and-pencil assessment instruments in making one's determinations.

## THE INITIAL REFERRAL

The intake evaluation may vary depending on whether the evaluation is a prelude to treatment (either pharmacological or psychosocial) or whether a second opinion has been requested by another clinician who will do the treatment. When evaluating patients who may have bipolar disorder, it is useful to obtain as much information as possible from the referring source about the reasons for the evaluation. If a colleague says she is treating "a depressed patient who I'm now thinking may be bipolar," the issue may be that conventional treatments for depression have not worked well. A referral that asks "whether this is bipolar or a personality disorder" may mean that patient has been difficult to treat, confrontational, or inconsistent in drug adherence.

As with any patient, the clinician should consider whether anyone else is already treating this patient and make contact with that provider. Patients who self-refer—and often those referred by another doctor— may have never notified the existing therapist or psychopharmacologist that they are seeking a second opinion (see also the Chapter 11 discussion of split treatment). It is almost always a good idea to obtain Health Insurance Portability and Accountability Act (HIPAA) releases for all relevant treatment personnel, even if there won't be any immediate contact.

## INVOLVING COLLATERALS
## IN THE DIAGNOSTIC INTERVIEW

In our experience, involving a spouse, parent, sibling, or even a close friend in the intake evaluation is nearly always worth the time and trouble. In instances in which the clinician needs the perspective of a family member, it may make sense to hold up the treatment until the communication occurs. For example, one 17-year-old boy with bipolar I disorder was not responding to mood stabilizers or antipsychotics. A parent finally divulged that his son smoked marijuana almost every day, and that the parent sometimes joined in, not realizing that marijuana could significantly reduce the impact of psychiatric medications.

Collateral informants have a different view of the history of the patient's disorder and often see things that the patient can't see (e.g., irritability, grandiosity, rapidity of speech, a new subtle pessimism, social withdrawal, psychomotor retardation). Family members are especially helpful in clarifying whether the patient has had prior hypomanic or mixed episodes. Since hypomanic episodes are often ego-syntonic for patients, consistent with their view of themselves as highly energetic, creative, and productive, they may forget events that occurred during hypomania or mania, particularly if they are depressed when trying to recall these events.

A good rule of thumb is to ask patients to bring in one family member or friend, ideally someone who spends at least 4 hours a week in their company, regardless of whether they live together. Patients have variable reactions to this request. Many are delighted that a family member can provide input given that many practitioners avoid contact with family members. Others may become defensive, saying "I don't want my wife's view of me to dominate," or "I've spent my life trying to get away from my parents." Tell the patient, "You can be in the room or not when I talk to them," and "My diagnosis is going to be based on a synthesis of what you and they say, not just what they say." Nonetheless, if a patient adamantly refuses, it is generally better to wait until one has established a rapport with the patient and involve family members later.

## COLLECTING INFORMATION ABOUT MOOD EPISODES

Many structured interview protocols instruct clinicians to ask "stem" questions followed by "associated symptom" questions. For example, the instructions for the Structured Clinical Interview for DSM-IV[1] suggest asking about whether depressed mood or loss of interests (criterion A symptoms) have been present for 2 weeks or more (at some point in the past), and only to follow up with questions about sleep changes, appetite changes, fatigue, psychomotor retardation, and suicidality (criterion B symptoms) if the patient endorses one of the two "A" symptoms.

These methods can be problematic for a number of reasons. Structured interviews teach interviewers to be systematic in asking about symptoms but may miss nuances that can be elicited by more experienced clinicians. As an example, patients do not tend to think about illness periods in durations of 2 weeks or more and may decide that the clinician doesn't want to hear about shorter episodes. Additionally, many individuals will say "no" to depressed mood or loss of interests, but then describe a clear period in which their sleep was disturbed and they felt fatigued, slowed down, worthless, and suicidal. If the interviewer then "circles back" to the depressed mood or loss of interests question, patients may well endorse it the second time.

As a general framework for assessing whether a patient has had one or more past episodes of depression or (hypo)mania, we suggest the following: Describe to the patient a *template* for that type of episode first, a brief statement describing what a depressive or manic/hypomanic episode generally looks like. Then, follow it up with "Has there been a period of time like this? Could you have had something like that? [If so,] How long did that period last?" Once evidence has been obtained indicating that the patient has had such a period, the associated "A" and "B" symptoms that occurred during that same interval can be confirmed. It is critical to be able to describe episodes with onsets and offsets, acknowledging that patients frequently distort episode time frames.

Compare the following two interviews:

CLINICIAN: Has there ever been a 2 week or more period where you felt depressed nearly every day, for most of the day?

PATIENT: No, probably not every day.

CLINICIAN: Or 2 or more weeks when you lost interest in things? Nothing felt like any fun?

PATIENT: Can't think of anything.

Manuals for structured interviews might ask the clinician to probe more deeply, but basically, once the patient has answered "no" to the two stem questions, it is time to move on to the next disorder. Now, consider this approach:

CLINICIAN: As you may know, when people get depressed, they get intensely sad and lose interest in a variety of things. They may be unable to sleep or sleep too much, have changes in appetite, feel sluggish and slowed down, feel bad about themselves, even feel like hurting themselves or ending their lives. Has there ever been a period of time like that for you?

PATIENT: Yeah. Last winter.

CLINICIAN: How long did that last?

PATIENT: I'm guessing for most of the winter. Started right after the holidays.

CLINICIAN: How was your mood that winter?

PATIENT: Very sad, really apathetic, didn't care about anything . . . you know, like, time to check out.

CLINICIAN: Check out?

PATIENT: Yeah, you know, like [pauses] . . . cash my check. End it.

CLINICIAN: How did it start?

PATIENT: Not really sure, I just remember not wanting to go to work, staying inside a lot.

CLINICIAN: Sounds like a difficult time. What was your sleep like that winter?

Patients may also not respond well to questions like "Was there a 1-week or longer period where you felt unusually high, happy, or cheerful?" They may remember being full of energy or not needing to sleep, but they may have little recollection of their mood without this context. When trying to determine the duration of episodes, ask questions like these:

CLINICIAN: Some people get very high or wired for periods of time, where they don't feel like they need to sleep because they don't get tired. At those times they may feel powerful, like they can do anything; full of energy, thoughts going a mile a minute, doing too many things. Ever felt like this?

PATIENT: Definitely.

CLINICIAN: When was the last time?

PATIENT: Probably end of spring semester.

CLINICIAN: Do you remember when it began? What was the first sign?

PATIENT: During finals week, I was like staying up and partying almost every night. And yet I totally aced all my classes! I felt, like, invulnerable.

CLINICIAN: How long did it last? What brought it to an end?

PATIENT: When I went back home to New Jersey. That'll put an end to any party. Maybe a few weeks all together.

CLINICIAN: Do you remember what your mood was like at the time?

PATIENT: I dunno, fine, I guess. Good maybe at first, but then I started feeling pissed off when no one else wanted to mess around.

Additional questions would include how much sleep was lost and whether the patient felt tired the next day; whether he felt full of energy and ideas; and whether he engaged in any impulsive or risky behavior. Finally, we would want to know whether the activated phase got him into trouble. From the previous dialogue, it appears that his behavior did not affect his grades, but we do not know yet whether it damaged his relationships.

## GETTING THE STORY OF THE DISORDER

### Assessing the Prior Course of Illness

It is very easy to get stuck in a cross-sectional mind-set when interviewing a patient. We can get very wrapped up in whether the patient has met DSM-5 criteria for mania or depression in the last month or even in the last week. Instead, try to get the *story of the disorder*: when it started, when past episodes began and ended, what level of functional impairment occurred, and whether mood episodes were associated with any obvious stressors.

The prior course of the patient's illness may be more informative than the presenting symptoms. For example, it can be puzzling when a 20-year-old reports feeling irritable, activated, and goal-driven but also has clearly delusional thinking. In distinguishing bipolar disorder from schizoaffective disorder, one can spend considerable time trying to ferret out whether the manic or the psychotic symptoms came first, or whether they have truly co-occurred during the most recent episode. While this is all valuable information, it may not be as helpful as asking some of the following questions:

"When you've had your high periods in the past, have they always gone along with feeling that people can read you mind? Can you think of any times when you felt high and didn't think about this?"

"In the past, which would people have noticed more—your being sped up, irritable, and not sleeping, or your thinking about radio waves and extrasensory perception? Which seems more prominent to you?"

Part of the reason to clarify the story of the disorder is to determine whether the illness has been episodic versus chronic. Many patients and their relatives describe the patient as "always irritable," "always pessimistic," or "chronically moody." It is important to clarify what the patient and/or relative means: Is "chronically moody" synonymous with day-to-day or hour-to-hour mood fluctuations? Or is it a description of someone who has multiple discrete episodes, but with clear euthymic periods in between? As described in Chapter 2, the diagnosis of bipolar disorder versus personality disorders (notably, borderline personality disorder) often hinges on whether there have been episodes with a beginning, a middle, and an end. We will say more about personality disorders shortly.

Although not technically relevant to the diagnosis, information about the "topography" of the episode (i.e., its prodromal, active, and residual phases) may be helpful in instructing the patient or family to recognize early warning signs of new episodes. Once again, try presenting the following scenario to help elicit more of the story of the disorder:

"Many people have manic episodes that build over time, and start with symptoms that aren't that severe, like mild increases in energy, irritability or snappiness, or feeling like your mind is racing. We call this the prodromal period. Then, things get very intense and the person may not be sleeping much at all, and may be bitterly angry; driving recklessly on the freeway or spending all their money, and talking a mile a minute. Do your episodes look like that? If not, what are they like?"

Once it has been established that there has been at least one prior manic or hypomanic episode, the clinician can move to questions like "How many of these do you think you've had over your lifetime? What is your functioning like between episodes? How long do they ordinarily last before you're back to your usual self?" If the patient reports having hundreds of manic episodes, one can add, "Let's just consider those that have lasted at least a week."

### Problems That Arise in Assessing Depression and Suicidality

Patients often give a history of clear-cut manic or hypomanic episodes but are vague about the onset–offset pattern of depressive episodes. The patient may have long periods of dysthymia that occasionally worsen and become major depressive episodes ("double depression"). If a patient says that she has always been depressed, it is a good idea to ask questions such as "When does it get worse? Any particular time of year [seasonality]? Does it always have the same effects on your ability to work? Ever make it impossible to work?"

It is helpful to distinguish between the daily rhythms of weekends versus weekdays. If the depression is not too severe and the patient is particularly committed to her work, she may be able to get up in the morning during the week but spend most of the unstructured weekend time in bed. Thus, she may still meet DSM-5 criteria for a major depressive episode.

Be aware of the depressive symptoms that most often characterize bipolar depressions: hypersomnia, hyperphagia (and weight gain), psychomotor retardation, and psychotic symptoms. Typically, the latter include depressive themes (e.g., somatic delusions such as "My body is rotting"; "I have an undiagnosed cancer"; or "I feel like I'm being punished for my sins"). Also, determine whether the first depressive episode occurred during the adolescent years; early-onset depression is more likely to convert to bipolar I or II disorder than is adult-onset depression.[2,3] A good way to ask this is "Many people get depressed when they're teenagers. Do you think you had worse depressions than your peers? If so, when was the first one?"

Bipolar depressions are often nonresponsive to antidepressants, so the patient's response to SSRIs or other agents during prior depressive episodes should always be assessed. Although it is well established that antidepressants can cause switches from depression to mania or mixed disorder, they are often blamed for manic or hypomanic episodes that might have occurred even without antidepressants. Ask about the timing of antidepressant treatment in relation to any new (hypo)manic episodes, and pay particular attention to those episodes that occurred within 2–3 months after initiating these agents. Furthermore, ask whether the patient was taking a mood stabilizer or second-generation antipsychotic when the antidepressant was initiated; combination treatment is less likely to result in manic switches than is antidepressant monotherapy.[4]

### Assessing Prior Suicidal Behavior

Many clinicians, especially those less experienced, are nervous about assessing suicidal behavior. We devote a considerable amount of discussion to managing suicidal behavior in Chapter 10; here, we limit our discussion to its assessment.

As may seem obvious, the best predictor of future suicidal behavior is past suicidal behavior in both adults and children, and including those with bipolar disorder.[5] Thus, we prefer to be reasonably direct in asking about suicidality, keeping in mind the differences between active suicidal behavior, past suicidal behavior, suicidal thinking (with or without serious intent), and nonsuicidal self-injurious behavior (e.g., self-cutting without suicidal intent).

One can ease into the topic when evaluating current or past depressive symptoms. Patients have an easier time with questions about suicide when they are framed as part of the depressive syndrome, in the same category as insomnia. Start with "Did you [or do you] have dark and morbid thoughts, like life isn't worth living? Or even wishing you were dead? Are you feeling that way now?" After obtaining a response, go further: "Have you thought of a specific method? Did you ever try to carry it out?" If the patient has never attempted suicide but thinks about it, ask "Were you ever worried about acting on it? Was anyone else ever worried that you would, or did anyone think you should be in the hospital?" Ask about family history as well: Those with first- or second-degree relatives who have committed suicide are at increased risk.

Ask about nonsuicidal self-injurious behavior, especially when interviewing adolescent or young adult patients, for whom this behavior is more common. The most prevalent self-injurious behaviors are self-cutting, burning oneself with cigarettes, or banging one's head against a wall. There may or may not be suicidal intent. Many bipolar patients (and not just those with comorbid borderline personality disorder) say that self-injurious behavior relieves their inner suffering for a short time. Ask about the relationship between self-injuries and mood episodes. Some patients self-harm even when not in a mood episode, implying the presence of comorbid personality disorders or untreated mood symptoms; for others, self-injurious behavior occurs exclusively during depressive episodes.

In Chapter 10 we offer additional suggestions on conducting a suicide risk assessment. For now, note the difference between patients who admit to wishing they were dead but "I would never do it" to those who have harmed themselves in what appear to be impulsive and "communicative" gestures, and those that have hatched a specific plan or looked online for specific methods.

## DIAGNOSTIC CHALLENGES

In Chapter 2, we described the difficult diagnostic differential decisions that need to be made between bipolar disorder and "near-neighbor" conditions. Here, we describe methods of assessing symptoms that are often at the root of these challenges.

### *Irritability and Hypomania*

Irritability, a symptom of both mania and depression and many other disorders (e.g., anxiety disorders, psychosis), has caused considerable confusion in the diagnostic nomenclature. Indeed, irritability comes in many different forms: the manic, "Don't get in my way" irritability that often accompanies attempts by others to limit the patient's access to a goal; the "Leave me alone" type that accompanies depression; and chronically irritable temperaments that are in evidence between episodes but may worsen when the patient is ill.

The key to placing irritability in the context of bipolar illness is to remember that (1) irritability is a nonspecific symptom that occurs in many different disorders; (2) it must worsen from a baseline state in order to qualify for the DSM-5 "A" mood component of the hypomanic or manic syndrome; and (3) it must coincide with the development of increased activity (for mania or hypomania) or the onset or worsening of sadness or loss of interests (for depression). When a patient describes an episode of irritability and increased activity, he must have four associated "B" symptoms to meet DSM-5 hypomania or mania criteria, and only three if the mood is elated. If the mood is only irritable, the clinician will need to obtain more examples of "B" manic symptoms than if the mood was elated.

Consider the following two presentations of irritability:

---

Candido, age 47, described himself as having a "grouchy personality." His wife gave many examples of how he yelled at their children for tiny infractions. She said that his outbursts had worsened since the kids were out of school for the summer. He denied changes in sleep but described various plans to "blow it on out of here, get on the road, don't look back." He denied increases in energy and did not feel depressed, except to say that he felt like a failure since having been laid off from his job.

Ian, age 41, said that he had grown more angry since the beginning of summer, when he was free from his academic year teaching job. He had been staying up later than usual, and also getting up earlier, averaging 4–5 hours of sleep per night. He described feeling more energetic and his thoughts moving more rapidly, but denied grandiosity. His wife said that his mood seemed quite different from the way it had been during the school year. For example, she said that Ian had "barked" an order to a waitress at a local restaurant and had whistled at a girl who was standing at a crosswalk, both of which he denied.

Ian's episode meets criteria for hypomania, whereas Candido's does not. Candido is chronically irritable, with a worsening due to environmental influences (kids out of school); he may meet DSM-5 criteria for persistent depressive disorder (formerly dysthymic disorder), but the history is not consistent with an episodic mood disorder. Note that Ian's symptoms represent a more dramatic change from his baseline mood.

In summary, when assessing the role of irritability in bipolar disorder, ask whether it increased at the same time as other hypomanic or manic symptoms, such as decreased need for sleep or increased energy. Try to determine whether irritability is associated with impatience when trying to achieve a goal (a manic symptom) or a desire to be left alone (usually a depressive or anxiety symptom). Determine whether recent environmental stressors explain the patient's irritable moods to a greater extent than do other manic or depressive symptoms.

## Mixed Presentations

Confusion among clinicians about the role of irritability often underlies disagreements about whether patients are experiencing mixed states. As described in Chapter 2, a bipolar patient meets criteria for the DSM-5 mixed course specifier only if she is fully manic or hypomanic and has at least 3 symptoms of a major depressive episode during the same week. This definition does not match what many clinicians see in practice: patients who have major depression with only one or two coincident manic symptoms, or patients who are manic or hypomanic but have depressive thinking (e.g., pessimism) and/or are suicidal. Research suggests that there are actually varying levels of "mixity," particularly among women, such as hypomanic episodes with depressive symptoms that do not meet the full criteria for major depressive disorder.[6] Children and adolescents with bipolar spectrum disorders have more periods of mixed symptoms than do adults.[7]

When assessing whether the patient meets the criteria for a DSM-5 mixed episode specifier, make sure that she is describing simultaneous depressive and (hypo)manic symptoms, not symptoms that alternate over the course of several days. Other specifiers or diagnostic options may include ultrarapid cycling (four or more episodes in one month), ultradian cycling (within 24 hours), or personality disorders. Consider the following interchange between a clinician and patient, in which the clinician tries to pin down the exact timing of mixed symptoms.

CLINICIAN: You've described several periods of depression. Some people feel depressed and also high at the same time, what we call "mixed." They feel like their thoughts are going fast, get very irritable, and have more energy, but they also feel very fatigued, bad about themselves, and have insomnia. Did that ever happen to you?

PATIENT: Most definitely.

CLINICIAN: When was the last time?

PATIENT: Just recently! I was up all night, jamming on my Les Paul, writing songs, looking at record company websites, and the next day I was totally exhausted.

CLINICIAN: And when you were exhausted, did you go back to sleep?

PATIENT: That's the thing, I didn't really need to! I felt like I could get along on just a few hours or just catnaps during the day.

CLINICIAN: How would you describe your mood at those times?

PATIENT: Probably pretty good. Or maybe pissed off. Yeah, more like pissed off. If my wife told me to get to bed I'd be like, down her throat.

CLINICIAN: How about feeling any sadness?

PATIENT: (*Pauses.*) No, not that I can remember . . . maybe just feeling bad about what I was doing to my family.

CLINICIAN: You felt bad about your family when?

PATIENT: That came later. After I got fired.

This patient is probably describing a hypomanic or manic episode without mixity. There is not much evidence of depressive symptoms, even though he heartily endorses the "vision" of the mixed episode presented by the clinician. Now, consider this next patient:

CLINICIAN: So you'd be up all night and still be able to go to work the next day?

PATIENT: Yeah, I just couldn't stop my mind. Too many ideas, too many threads to follow.

CLINICIAN: So, did you feel like you needed to sleep?

PATIENT: I desperately needed to. I felt like I was dying. I couldn't sleep at all, kept waking up, thinking again, waking up, and then, bam! . . . 5:00 A.M. rolls around and I'm up for work.

CLINICIAN: Sounds pretty awful. And how did you feel the next day?

PATIENT: Horrible. Drifting off to sleep in the middle of meetings. Sending a text message felt like a major accomplishment.

CLINICIAN: What about your mood?

PATIENT: Usually mad, angry, sometimes sad, but definitely not that "up" feeling.

This patient is more likely to meet criteria for a mixed episode specifier. Note the presence of a decreased need for sleep in the first patient and insomnia in the second. The feeling of being exhausted the next day is rare among truly manic or hypomanic persons.

If the patient has had a major depressive episode and only one or two manic or hypomanic symptoms, check:

1. When was the onset of her first depressive episode?
2. Do any first- or second-degree relatives have bipolar disorder?
3. Is there a history of antidepressant-induced mood switches?

Patients with early-age illness onset (i.e., under age 18), a family history of mania, and a history of antidepressant-induced mood switches are at greater risk for converting to bipolar I or II disorder than depressed patients without these features.

### Chronic Irritability versus Mixed States

Some clinicians diagnose persistent, nonepisodic irritability as a "chronic mixed state" (implying a bipolar diagnosis), but there is little research to suggest that bipolar patients have persistent mixed states. The few studies that have distinguished episodic irritability from chronic irritability have concluded that chronic irritability is more likely to be a sign of major depression than of mania (e.g., Brotman et al.[8]). Patients with chronic irritability may also have a persistent depressive disorder, an anxiety disorder or a personality disorder.

Ask whether the patient has increased irritability that goes along with increased energy, activity, and speed of thinking, or a decreased need for sleep. Irritability should also be tied to observable changes in functioning (hypomania) or a clear deterioration in functioning (mania). A patient who shows most of the signs of major depression and has irritability that "tracks" with the other depressive symptoms, but no other hypomania symptoms, is probably best conceptualized as having a depressive disorder. As discussed in Chapter 2, there are disagreements in our field as to the boundaries of "depressive–mixed" disorders and whether these are on a continuum with bipolar disorder, but there is general agreement that chronic irritability alone (even if accompanied by dramatic temper outbursts and violence) does not in itself point to a bipolar course of illness.

### Sleep Disturbances

A common error in assessing bipolarity is the confusion between decreased need for sleep and insomnia. Thus, when interviewing a patient, it is important to get specifics on the nature of sleep disturbance in manic, hypomanic, and depressed episodes. Insomnia can be conceptualized as initial (trouble falling asleep), middle (awakening several times in the middle of the night), or terminal (waking up too early and being unable to get back to sleep). These are generally symptoms of depression rather than hypomania or mania. During the depressive phases of bipolar disorder, patients may also be *hypersomnic*, where they sleep many hours during the day, then complain of being unable to sleep at night, or they sleep through the night, then for most of the day.

In almost all of these instances, the patient will complain of fatigue and the desire to sleep. The "smoking gun" for mania is the presence of a decreased *need* for sleep. The patient with (hypo)mania will (1) purposely not go to sleep (because sleep is unnecessary, boring, or a waste of time), or (2) try to sleep, but complain of being too wired to actually fall asleep. These patients typically try to get work done at night and may even try to compose music, write poetry, or telephone long-lost friends. Creative individuals may ascribe not sleeping to the creative impulse, but often the nighttime activities are less creative, such as cleaning the closet. Importantly, the patient will not be tired the next day, and the cycle will repeat the next night. In these circumstances, mania/hypomania can be fairly easy to diagnose.

Start by asking, "How has your sleep been [or how was it at the time]?" Then, narrow it down further: "How long does it take you to fall asleep? Do you then wake up during the night? How many times? What time do you wake up? Is this later or earlier than you want? Do you feel rested? How long do these periods last . . . how many nights in a row? Now, what about the opposite, sleeping too much and not wanting to do much else?" To assess decreased need for sleep, ask, "When you're wired like that and don't sleep, how do you feel the next day? Can you get by with less than, say, 5 hours? Has that always been true of you, or only when you're also feeling wired [or racy, or high]?"

Many patients may not be able to describe their sleep patterns. Once again, a spouse's input may be helpful. If the symptom is currently occurring, suggest that the patient keep a daily sleep and mood log, such as those discussed in Chapter 7 (see *www.healthline.com/health-slideshow/top-iphone-android-apps-bipolar-disorder#1*).

## DIFFERENTIAL DIAGNOSIS AND COMORBID DISORDERS

This section is intended to complement parallel sections in Chapter 2, highlighting how to distinguish between disorders that overlap with bipolar disorder in symptomatology.

### Substance Abuse Disorders

Among the many challenges the clinician faces in diagnosing bipolar disorder, uncovering substance abuse is perhaps the most difficult. It can be quite difficult to determine the role of alcohol or illicit substances at the first meeting; sometimes, this information emerges later, once a working alliance has developed.

The primary principle in assessing the presence of primary substance use is to determine whether there have been any manic, hypomanic, depressive, or mixed episodes that cannot be reasonably attributed to substances. To have a diagnosis of bipolar disorder, there must be evidence that episodes have occurred without provocation by street drugs, alcohol, or prescription drugs, including antidepressants.

If a patient describes a number of past depressive episodes, and also describes drinking heavily, ask, "Were there any periods when you were depressed that hadn't been associated with drinking?" Other informative questions include "What is your mood like when you've been sober for awhile? What happens when you stop drinking [or using marijuana/other street drugs?]" Some patients describe a cyclothymic temperament when they are not using substances, characterized by up and down moods that are not debilitating. They may only have major episodes (with functional impairment) when they are using substances regularly.

If the issue is current use, urine toxicology screens, collateral reports, and prior medical records are usually helpful. Interviewing a significant other may be profoundly illuminating, both in obtaining a more accurate record of how much the patient is using and in establishing the pattern of mood swings and drug–alcohol use. Patients may describe prior psychiatric hospitalizations and manic behavior but neglect to mention that they were in a drug rehabilitation facility. They may also forget how much of a substance they used during past episodes.

Another way of collecting this information is to draw a mood time line. For example, draw time on the $x$-axis, and the patient's pattern of up and down cycling on the $y$-axis (from depressed to hypomanic or manic). Then, ask him to recount when during these cycles his cannabis use was at its height, when he began using cocaine, or when he started or stopped drinking. Nonetheless, some patients have a period of continuous use that is difficult to separate from manic or depressive episodes. In these cases, the patient may need a chemical dependency program before beginning treatment for bipolar disorder.

### Bipolar Disorder versus Borderline Personality Disorder

Often, the co-diagnosis of bipolar and borderline personality disorder is based on the same set of symptoms. Consider the following vignette:

Rosie, a 19-year-old female, was diagnosed with ADHD and "borderline personality features." The latter was based on her history of impulsive sexual encounters, rageful responses to her mother and father, rapidly shifting interpersonal attachments, poor peer functioning, and self-destructive behavior. A thorough diagnostic assessment revealed that Rosie had developed a major depressive episode at age 14, following the breakup of her first romantic relationship. During that time she began self-cutting with glass and razors, smoking tobacco and marijuana, and being truant from school. Her ADHD medication was increased to little effect, with the exception that her sleep became more disturbed. Her mother reported numerous short periods of hypomania in Rosie's mid- to late-teens, each lasting 1–2 days, in which she had elevated mood, increased energy, increased sexual drive, and decreased need for sleep.[9] (p. 14)

This case illustrates the significant overlap between these two disorders. The problem is magnified in bipolar II disorder (Rosie's eventual diagnosis) because borderline patients usually have major depressive episodes, leaving the clinician with the difficult task of distinguishing hypomanic episodes from personality-driven affective storms and impulsive behavior. Of course, a patient can be diagnosed with both disorders, but doing so does not help much with treatment planning. Instead, consider the following: How distinctive are the periods of hypomania or irritability/impulsiveness? Can the patient (or collaterals) distinguish a beginning and an end of episodes? Typically, patients with borderline personality disorder do not have episodes of decreased need for sleep along with periods of frenetic activity, grandiosity, or racing thoughts, even though any one of these symptoms may have been present at some point.

Bipolar disorder characterized by rapid cycling can look very similar to mood reactivity in borderline personality disorder. The classic definition of rapid cycling (four or more episodes per year) is fairly distinct from borderline personality disorder because there must be periods of remission in between episodes. A patient who describes ultrarapid cycling, however, may be describing the frequent affective shifts of borderline personality disorder. The mood swings of borderline patients tend to vary with day-to-day events, such as the ups and downs of a romantic relationship. Events in which a person with borderline personality disorder feels "invalidated" by others[10]—for example, feeling rejected by a close relative or romantic partner, then being dismissed for these emotional reactions—may lead to periods of rage and aggressive or self-destructive behavior (e.g., abruptly jumping into bed with another partner, self-cutting, binge eating). Usually, however, these periods of rage are not accompanied by increases in energy, activity, and speed of thinking, or a decreased need for sleep. Although a relationship breakup may disrupt a patient's sleep and circadian rhythms, it is less likely to trigger a hypomanic episode.

It is very difficult to distinguish a bipolar depression from a depression that may be tied to a personality disorder. Depressions associated with personality disorder tend to be more chronic and persistent, or what used to be called "dysthymic." Otherwise, symptoms of depression—such as insomnia, suicidality, or feelings of worthlessness—are not particularly useful in making distinctions between mood and personality disorders.

### Bipolar Disorder and ADHD

There has been considerable debate about how to distinguish bipolar disorder from ADHD, particularly in children and adolescents. On the surface, the two disorders sound almost identical. The diagnostic confusion derives largely from the overlapping "B" items in the DSM for mania and ADHD: distractibility, increased motor hyperactivity, impulsive behavior, and pressured speech. Moreover, children with ADHD are often irritable. In comparisons of clinical samples of children, these overlapping symptoms are far less useful in distinguishing between the two disorders compared to euphoric/elevated mood, grandiosity, hypersexuality, and decreased need for sleep.[11,12]

Some patients are diagnosed with both bipolar disorder and ADHD. Before deciding for certain that a patient has both disorders, ask the patient about the onset of the cognitive problems associated with ADHD (inattention, distractibility, disorganization, forgetfulness): If they began in childhood before the onset of problems with mood swings, and persisted throughout school, the ADHD diagnosis may be warranted. Look for recollections of classic childhood ADHD behavior, such as jumping out of one's seat in class, raising one's hand impulsively, forgetting to bring assignments back, and being frequently off-task. Once again, inquire about the episodic nature of these symptoms. Bipolar patients may show any of these behaviors during mood episodes, whereas the cognitive problems of ADHD tend to be chronic (unless treated).

Of course, it is difficult to tell whether these same behaviors—particularly hyperactive or impulsive behavior—might reflect early-onset mania. Children with ADHD usually do not get by with only a few hours of sleep and do not ordinarily express euphoric mood or grandiose ideas. Hypersexuality can be present even in a young manic child (e.g., drawing obscene pictures in class) but are rarely characteristic of ADHD. Another behavior—uninhibited people seeking—has also been described as distinguishing manic from ADHD behavior in childhood.[12]

As the child enters the teen years, periods of depression may be more informative than periods of mania. Adult bipolar patients often describe an adolescence filled with periods of social withdrawal, fatigue, suicidality, and psychomotor retardation, although they may also have had ongoing problems with concentration and inattention that did not coincide with mood swings. In some of these cases, the co-diagnosis of bipolar disorder and ADHD may be justified. However, many children with ADHD develop major depressive episodes and suicidal behavior in adolescence (especially girls).[13] For this reason, the mere presence of low mood alongside ADHD does not necessarily indicate bipolar disorder.

Some adult patients say that they had undiagnosed and untreated ADHD as children. Check as to their recollection of the onset of their cognitive problems. Can they recall a period of time in which their cognitive functioning appeared to be normal, even though they were not taking any medications? Have they had problems with job performance as adults, even when sleep and other indicators of mood disorder were normal? Neuropsychological testing may be a helpful supplement to the diagnostic evaluation. Tests that tap attention, processing speed, cognitive disorganization, and working memory may be more informative than self-report or informant reports. Testing should be scheduled when the patient is in remission from the mood disorder for at least a few weeks.

## EVALUATING THE PSYCHOSOCIAL CONTEXT

In the foregoing discussions, we have focused on the symptomatic picture of the disorder. This level of evaluation informs the psychosocial context of the patient's pattern of mood cycling, but direct questions about the family and social environment are usually essential in treatment planning given their prognostic value.[14] Thus, the intake interview should include some focused questions about psychosocial context.

Begin by asking whether the most recent symptoms were precipitated by major *life events*. It may be helpful to think of life events in terms of several dimensions: negative versus positive, dependent versus independent (i.e., potentially caused by the patient's behavior or not), and degree of social rhythm (i.e., daily and nightly routine) disruption. Frequently, patients say that their recent depressed or mixed episode was caused by job loss, but careful questioning may reveal that the mood symptoms occurred first and accelerated the patient's job termination.

Events can be positive in valence but also disruptive to social rhythms. Examples of these may include new romantic relationships, which often are paired with significant changes in sleep–wake rhythms; birth of a baby; or a job promotion. Life events that promote *goal attainment* may be especially likely to promote excessive confidence, motivation for reward, and manic or hypomanic symptoms.[15]

A second dimension to consider is the current family or marital environment (see Chapters 7 and 8). Highly conflicted dyadic relationships characterized by intense criticism, hostility, or emotional overinvolvement (high "expressed emotion") can be associated with earlier recurrences, more severe symptoms, and poorer social functioning over a year or more of treatment.[16] There are self-report and informant-report scales that clarify the nature of family relationships (e.g., the

Conflict Behavior Questionnaire, available at *www.first5cc.org/sites/ default/files/conflict%20behavior%20questionnaire-teen-english%20v1. pdf*), but many of these scales assume that the patient is an adolescent or young adult living with his parents. Interviewing the patient and spouse or parent(s) together is often the most informative procedure. As Yogi Berra once said, "You can observe a lot by just watching."

Why are these distinctions in social triggers so important? The psychotherapy recommended will need to consider the context in which the most recent symptoms occurred. When working with a patient involved in a relationship with high expressed emotion, it is likely that the patient and relatives will benefit from a psychoeducationally oriented family therapy.[17] Knowing that certain events provoke goal attainment cognitions (e.g., "I can't lose") allows the clinician to be on the lookout for events that may precipitate manic symptoms, and to introduce cognitive restructuring early in the manic escalation.[18] Knowing that a change in routines is imminent (e.g., a graduate student is about to start school again) may help with the planning of social rhythm interventions that can help to stabilize moods.[19]

Finally, when hypomanic, many patients alienate employers, family members, or new romantic partners with arrogance or irritability. When patients and their close relatives become aware that these symptoms can represent early warnings signs of a recurrence, they have taken a first step toward better functioning in the social, occupational, and familial context.

## EVALUATING THE PSYCHIATRIC MEDICATION HISTORY

Obtaining an accurate and thorough psychiatric medication history is a critical part of the initial evaluation. Of course, if the patient has never been in treatment before, this is rather quick and easy, although here, too, it is always helpful to probe about medications that patients often do not see as medications, such as over-the-counter sleeping pills (e.g., diphenhydramine or Benadryl) or "natural" substances that have potential psychotropic effects, such as omega-3 fatty acids (fish oil) or s-adenosylmethionine (SAM-e), both of which may have some antidepressant effects.

For previously treated patients, the clinician obtaining the history can create an accurate list of current and past medications. As in so many other areas of a thorough evaluation, collateral information may be required. Often, patients are unsure of their current doses and, even more commonly, do not have a comprehensive list of prior treatments.

Other sources of information can be family members, past treating professionals, or hospital records. (The latter two sources, of course, require formal authorization for release of records.) Hospitals are notoriously slow in responding (if they respond at all) to record requests. It is frequently helpful to suggest to patients that they go to the hospital or previous clinic themselves and fill out the required release of information forms in order to expedite what is otherwise an excruciatingly slow process.

Just creating a list of prior treatments, however, is insufficient. The vital information needed by the treating psychiatrist—especially when patients say they did not respond to the prior treatments—is that of dose and duration of treatment. Even though it is not always possible to obtain this information, it is best to determine for each medication the maximum dose, the duration of treatment with it, and the side effects experienced. Very frequently, patients will remember a past medication that "did not work." Upon more careful examination, it becomes clear that the medication was taken only transiently, inconsistently, for too short a period of time, or at too low a dose for it to have been effective.

Jan, a 34-year-old woman with bipolar disorder, insisted that she had tried all the mood stabilizers available without effect, leading to a sense of frustration and discouragement. Her history was confusing as she conflated the current episode with past episodes. She remembered few details of her medication history, irritably repeating that "none of them helped a damn." With the aid of past treatment records (and reinterviewing Jan with this information in hand), it became clear that, for at least two medications, lithium and risperidone (Risperdal), treatment duration had been only a few days each. Moreover, it was not clear whether she had taken the medications during those days either. In both circumstances, Jan was hospitalized within a few days after starting the medication, and in both cases a different psychiatrist had changed her treatment regimen. After an extensive discussion about this issue, Jan reluctantly agreed to try lithium again. Ultimately, lithium was very helpful as a long-term mood stabilizer.

When patients are treated with multiple medications simultaneously (as frequently occurs in bipolar disorder), they make misattributions about side effects. Thus, as part of a history, a patient may say that lithium caused intolerable sedation, forgetting that olanzapine (Zyprexa), a highly sedating antimanic agent, was part of the regimen at that time. Collateral history, such as medical records, along with explicitly asking about other, simultaneously prescribed medications can help to avoid these errors.

## EVALUATING THE MEDICAL HISTORY
## AND LABORATORY TESTS

Taking a classical medical history is no different with psychiatric patients than with other medical patients. The core information to be obtained is *all* medications currently being taken, allergies to medications, a history of surgeries and/or hospitalizations, and a history of any significant medical disorder (currently or in the past). As noted in Chapter 2, a number of medications prescribed for nonpsychiatric disorders may cause psychiatric symptoms such as mania or depression. Whether the patient has had a recent (within the last few months) medical examination by a primary care doctor is also relevant.

There is significant disagreement as to the extent of appropriate laboratory testing when a bipolar patient presents for evaluation and treatment. A reasonable approach would be to obtain a chemistry panel that includes electrolytes, liver enzymes, and a measure of renal function, along with a thyroid-stimulating hormone (TSH) level as the most important screening test for thyroid function (assuming that these tests have not already been done by another physician within the last few months).

In contrast to the varied practices of administering laboratory tests, the vast majority of patients with mood symptoms do not need any neuroimaging test, such as computed tomography (CT), magnetic resonance imaging (MRI) or functional MRI (fMRI), or positron-emission tomography (PET) scans. Rarely do these tests—which range from costly to downright bank-breaking—add to the diagnostic evaluation or alter treatment recommendations. Therefore, unless there is a very specific reason, such as numbness or weakness on one side of the body, dramatic cognitive changes that are not consistent with mania or depression, or a first manic episode much later in life, imaging studies should not be part of the routine evaluation of mood disorders.

## SELF-RATED SCALES TO INFORM DIAGNOSIS
## AND FUNCTIONING

Many clinicians routinely collect self-report data from their patients, beyond the usual checklists of medication history, surgeries, and allergies. Reviewing standardized questionnaires before the evaluation may seem like quite an investment of time, but it may also speed up the interview process and help to focus the interviewer's lines of inquiry. For example, knowing beforehand that a patient has been considering suicide allows one to spend time in the first interview on prevention planning.

## Mood Disorders Questionnaire

With the consistent evidence that many, if not most, bipolar individuals are inaccurately diagnosed for many years, self-report screening measures that have been developed may help to ascertain a history of manic or hypomanic symptoms/episodes. Theoretically, these would be more likely to be helpful in the milder bipolar disorders, such as bipolar II or cyclothymic disorder. The most commonly used rating instrument is the Mood Disorder Questionnaire (MDQ),[20] a simple 13-item questionnaire, with two additional questions probing for concurrence of the manic symptoms and functional consequence of the symptoms (available at *www.dbsalliance.org/pdfs/mdq.pdf*).

Initial evaluations of the MDQ suggested that a score of 7 or more (more than half the symptoms endorsed), with symptom concurrence and at least moderate functional consequences, was consistent with a clinical diagnosis of bipolar disorder and excluded other disorders, suggesting that the MDQ had good sensitivity and excellent specificity.[20] However, there has been increasing controversy about the clinical usefulness of the MDQ for two reasons:

1. It was developed as a screening instrument and is not meant to substitute for a diagnostic interview. If it used as a guide to areas that the clinician should probe, then it has served a purpose. By itself, however, it should not be expected to yield a clinically reliable diagnosis of bipolar disorder.
2. The sensitivity and specificity of the instrument differs depending on the population studied. For example, patients with borderline personality disorder also score above the clinical cutoff for the instrument.[21] Using the MDQ in a group of patients in a mood disorders specialty clinic may yield very different results compared to using it in either a general medical clinic (in which the goal is to screen for bipolar disorder) or a dual-diagnosis clinic in which patients may have substance abuse disorders that give rise to mood symptoms that are *not* bipolar disorder.

In a recent study of patients in a dual-diagnosis setting, the MDQ did an excellent job of ruling out bipolar disorder; that is, those who had low MDQ scores were very unlikely to be deemed bipolar from a clinical interview. However, almost half of those screening positive on the MDQ did not have bipolar disorder.[22] When a clinician discussed MDQ items with patients directly, it became clear that patients endorsed manic/hypomanic symptoms that clearly referred to the effects of drug misuse, not bipolar disorder.

Thus, the MDQ should not be mistaken for a diagnostic instrument, but it may help to reduce *false negatives:* If patients score low on the MDQ, then they are unlikely to have bipolar disorder. Some patients, surprisingly, have never been asked these questions before.

### Self-Rating Scales for Depression

No single scale is necessarily better than all the others, but there are good reliability and validity data for the Beck Depression Inventory–II (BDI-II[23]) and the Quick Inventory of Depressive Symptoms (QIDS[24]). The BDI-II uses scores of 14–19 for mild depression, 20–28 for moderate depression, and 29 or above for severe depression. The QIDS distinguishes between subsyndromal (scores of 13–27) and syndromal depression (scores of 28 or higher). It can be useful to supplement these rating scales with the Beck Scale for Suicide Ideation,[25] which contains 21 groups of statements referring to various forms of suicidal ideation (thoughts, plans, or wishes to commit suicide; e.g., "I have periods of thinking about killing myself") during the preceding week. Patients may report passive suicidal ideation on the Beck Scale for Suicide Ideation to a greater extent than in direct interviews.

We have not been overly impressed with any of the self-rating scales used to rate mania or hypomania. Several such scales exist, and some have good reliability and validity data (e.g., the Altman Self-Rating Scale for Mania).[26] However, we are not convinced that having patients' scores on these scales adds to the information gained by asking patients questions about their mood, sleep, and activity, or by observing their behavior and thought processes within a session.

It is a good idea to get a rating of current psychosocial functioning to assess how much the symptoms of bipolar disorder have affected the patient's daily life. The Life Functioning Questionnaire (LFQ[27]) is a gender-neutral measure of social role functioning in four domains: work, duties at home, leisure time with family, and friends. Items under each domain cover the time spent in each role domain, the level of interpersonal conflict in each, enjoyment of the activity, and the perceived quality of social performance. Two UCLA-based studies found that among patients with bipolar disorder, subsyndromal depressive symptoms were closely associated with LFQ role impairment scores over time.[28,29]

## SUMMARY

Although we cannot emphasize strongly enough the value of a good intake evaluation, it is also important to recognize that illness data are collected from patients on a continuous basis. The initial evaluation is the start of one's treatment relationship with the patient. Patients' memories of prior episodes and prior life events may change, and they may begin to acknowledge the previous role of substance or alcohol abuse, or they may recall episodes of mania or depression only when they are in the corresponding mood state. So, like many of the recommendations in this book, think of the evaluation as a moving target, and the initial diagnostic impressions as hypotheses that can be retained, revised, or thrown out altogether.

In Chapters 4 through 9, we address treatment considerations at different phases of the illness or when treatment nonadherence, nonresponse, or suicidality appear. Some of the information gleaned from the intake, while not immediately usable, becomes essential later on. Let us now consider treatment considerations in the first phase of treatment: the acute manic episode.

# CHAPTER 4

## Treatment of Acute Mania and Hypomania

Despite the 21st-century explosion of medications shown to be effective in treating acute mania, the overall treatment of manic and hypomanic states continues to be difficult. The management strategies vary by setting (i.e., inpatient vs. outpatient), therapeutic alliance, patients' insight, treatment adherence, comorbid disorders, and the involvement of families. These variables can make what at first glance looks to be simple, exceedingly complex.

### THE CLINICAL SETTING

The first clinical question to address in evaluating and treating acutely manic and hypomanic states is whether the patient can be treated in an outpatient setting or needs hospitalization. By definition, all hypomanias are treated in an outpatient setting (since if the episode is severe enough to require hospitalization, the DSM-5 diagnosis must be mania, not hypomania). Some individuals with mania can also be treated as outpatients. However, a substantial proportion of manias require a protective treatment setting. The decision to hospitalize depends on a number of factors, some of which may have to be determined by the treating psychiatrist who is arranging the admission (see Table 4.1). Among all these factors, the two core issues are (1) whether the bipolar individual is acting in ways that may be destructive or dangerous and (2) whether the individual has sufficient insight to cooperate with treatment.

**TABLE 4.1. Factors to Consider in Hospitalizing Manic Individuals**

- Destructive behavior
  - In the work setting (inappropriate verbal behavior, aggressiveness)
  - Inappropriate sexual behavior (e.g., multiple partners)
  - Uncontrolled spending
  - Dangerous or erratic (e.g., driving recklessly)
  - Drug–alcohol use
  - Suicidality or homicidality
- Psychosis
- Degree of insight
- Willingness to adhere to treatment
- Quality of social network (family and/or friends)
- Legal considerations regarding involuntary hospitalizations (state-specific)

It is particularly frustrating when it is obvious to the treating professionals, as well as family members, that the manic individual is doing real damage to his life but has no insight into the consequences of his behavior. Moreover, the laws of the state may make involuntary hospitalization impossible. If the patient's manic episode is his first, families are typically frightened, confused and simply have no idea who to call or what to do. If the individual has had prior episodes, families are generally far more helpful and proactive in managing a difficult and potentially dangerous situation, but the patient may still lack insight and be highly uncooperative with treatment.

Gil, a young adult who lived with his parents, had had mild chronic depression for years. Over a 48-hour period, he showed a dramatic increase in his activity level and decreased sleep. He described a new life plan to become a rap star. Prior to this point, he had never shown any particular interest or talent in music or performing. Highly irritable with his parents, he ended up shoving his father and threatening to hit his mother, neither of which had ever happened before. His parents were befuddled as to how to understand the dramatic change in their son. Gil refused to see a psychiatrist or therapist, insisting that he felt well for the first time in years. Luckily, Gil's parents discussed their concern to a friend who was a mental health professional. He counseled them to call the police if Gil became violent again. When Gil shoved his father the next day, the police were called and Gil was involuntary hospitalized for his first acute manic episode.

If a person has already been diagnosed as bipolar, the therapist and/ or psychopharmacologist can be most effective by collaborating with the family in assessing whether the individual can be treated outside the hospital. If hospitalization is necessary, the treating professionals can help guide the family as to when to call the police, 911, or the local psychiatric emergency team.

---

After multiple, destructive manic episodes, Ramon created a plan with his close friends: If, in their opinion, he became manic, they would call his psychiatrist so he could be reevaluated. Ramon trusted his friends and the agreement was made. A year later, after Ramon bought a $6,000 couch, voiced plans to renovate his apartment in a "faux Romanesque" style, and placed many late-night calls to people, his friends called his psychiatrist. After speaking with Ramon and confirming the acute mania, the psychiatrist recommended increasing his lithium dose and adding a new agent, olanzapine (Zyprexa). Although Ramon disagreed with the mania diagnosis, he reluctantly agreed to the plan given his pact with his friends. The mania resolved over 4 weeks and Ramon was able to cancel the couch order (although he did lose some of his deposit).

---

As Ramon's case illustrates, friends and family members can play a critical role in preventing the escalation of mania. In Chapter 7, we discuss the development of a relapse prevention plan, in which patients, family members, or significant others and therapists/physicians make a list of prodromal symptoms, stress triggers, and preventative strategies in the event that these symptoms appear.

---

Brent, age 33, had a very consistent early symptom of mania: a preoccupation with television game shows, which he watched incessantly, thinking his name would be called. His sister, Sonia, identified an increase in the amount of time Brent spent in front of the TV as a warning sign, especially if it was accompanied by staying up late and making "lists of incoherent equations and probabilities." Her strategies were not limited to calling his psychiatrist, however. She worked with Brent on implementing a common bedtime, and insisted that he spend the majority of the evening away from the TV, which had become a trigger for his symptoms. She also helped him control his bank account when he started purchasing unnecessary items from television auctions.

---

As previously noted, hypomanic states are not associated with behaviors that are as dangerous as those seen in manias. Nonetheless, insight during hypomanias is quite variable. Some individuals are keenly aware of their mood states and are willing to cooperate with treatment, whereas others either lack insight or can acknowledge the hypomanic symptoms but enjoy the euphoric, energized state too much to agree to its treatment.

## PRETREATMENT EVALUATION

If a thorough history can be obtained with the help of collateral information, no special lab tests are needed for an individual in a first manic/hypomanic episode. The standard premedication tests of a chemistry panel (electrolytes, liver enzymes, creatinine [renal function], and glucose), a TSH (thyroid-stimulating hormone) level, which measures thyroid function, and possibly a lipid profile (cholesterol and triglycerides) to establish a baseline are usually sufficient. As discussed in Chapter 3, neuroimaging tests such as a CT scan or MRI are not usually necessary.

Evaluation of drug use is mandatory unless it is well known to the clinician or to family members that the patient is not a drug user. As noted in Chapter 2, drug abuse can mimic or exacerbate mania. Because patients are not always forthcoming or accurate about their use of illegal substances or alcohol, blood and urine tests are critical.

## TREATMENT OF MANIA

Before instituting a new medication regimen, a clinician should always address a few clinical issues in the circumstance of an acute mania. They include sleep deprivation, recent medication prescriptions, drug abuse, ongoing use of antidepressants, and medication adherence. Sleep disruption has been demonstrated to be a trigger for manic episodes, as well as being a core symptom of mania.[1] For patients with manic episodes that may have been precipitated by sleep deprivation (e.g., a student studying all night, or flying on a red-eye flight and losing a night of sleep), particular attention must be paid to restoring sleep as part of the antimanic regimen. A review of recently added medications is also critical, since some agents (e.g., corticosteroids and SAM-e, sold over the counter) may be capable of precipitating mania. Discontinuing these medications should be considered.

Drugs of abuse—especially stimulants—should always be considered as a potential precipitant of a manic episode. Patients who have recurrences despite seemingly optimal treatment may be abusing drugs. Urine toxicology screens are often needed before major changes in treatment are undertaken. Discontinuing the drug of abuse is, of course, a mandatory part of treating the mania, and one of the major reasons that mania is often treated in an inpatient setting.

When antidepressants have triggered a manic episode, they should be discontinued. This strategy is recommended regardless of whether the antidepressant was prescribed at constant doses for a long time (e.g., many months or years) or it is a recent addition to the manic individual's medication regimen. Different considerations apply with hypomanic (vs. manic) states, as discussed below.

Finally, if the manic patient was on a mood stabilizer regimen, it is important to ascertain whether she has been taking the medications as prescribed (a "breakthrough" episode) or taking less or none of the previously prescribed medications (a nonadherence-precipitated episode), since the direction of treatment will differ. It must also be recognized that this distinction may be blurred in reality. As an example, consider a patient with bipolar I disorder who becomes hypomanic, then becomes less adherent to his medication regimen *because of the hypomania*, leading to a full blown mania. In this situation, the manic episode is only partly due to nonadherence, since the original hypomania triggered the inconsistent medication adherence.

### Inpatient Treatment of Manic States

The choice of available treatments is the same for inpatients and outpatients with mania. The major difference is the choice of how the medications are administered. In outpatient settings, medications are virtually always taken orally, with rare use of long-acting intramuscular mood stabilizer agents during maintenance treatment (discussed more in Chapter 6). Thus, the bipolar individual must agree to take medications for maintenance treatment to be successful.

In inpatient settings, because of the inherently greater severity of the manic state, patients may be given intramuscular preparations to induce rapid behavioral calming in dangerous situations, such as when escalation of agitation and violent behavior is either a possibility or has already occurred. Both intramuscular injections of benzodiazepines, such as lorazepam (Ativan), or intramuscular antipsychotics, such as olanzapine (Zyprexa), ziprasidone (Geodon), or aripiprazole (Abilify) are typically prescribed, often in combination, with good results in calming the patient in a potentially hazardous situation. Once the manic individual agrees to treatment, oral preparations are used.

Given that acutely manic individuals are frequently ambivalent (at best) about treatment, a universal concern in inpatient units is whether the patient is actually swallowing the medications or is "cheeking" the pill, hiding it in her mouth, then spitting it out later. In response to this appropriate concern, a number of antipsychotics—for example, olanzapine, risperidone (Risperdal), and aripiprazole—are available in forms that dissolve instantly when exposed to saliva, making cheeking essentially impossible. Often, these preparations are used in the initial treatment of mania on inpatient units until there is more of a therapeutic alliance with the patient and some reason to believe that the manic patient is actually swallowing the pills. Of course, these preparations hold no value in treating patients outside hospitals. Any individual outside a hospital who does not want to take medications simply will not take the pills.

## Overall Considerations

Without a doubt, mania can be effectively treated with medications, as is evidenced by the number of different treatments with approval by the U.S. Food and Drug Administration (FDA) for this purpose, which means that they show significantly greater efficacy than placebo in double-blind studies. However, currently available antimanic agents are neither as effective as we would like nor do they work nearly as quickly as would be optimal. Most treatment studies of acute mania, virtually all of which involve hospitalized patients, measure outcome after 3 weeks of treatment. At that time, around 50% of patients have shown a response, defined as a 50% decrease in scores on the Young Mania Rating Scale (YMRS)[2] or a similar measure. Thus, half the treated patients are not even 50% better after 3 weeks. Furthermore, the average YMRS score after 3 weeks of treatment is often higher than the minimum score required for entry into an acute mania study. Finally, if we raise the bar, examining the rate of remission—meaning patients are mostly all better—that rate is 20% after 3 weeks of treatment.[3] In contrast, average hospital stays in the United States for acute mania are substantially shorter than 3 weeks. Therefore, many, if not most, individuals hospitalized for mania leave the hospital in significantly symptomatic states.

Once the choice of inpatient or outpatient treatment setting has been made, the most important factor in deciding among the different treatment options is the clinical urgency of the situation. When treating a patient who is hospitalized *or* has mania of sufficient intensity that hospitalization should be considered *or* a patient who is escalating quickly toward an unmanageable state, a good psychopharmacologist errs on the side of "overtreating": Treatments are prescribed with relatively rapidly increasing doses. In these situations, the goal of preventing dangerous behavior or hospitalization justifies a more aggressive approach. Conversely, if the individual is an outpatient and the manic symptoms are relatively static and not becoming worse by the day (even if the patient is bipolar I), a less aggressive treatment stance with slower dose increases makes more sense. For example, a manic state of relatively greater intensity might be appropriately treated with quetiapine (Seroquel), with daily doses rapidly increasing to 300–400 mg, or olanzapine at doses of 10–20 mg daily.

If the manic individual is already taking a mood stabilizer and has a manic breakthrough episode (despite reasonable adherence), the simplest strategy would be to increase the dose of the mood stabilizer, if possible. (Unfortunately, no study has ever examined this approach to treating a mania, but common sense suggests it highly.) This strategy is less likely to be helpful if the patient is already taking relatively high doses of the mood stabilizer, in which case raising the dose would likely cause only side effects, not more therapeutic effects. If the patient already has significant side effects, he will be unlikely to tolerate higher doses.

An extraordinary variety of medication options are available to treat acute manic states. These range from lithium to some anticonvulsants, to all the antipsychotics. Table 4.2 lists the treatments for acute mania with the usual dose ranges and most common side effects of each.

Lithium is not usually the first medication prescribed for a severe mania (at least as a solo antimanic agent) because of the greater difficulty in finding the optimal dose and relatively slow onset of efficacy. When antipsychotics are used for initial treatment of a milder mania, doses might start with quetiapine 50–200 mg or olanzapine 5–10 mg daily. In treating milder manias, lithium or valproate (Depakote) are appropriate treatments.

### Choosing a Treatment

Table 4.3 lists the factors that we might consider in choosing one or another of these antimanic medications. In choosing a first treatment, a past history of a positive treatment response, along with tolerability for that treatment, should always be considered strongly. As an example, acute lithium responders who discontinue treatment are very likely to respond if the lithium is restarted for a later manic episode.

Given that (1) all antimanic treatments listed are more effective than placebo, (2) the antimanic agents differ slightly but not dramatically from each other in efficacy, and (3) adherence to treatment is so critical in the short-term and especially the long-term treatment of bipolar disorder, it makes sense to consider patient input in the choice of a specific agent. A patient who insists that one antipsychotic would be more acceptable than another (or more than lithium) should be given that antipsychotic or any other of the first-line medications listed in Table 4.2.

**TABLE 4.2. Medication Options for Treating Acute Mania**

| Medication[a] | Usual starting daily dose | Typical full daily dose | Comments |
|---|---|---|---|
| lithium (Eskalith-CR) | 600–900 mg | 900–2,400 mg | Plasma levels 0.6–1.2 mEq/liter |
| valproate (Depakote, Depakote-ER) | 750 mg | 1,000–3,000 mg | Plasma levels > 94 µg/ml |
| risperidone (Risperdal) | 2 mg | 4–6 mg | |
| olanzapine (Zyprexa) | 5–10 mg | 10–30 mg | Sedating |
| quetiapine (Seroquel) | 100–200 mg | 300–800 mg | Sedating |
| ziprasidone (Geodon) | 40–80 mg | 120–160 mg | Infrequently prescribed |
| aripiprazole (Abilify) | 5–10 mg | 10–30 mg | |
| asenapine (Saphris) | 10 mg | 10–20 mg | |
| carbamazepine (Equetro) | 200–400 mg | 600–1,600 mg | Slow onset, rarely prescribed |
| haloperidol (Haldol) | 2–5 mg | 5–20 mg | First-generation antipsychotic |

[a]Trade names are in parentheses.

**TABLE 4.3. Factors to Consider in Choosing an Antimanic Treatment**

- Necessity for speed of onset
- Severity of mania
- Complexity of regimen affecting treatment adherence
- Prior treatment history
- Patient preference
- Specific symptom complexes
  o Atypical manic features (including mixed states vs. classic euphoric mania)
  o Psychotic features
  o Profound insomnia or agitation
- Family history of response
- Side-effect profile

Clinical features, including psychosis, atypical manic features, or profound agitation/insomnia, may also sway the choice of antimanic treatments. Not surprisingly, antipsychotic medications are usually prescribed for patients with overtly psychotic manias, with dominant delusions or hallucinations. Mixed mania features (vs. classic euphoric mania) seem to predict a poorer response to lithium compared to valproate or to antipsychotics.[4] Finally, manic individuals who are profoundly agitated and/or barely sleeping are typically given more sedating antipsychotics such as olanzapine and quetiapine, since, beyond their antimanic qualities, these medications slow patients down and help to ensure sleep.

Another option to enhance sleep and tranquilization is to use a less sedating antimanic agent, such as lithium or aripiprazole, plus a benzodiazepine such as clonazepam (Klonopin) or lorazepam. When prescribing these combinations, the benzodiazepine provides the necessary tranquilization to ensure sleep and some behavioral slowing until the antimanic agent can take effect.

Family history of treatment response to antimanic agents generally is far less important than the other factors listed in Table 4.3. However, lithium response may run in families and sometimes plays a role in treatment decisions.[5] Whether response to other antimanic agents such as valproate or antipsychotics is familial has not been established.

Finally, consider side-effect profiles in constructing a long-term maintenance regimen since a number of these are far more relevant over months and years than over the first few weeks of acute antimanic treatment. When a patient is acutely manic, however, the need to gain control over emergent symptoms may increase the importance of rapid efficacy and behavioral control over adverse side effects.

## First- and Second-Line Agents

If one assumes that the manic individual is not already on some mood stabilizer and the factors described in Table 4.3 do not provide a clear and obvious treatment choice, then the first-line antimanic agents are lithium, valproate, an antipsychotic, or the combination of lithium or valproate plus an antipsychotic. Lithium, the first antimanic agent discovered,[6] and valproate, which has been used effectively to treat mania for 20-plus years, work very well in treating acute mania.[7] All antipsychotics seem to be effective in treating acute mania.[8] Furthermore, meta-analyses, in which drug–placebo differences for the antipsychotics are compared, suggest that antipsychotics, including all the second-generation antipsychotics (SGAs) and haloperidol (Haldol, a first-generation agent), are somewhat more effective than lithium or valproate.[9] Few consistent differences in efficacy are seen when comparing one antipsychotic to another.[10]

Given tolerability issues, SGAs, which include all antipsychotics released since 1990, tend to be prescribed far more frequently than first-generation antipsychotics, although no evidence suggests that they are more effective than first-generation agents such as haloperidol. With many of these "new" antipsychotics available in generic form, the cost savings for older medications such as haloperidol are diminishing.

Among the medications listed in Table 4.2, carbamazepine (Tegretol) is prescribed least often as a first-line agent. This reflects both its relatively slow onset of efficacy and its difficult side-effect profile, which make the rapid dose increases that are vital in treating acute mania rather difficult.

When patients are acutely ill, they are often treated with a combination of antimanic agents, classically, either lithium or valproate combined with an SGA. Multiple studies have consistently shown that an antipsychotic added to either lithium or valproate increases response rates by 20–25%, regardless of which antipsychotic is prescribed.[11] Unfortunately, we do not know whether lithium or valproate add antimanic efficacy to SGAs, since no study has addressed this question. Thus, in situations with greater clinical urgency, combination antimanic treatment is often recommended. For manic outpatients, however, with greater treatment complexity comes greater difficulty in treatment adherence.

In order to ensure adequate sleep in a manic patient, the two most commonly prescribed options are either a sedating antimanic agent, such as olanzapine or quetiapine (clear favorite strategies on inpatient units) or a less sedating antimanic agent, such as lithium or aripiprazole plus a hypnotic (sleeping pill). The hypnotic, typically zolpidem (Ambien), lorazepam, or clonazepam, helps to ensure adequate sleep, since, as noted earlier, decreased sleep is both a symptom of mania and a factor in worsening mania. Then, when the patient improves, the hypnotic can be tapered and discontinued.

## Strategies for Prescribing Medications and for Managing Side Effects

### Lithium

Although lithium is our oldest, established antimanic agent, in the United States it is prescribed much less, certainly as a solo treatment, than antipsychotics. In Europe, lithium continues to be prescribed a great deal, far more than in the United States. This assuredly reflects both cultural factors and the lower financial cost of lithium compared to antipsychotics in countries with more centralized health service systems.

Prior to starting lithium, blood tests measuring renal (kidney) function (serum creatinine) and thyroid function (TSH) should be obtained. Some psychiatrists also measure serum calcium (since lithium occasionally increases calcium), a blood urea nitrogen (BUN) test (another test of kidney function, but one that adds little to the serum creatinine measurement), an electrocardiogram (EKG, for those over 40 years old), and a pregnancy test (see Chapter 9 for treating bipolar disorder during pregnancy). In an outpatient setting, when a manic patient balks at getting blood drawn, lithium can be started, and the initial blood tests may be drawn a few days later. This is less than optimal, but it should be done when initiating treatment is urgent and the patient refuses to have his blood drawn immediately.

Starting doses of lithium treatment are 600 mg (typically two capsules, 300 mg each) with outpatients and 900 mg with inpatients. Age is a central determinant of lithium doses, since it is excreted unchanged by the kidneys. Since decreased renal function is a universal consequence of normal aging, older manic patients need less lithium to obtain the same lithium blood levels than do younger patients. For older bipolar individuals, a starting dose should be 150–300 mg daily. Based on side effects (see below) and therapeutic response, after a few days the dosages can be raised by 300 mg daily in younger adults and by 150–300 mg in older adults. If possible, it is optimal for lithium to be administered on a once-daily regimen, since it is both more convenient and (compared to divided-dose regimens) safer for the kidneys when prescribed over months and years.[12] In the beginning of treatment, however, nausea may necessitate divided-dose regimens until there is accommodation to this gastrointestinal side effect. If nausea persists, switching to a slow-release lithium preparation, such as Eskalith CR, may reduce this side effect, but it increases the risk for diarrhea.

More than any other medication in psychiatry, lithium doses are regulated by blood levels, measured as a concentration in the blood (or more accurately, the serum part of the blood). For treatment of acute mania, optimal lithium levels in younger adults are 0.8–1.2 milliequivalents (mEq) per liter. Generally, lithium levels > 1.2 mEq/liter do not provide any further benefit and are associated with increased side effects. When conducted properly, lithium levels should be drawn approximately 12 hours (10–14 hours is acceptable) after the last ingestion of lithium. Food does not interfere with lithium absorption and therefore the patient does not need to fast for lithium levels. Most commonly, patients take lithium at night and have samples to measure their lithium levels drawn in the morning.

After beginning lithium or, after a dose increase, lithium levels in younger adults achieve steady state, meaning they will no longer change if the dose remains constant after 4 days. Therefore, at all doses, lithium levels should be drawn after 4 days. However, in an urgent clinical situation, such as treating acute mania, the lithium level may be estimated at 3 days by adding another 20% to the measured level. Thus, a lithium level of 0.6 after 3 days of treatment equates to a true (i.e., steady state) level of 0.7.

With older manic adults, optimal lithium levels are lower, since they both respond to lower doses/levels and are far more sensitive to side effects at any dose/level. Therefore, in treating an older manic individual, target lithium levels are 0.5–0.8 mEq/liter. Because of the slower excretion of lithium in older adults, achieving steady state takes a longer period of time, typically 6–8 days. As in the treatment of younger adults, a lithium level may be obtained after 4–5 days with an approximation made as to the true lithium level.

Lithium's efficacy in treating acute mania is relatively slower than that of antipsychotics. Thus, when the clinical situation is urgent, manic patients are frequently treated with an antipsychotic plus lithium for a number of weeks, until, it is hoped, lithium begins to take effect and the antipsychotics can be withdrawn. Alternatively, a benzodiazepine tranquilizer such as clonazepam or lorazepam may be used in addition to lithium. However, the latter medicines are useful for simple calming; they do not have the same efficacy in treating true mania as the antipsychotics or lithium. With usual dose increases, one expects to see lithium's efficacy within a few weeks. If a positive effect is not seen after 3 weeks, a different treatment strategy should be employed.

The most common acute side effects of lithium are nausea, diarrhea, tremor, increased urination, thirst, and cognitive dulling.[13] Cognitive dulling as a side effect is very real, but some manic patients mislabel the loss of their manic intensity and sharpness as a side effect of lithium. Lithium side effects are typically dose related. An obvious treatment strategy for distressing lithium side effects is to decrease the dose. Weight gain that may be seen in the initial phase of treatment is more problematic during maintenance treatment. Longer-term side effects are discussed in Chapter 6.

## Valproate (Depakote, Depakote-ER)

Valproate is equivalent to lithium in effectiveness in treating acute mania and is still commonly prescribed for this reason.[7] Before instituting valproate, chemistry panels that include liver function tests and a complete blood count (CBC) should be obtained.

Valproate treatment can be started in a number of ways. The most rapid and aggressive of these methods is to begin at a dose of 20 mg/kg/day, yielding a starting dose of 1,500 mg for a 150-pound person. This method, called a *loading strategy*, is used almost exclusively in hospital settings where patients can be closely monitored and the consequences of early side effects are less problematic. A more common approach, used in both inpatient and outpatient settings, is simply a rapidly escalating dose, usually starting with 750 mg daily and increasing over a few days to a week to 1,500 mg in most patients. In the beginning of treatment, valproate is usually given in divided doses, to reduce the nausea that is relatively common early in treatment. Later on, if side effects are not excessive, the entire dose can be given at night.

Serum valproate levels are monitored less consistently than lithium levels. However, in the one good study in this area, valproate levels showed a reasonably linear relationship with efficacy, with higher levels associated with better response.[14] Overall, the recommendation based on the results of this study is to target valproate levels > 94 µg/ml. Valproate levels above 125 tend to be associated with a greater side-effect burden and treatment intolerance.

The speed of onset of valproate's efficacy is similar to that of lithium and somewhat slower than that of the antipsychotics. Because valproate is more sedating than lithium, there can be less of a need for a second medicine to reduce agitation and ensure sleep.

The most common short-term side effects seen with valproate are nausea, vomiting, diarrhea, sedation (which may be therapeutic in acutely manic patients), and tremor. Increase in liver enzymes or thrombocytopenia (low platelet counts) may occur as side effects. Weight gain, alopecia (diffuse hair loss), and polycystic ovarian syndrome may be seen during longer-term treatment (see Chapter 6). Overall, in acute mania, valproate is somewhat better tolerated than lithium.

### Second-Generation Antipsychotics (Atypical Antipsychotics)

As noted earlier, antipsychotics have become primary treatments, either as solo agents or in combination with lithium or valproate in treating acute mania. Despite the equal efficacy between the older antipsychotics such as haloperidol and these newer agents, the SGAs now dominate the treatment of mania due primarily to tolerability issues, although the relentless marketing of these agents by pharmaceutical firms has assuredly contributed at least somewhat to their popularity. Initially, these medications were described as "atypical" antipsychotics, since they were biologically different than the older agents in that they affected other neurotransmitter systems in addition to blocking the dopamine 2 receptor (a quality common to all antipsychotics). Additionally, they did not show the "typical" side effects of antipsychotics as frequently compared with the older agents. However, these medications should more properly be described as "second-generation" agents, since they were released after all the earlier agents. Nowadays, their dominant place in prescribing practices makes the term *atypical* seem incongruous because they are now more commonly prescribed than the typical agents.

All SGAs that have been evaluated have shown clear efficacy for acute mania. Most of these have received FDA approvals for this purpose. As of now (2014), these include olanzapine, risperidone, quetiapine, ziprasidone, aripiprazole, and asenapine (Saphris). Other antipsychotics are also likely to be effective. As an example, paliperidone (Invega) has been shown to be effective in acute mania but does not have the FDA indication.[15] Overall, these medications are equally effective in treating acute mania in both inpatient and outpatient settings. However, their side effects differ significantly, such that there are valid reasons to prescribe one or another of these agents with individual patients. Table 4.2 presents the starting dose, usual dose, and most important side effects associated with each of these medications.

## RISPERIDONE (RISPERDAL)

For treating acute mania, risperidone, released in 1994, should be started at 2 mg daily for inpatients or 1–2 mg for outpatients. Mean doses are 4.0–4.5 mg, with the usual range of 1–6 mg.[16,17] The entire dose may be prescribed once daily or be divided for the therapeutic use of its calming/sedating properties. Doses beyond 6 mg are associated with substantial extrapyramidal side effects, such as *akinesia* (motor slowing) and *akathisia* (motor restlessness), similar to what is seen with first-generation antipsychotics. Risperidone causes a moderate amount of sedation, occupying a middle ground between relatively sedating agents, such as olanzapine, and quetiapine and the relatively less sedating agents, such as aripiprazole and ziprasidone. Longer-term side effects include weight gain and *galactorrhea* (inappropriate breast milk production).

## OLANZAPINE (ZYPREXA)

Olanzapine is the most popular SGA in the United States for treating acute mania, despite its problematic side-effect profile with long-term use, and the lack of evidence that it is more effective than other agents. Antimanic doses begin at 5 mg, whereas the targeted daily doses are 15–20 mg, with higher doses prescribed for poorly responsive manias.[18,19] As with most of the other SGAs, olanzapine may be taken once daily or in divided doses if daytime sedation would be helpful. Olanzapine's popularity with psychiatrists, especially hospital-based practitioners, assuredly reflects the ease of prescribing a full antimanic dose quickly and the therapeutic use of the side effect of sedation.

For acutely manic patients, especially inpatients, olanzapine is able to slow hyperactivity, irritability, and overall activation, making clinical management easier. In very hyperactive patients, the considerable sedation associated with olanzapine use is generally well tolerated. Aside from sedation, increased appetite and weight gain are the most common side effects, even in short-term acute mania treatment. Weight gain and the health risks associated with olanzapine, called the *metabolic syndrome*, form the greatest difficulty in the long-term use.

### QUETIAPINE (SEROQUEL)

Quetiapine is usually started at 100–200 mg daily, with full antimanic doses ranging from 300–800 mg daily.[20,21] As with most other medications in this class, once-daily dosing of quetiapine, typically at night, or divided-dose regimens may be used. Quetiapine's side effects are similar to those of olanzapine but with somewhat less sedation and less weight gain. Other side effects associated with quetiapine are dizziness (probably due to orthostatic hypotension, a lowering of blood pressure when the patient stands), dry mouth, and constipation.

### ZIPRASIDONE (GEODON)

Although it shares the same FDA indication as the three antipsychotics just described, ziprasidone is prescribed far less frequently than these other medications for treating acute mania. Starting doses are either 40 mg or 40 mg twice daily, with full doses of 120–160 mg.[22,23] Ziprasidone is one of only two SGAs recommended to be given in divided doses. Additionally, ziprasidone's absorption is enhanced by food; therefore, doses should be taken with or right after meals.

The relative unpopularity of ziprasidone reflects its unpredictable side-effect profile. It can cause either sedation or activation/akathisia, and these side effects can be mild or significant—and they are impossible to predict. Ziprasidone is associated with little to no weight gain. When ziprasidone was first released, there was an additional concern that it prolonged cardiac conduction as measured by the QT interval (a measurement derived from EKGs). In retrospect, however, this risk was overstated, since postmarketing studies have not indicated higher rates of clinically relevant cardiac difficulties.[24] EKGs are not required prior to ziprasidone prescription unless other cardiac risk factors are present.

## ARIPIPRAZOLE (ABILIFY)

Similar to ziprasidone, aripiprazole is prescribed much less frequently than olanzapine or other, more sedating SGAs in treating acute mania, especially in the inpatient setting. This preference again reflects the habit of prescribing sedating medications to slow down hyperactive manic individuals. (As noted earlier, response rates to aripiprazole in treating acute mania are similar to the more sedating antipsychotics.) Usual doses of aripiprazole for mania begin at 5–10 mg, with full doses ranging from 10–30 mg.[25] In the early acute mania studies, aripiprazole was started, idiosyncratically, at 30 mg, with doses lowered if needed. Good clinical psychopharmacology practice is characterized by starting at lower doses and raising the dose if needed, not the opposite tactic.

Common side effects with aripiprazole are sedation, akathisia/restlessness, and constipation. Relative to other antipsychotics, aripiprazole has a low liability for weight gain.

## ASENAPINE (SAPHRIS)

Asenapine is the most recent SGA approved for acute mania.[26] Starting doses are 5 mg twice daily, increasing to 10 mg twice daily, if needed. Alone among the antipsychotics, asenapine is poorly absorbed through the gastrointestinal tract. Therefore, it is taken sublingually, absorbed through the salivary system.

Asenapine's most common side effects are somnolence, dizziness, akathisia, and mild weight gain. A subgroup of individuals treated with asenapine complain of an unpleasant taste; this can often be effectively treated by switching to black cherry–flavored (!) asenapine, formulated specifically for this reason.

## CARBAMAZEPINE (TEGRETOL, EQUETRO)

Although carbamazepine only achieved an FDA indication for acute mania (in the form of the extended release capsule formulation Equetro) in 2004, it was the first anticonvulsant and the second antimanic agent used with bipolar patients. Its first studies emerged over 30 years ago.[27]

Systematic reviews of antimanic medications all show that carbamazepine effectively treats mania (as defined by 3-week response rates) and is crudely equivalent to both lithium and valproate.[9] Despite this, carbamazepine is essentially never prescribed as a first-line treatment nowadays and infrequently prescribed for acute mania because of its relatively slow time to efficacy, side effect considerations, and drug–drug interactions (see below).

Prior to prescribing carbamazepine, a CBC and a general chemistry panel, which includes liver function tests and electrolytes, should be obtained. It is difficult to prescribe a specific schedule for implementing carbamazepine in the setting of acute mania since, for many patients, its side effects preclude the rapid increase in dose that is clinically necessary. Therefore, carbamazepine should be started at doses of 200–400 mg daily, with 200-mg dose increases as tolerated. Usual doses of carbamazepine range between 600 and 1,600 mg daily, with mean doses hovering around 900 mg.

Carbamazepine levels are available (and used in neurology when the medication is used for seizure control). However, no study has yet shown a correlation between carbamazepine levels and efficacy in acute mania.[28] Thus, the anticonvulsant therapeutic range of 4–12 µg/ml should be utilized as a broad range that establishes usual blood levels, not therapeutic levels.

The side effects that are most problematic with carbamazepine are primarily neurological: dizziness, ataxia (poor balance), a general feeling of being unwell, diplopia (double vision), and blurred vision, along with fatigue and nausea. More patients experience significant side effects with carbamazepine than with either lithium or valproate. Additionally, carbamazepine is associated with a number of other medical side effects, such as hyponatremia (low sodium), a mild increase in liver enzymes, or thrombocytopenia (low platelet count). Carbamazepine can also cause a very rare but potentially life-threatening agranulocytosis, in which the bone marrow stops making blood cells. In these circumstances, the lack of white blood cells makes the patient vulnerable to overwhelming infections and may be fatal. Most clinicians monitor sequential white blood cell counts by blood tests, although these are unlikely to diagnose the very rare cases of agranulocytosis.

The final complication making carbamazepine a difficult antimanic medication to use (compared to the other available treatment options) is its ability to lower the blood levels of many other medications by increasing their hepatic (liver) metabolism.[29,30] Since most manic patients are taking multiple medications, this feature makes monitoring of doses far more difficult.

## Other Medications for Acute Mania

A number of other medications are sometimes considered to treat acute mania, typically because of their similarity to the established effective agents we have described. However, similarities in chemical structure or treatment class do not necessarily imply similarities in efficacy. As the most glaring example, not all anticonvulsants effectively treat mania even though valproate and carbamazepine, two agents in the class, do so. Lamotrigine (Lamictal), an anticonvulsant that is an effective maintenance treatment in bipolar disorder (see Chapter 6) and also used to treat acute bipolar depression (see Chapter 5), is ineffective in treating acute mania and should not be used for this purpose.[31] Similarly, topiramate (Topamax), another anticonvulsant, has been evaluated in a number of studies and has no demonstrable efficacy for acute mania.[32] Gabapentin (Neurontin), another anticonvulsant, is ineffective in treating acute mania,[8] but is sedating and can sometimes be added adjunctively to an antimanic agent just for antianxiety purposes, analogous to the use of benzodiazepines.

Benzodiazepines, the commonly prescribed class of antianxiety agents, frequently form part of a medication regimen to treat acute mania. The two agents in this class most commonly prescribed for this purpose are lorazepam and clonazepam. Overall, benzodiazepines are only weak antimanic agents. However, they may be more helpful as adjunctive medications that calm agitation and ensure better and more sleep, as well as decrease anxiety. The usual lorazepam dose ranges between 1 and 8 mg daily, almost always in divided doses given its relatively short half-life. In contrast, clonazepam, with its somewhat longer half-life, may be prescribed either once or twice daily, with a typical dose ranging between 1 and 4 mg per day. Typical side effects with benzodiazepines are as expected: sedation, ataxia (unsteady balance) and mild cognitive impairment.

### Partial Hospital Programs

Because of the expense of inpatient hospitalizations and the ruthlessness of insurance programs in insisting on early discharges from the hospital, many, if not most, manic individuals are discharged from hospital when they are somewhat better but very far from well. (Because of their different health care systems, the average length of stay in European psychiatric hospitals is consistently longer than in the United States.) Therefore, the situation frequently arises in which a manic individual is out of the hospital, still manic—albeit less so—but not well enough to be treated with once-weekly psychotherapy plus medication management. *Partial hospital programs* (also known as *day hospitals*) are excellent settings for this transitional time between inpatient hospitalization and classic outpatient treatment.

In partial hospital programs, individuals are seen 3–5 days weekly, typically for 4–8 hours daily, but they sleep in their own homes. The programs are usually not open on weekends. Partial hospital programs provide for greater structure than is available in classic outpatient treatment, are less expensive than inpatient programs, and provide family members with respite from excessive proximity to someone who is still manic and needs more direction and guidance than most families can provide. Partial hospital programs have indefinite time frames, but a typical stay would be 2–6 weeks during a resolving manic episode.

---

Bill, 25 years old and living with his parents and younger sister, experienced another round of his hyperactive manias that required hospitalization. He elected to be hospitalized and, after 8 days, was sufficiently improved and discharged. At the time he left the hospital, however, Bill was still hypomanic. During his first weekend home, he talked incessantly and "got in everyone's business." By Monday after discharge, he started in the partial hospital program 5 days weekly. Initially, evenings were rather difficult for the family, but during the day, Bill's parents went to work and his sister went to school. By the second weekend home, his family could leave Bill alone for a number of hours, and by the third weekend, he was able to drive to his friends' houses without supervision. Approximately 1 month after discharge from the hospital, Bill left the partial hospital program, well enough to continue less intensive treatment.

---

## TREATMENT OF HYPOMANIA

Treatment studies specifically targeting hypomania and excluding mania essentially do not exist. The range of treatments for hypomania is identical to that available for mania. However, since there is less inherent urgency in treating hypomania, doses and dose escalations are generally less aggressive. A number of rather "gentle" strategies, shown in Table 4.4, might be considered, but these interventions would be inadequate to treat a full-blown mania. These strategies are more likely to be employed in patients with bipolar II disorder, for whom the risk of activation evolving into a full-blown mania is far lower than that for an individual with bipolar I disorder, for whom the hypomania may represent the early evolution of a full manic episode.

First, some bipolar experts have suggested that not all hypomanias even need to be treated. If the symptoms are mild and the patient is insightful and able both to self-monitor and to work collaboratively

**TABLE 4.4. Treatment Strategies for Hypomania in Bipolar II Individuals**

- More careful monitoring
- Ensuring adequate sleep via transient prescription of a hypnotic
- Transient increases in maintenance mood stabilizer doses
- Transient addition of low-dose antipsychotic
- Discontinuing or lowering the dose of an antidepressant (if it is part of the maintenance regimen)

with mental health professionals, watchful monitoring may suffice. Second, some hypomanias can be treated by optimizing sleep, since, as noted earlier, sleeping less is both a symptom of hypomania and a driver of the syndrome. For some patients, simply increasing sleep time from 5 to 7 hours nightly can result in the diminution of hypomanic symptoms. Third, increasing the dose of a mood stabilizer—such as lithium, an anticonvulsant, or an antipsychotic—that is already part of the treatment regimen may be considered, despite the lack of any systematic study of this logical strategy. (This would not be an effective strategy if the mood stabilizer is lamotrigine, since it has no demonstrated efficacy in treating acutely manic/hypomanic states.) If the hypomania settles down, the medication dose can then be lowered to the usual maintenance dose after a few weeks to 1 month. Fourth, assuming the patient is not taking such an agent as a maintenance treatment, a temporary addition of a low-dose antipsychotic such as 0.5–2.0 mg risperidone, 2.5–10.0 mg aripiprazole, or 2.5–5.0 mg olanzapine can quickly and effectively diminish the raciness of hypomanic symptoms. Here, too, the low-dose antipsychotic may be withdrawn within a number of weeks.

Finally, as with the treatment of manias described earlier, antidepressants may "drive" hypomanic states or make treatment of the hypomania more difficult. The classic recommendation to discontinue a maintenance antidepressant immediately when a bipolar patient becomes manic may not always apply with a bipolar II individual who becomes hypomanic. In this circumstance, simply lowering the antidepressant dose may suffice. Additionally, for some bipolar II patients for whom depressions are far more common and more problematic than their hypomanias, the antidepressant can sometimes be continued, with a low-dose antipsychotic added to treat the hypomania.

Donna is 42 years old and has bipolar II disorder. Her maintenance treatment regimen is lithium 900 mg daily and sertraline (Zoloft) 75 mg. In the past, when attempts were made to taper and discontinue the sertraline, Donna became more depressed. Four years ago, during a hypomanic episode, Donna's sertraline was discontinued and low-dose aripiprazole (5 mg) was added.

The hypomania quickly resolved, but Donna became depressed just as quickly. Her depression resolved with the reinstitution of the sertraline. Because of this pattern, when Donna had another hypomania this past year, she and her psychiatrist agreed to continue the sertraline, use a mild sleeping pill (zolpidem) for sleep, and start aripiprazole 2.5 mg daily. The hypomania resolved within 2 weeks, and the aripiprazole and zolpidem were discontinued within 4 weeks without problems.

## TREATMENT-RESISTANT MANIA

In evaluating a manic episode that seems to be refractory to treatment, the first question to ask is whether the manic individual is actually taking the medications prescribed and at the proper dose. Psychological resistance to treatment is common, and ambivalence toward treatment is even more common. Combined with the frequent cognitive disorganization found in mania, nonadherence or partial nonadherence should always be considered as a cause of treatment nonresponse, especially in outpatients with mania. In inpatient settings, of course, it is somewhat easier to monitor medication adherence. For at least some medications—lithium, valproate, carbamazepine, and lamotrigine—obtaining blood levels may be helpful in ascertaining treatment adherence. Of course, a clever manic outpatient can always swallow a few pills of the prescribed medication just before getting his blood drawn; this will result in a blood level of the medication that the patient is, in fact, not taking regularly.

Beyond treatment adherence considerations, there are two other issues to consider in treatment-resistant acute mania: (1) The patient may be surreptitiously taking street drugs, from marijuana to stimulants to hallucinogens; and (2) the ongoing use of an antidepressant may have been missed. Discontinuing street drugs and antidepressants is mandatory in treatment-resistant mania, although the former is, of course, very difficult to do on an outpatient basis.

If the manic individual is truly not responding to classic, established treatments for acute mania—monotherapy with lithium or valproate (or less commonly, carbamazepine), an antipsychotic or a combination of lithium or valproate plus an antipsychotic—then other, less well-established treatment strategies should be considered. First, different mood stabilizers should be considered: Some manias respond to lithium plus an antipsychotic, whereas others may respond best to valproate plus an antipsychotic. Similarly, some patients respond better to one antipsychotic than to another. Second, a treatment that is frequently prescribed but has never been systematically evaluated by any controlled study is the combination of three or more of the previously mentioned well-established agents. Typically, the combination would consist of lithium, valproate, and an antipsychotic; using two antipsychotics simultaneously is less common. Oxcarbazepine (Trileptal), a congener of carbamazepine, may be effective in its usual anticonvulsant doses of 600–1,800 mg daily, although it is unclear whether carbamazepine nonresponders are likely to show benefit from oxcarbazepine.[33] Tamoxifen (Nolvadex), the estrogen receptor antagonist frequently prescribed in estrogen-positive breast cancer, is also a protein kinase C inhibitor. It has shown clear efficacy in treating acute mania both as monotherapy and as an adjunct to lithium at a dose of 40–80 mg daily.[34,35]

The last two treatments to consider for treatment-resistant acute mania are clozapine (Clozaril) or electroconvulsive therapy (ECT). (Clozapine is discussed more fully in Chapter 6 as a maintenance treatment for bipolar disorder; ECT is discussed at greater length in Chapter 5 as a treatment for bipolar depression.) Although no controlled studies are available that evaluate clozapine for acute mania, general clinical experience indicates its efficacy in treatment-resistant cases.[36] Its tolerability profile—including marked weight gain, sedation, and the potentially life-threatening side effect of agranulocytosis (also seen much more rarely in association with carbamazepine; see earlier discussion)—makes clozapine an infrequently chosen treatment in bipolar disorder.

In the few systematic studies evaluating its efficacy for mania, ECT seems to be as effective as it is for bipolar depression.[37] In general, the same number of treatments is required to treat both acute mania and acute depression. However, as one would anticipate, compared to depressed patients, far fewer manic patients consent to ECT, resulting in its far less frequent use. Involuntary ECT is rare due to laws in most states.

## CONTINUATION TREATMENT FOR ACUTE MANIA

*Continuation treatment* is the transitional phase between acute treatment and maintenance treatment. It begins when the patient's acute manic symptoms have markedly improved. The goal of continuation treatment is to prevent a relapse into the same episode for which treatment was begun. The concept of continuation treatment is predicated on the awareness that clinical improvement frequently precedes biological improvement. As an example, antibiotics are typically prescribed for a 1- to 2-week course even though infectious symptoms usually disappear within days of beginning the antibiotics. If antibiotics are discontinued right after the infectious symptoms disappear, the disease often recurs quickly. Similar considerations apply in treating psychiatric disorders, with the obvious difference being that everything takes longer in psychiatry. In bipolar disorder, symptoms may go underground briefly because of the natural cycling of the illness, not because the treatment has brought about a sustained recovery.

The optimal length of continuation treatment for a manic episode has never been studied. Of course, if the patient agrees to stay on long-term maintenance treatment, the question is mostly irrelevant, since the acute treatment will evolve directly into maintenance treatment. After first-episode manias—assuming the patient has refused indefinite maintenance treatment—the question of how long the acute antimanic treatment should continue after improvement becomes relevant. In the absence of data to guide the length of postmanic continuation treatment, consensus recommendations are for a 3- to 6-month continuation period before the agents are tapered and discontinued. In these situations, it is critical to taper the medications (as opposed to rapidly stopping them), since it is clear that when lithium is stopped rather suddenly—over a 2-week period, for example—patients are at very high risk for an emergent manic episode, far more quickly than one would expect from the natural cycling frequency of the disorder when treatment is withdrawn.[38] Whether these discontinuation-rebound manias would similarly occur after discontinuation of anticonvulsant mood stabilizers or antipsychotics is not known, but logic would dictate a similar strategy. Thus, tapering the acute mania treatment should be accomplished over a minimum of 4 weeks.

## SUMMARY

In this chapter we have emphasized pharmacological treatment of acute manic episodes. There are now more options available for manic patients than ever before, although many choices, each with different advantages and disadvantages, preclude one treatment algorithm. Furthermore, whether one works in an inpatient or outpatient setting, clinicians often face patients who develop severe depressive episodes after manic episodes, or who cycle regularly from one pole to the other. In these cases, treatment regimens need to be reevaluated, and a different set of clinical decisions considered. In Chapter 5 we address the pharmacological treatment of depressive episodes in bipolar I and II disorder.

# CHAPTER 5

## Pharmacological Treatment of Bipolar Depression

The treatment of bipolar depression is a clinical conundrum. In contrast to unipolar (i.e., nonbipolar) depression, for which there are hundreds of controlled studies, there is an astonishing paucity of well-done, controlled treatment studies for bipolar depression. This assuredly reflects a number of factors: the greater prevalence of unipolar disorder leading to more research in that area; the many years (the 1960s through the early 1990s) during which few medications for bipolar disorder other than lithium were vigorously evaluated; the concerns about antidepressants potentially worsening the course of bipolar disorder, thereby discouraging the evaluation of their efficacy; and the general notion that bipolar depression was sufficiently different from unipolar depression that psychotherapeutic approaches were not evaluated. Over the last 20 years there has been a long-needed increase in evaluating treatment approaches—both psychopharmacological and psychotherapeutic—for bipolar depression. Yet even now we have too few studies and insufficient consensus to construct an accepted treatment algorithm for bipolar depression. As we discussed in Chapter 2, this is particularly frustrating given the dominance of depressive times (vs. manic/hypomanic times) in the overall course of bipolar disorder, as well as the evidence that depressive symptoms are more clearly associated with functional impairment than are manic symptoms.

One other central factor contributing to the difficulties in treating bipolar depression concerns the role of antidepressants. From early on in the antidepressant era, it was clear that some bipolar patients became manic/hypomanic on antidepressants. This created a rare situation in which the question was not just whether a treatment (in this case, antidepressants) was effective but did this treatment make the disorder worse? As noted earlier, because of these concerns, there has been very little research into both the efficacy and the dangers of antidepressants for bipolar depression. Even now, with at least a number (albeit still rather small) of studies evaluating antidepressants for bipolar depression, there is still enormous controversy. Some influential researchers in the field view antidepressants as ineffective and frequently harmful, and recommend that they be prescribed only after many other treatments have been tried. Other researchers who rely on the same database of studies (which is easy to do given the paucity of studies) draw diametrically opposite conclusions, perceiving the risk of antidepressants to be small and easily managed, and recommend their use more frequently. It is no wonder that consensus recommendations on treating bipolar depression have been difficult to create!

In this chapter we focus on the treatment of acute bipolar depression. Later in the chapter, we briefly discuss continuation treatment of bipolar depression (i.e., how we keep patients well in the first months after successful acute treatment). Chapter 6 provides recommendations on maintenance treatment, including prevention of bipolar depressive episodes.

This chapter and the next focus on the pharmacological options for the treating physician. We favor close communication between the physician and psychotherapist throughout all phases of treatment, but many patients are seen by the physician infrequently. Because psychotherapists usually see the patient more frequently, they are often the first to observe early warning signs of new episodes or new treatment side effects, and may be in a good position to discuss treatment options with the patient before the next pharmacological appointment (see further discussion of split treatment in Chapter 11). Thus, the information in these chapters is very relevant to psychotherapists working with individuals with bipolar disorder.

## THE CLINICAL SETTING

As in the treatment of acute mania, the first clinical question to address is whether the patient can be adequately treated as an outpatient, or whether a higher level of care—a partial hospital program or an inpatient setting—is required. The clinical criteria that should be used to make this decision do not differ from those used for unipolar depression. For most patients, the three reasons to consider a higher level of care than outpatient treatment are (1) the level of suicidality of the patient; (2) the inability of the patient to cooperate with outpatient treatment; and (3) the inability of the patient to take care of the basics of self-care—eating, clothing, showering, and so forth. We devote Chapter 10 to the evaluation and management of suicidality, since suicide risk can occur in any phase of bipolar disorder.

Cooperation with treatment is relatively easy to evaluate: Can the patient come to clinical appointments? Can she take the medications that are prescribed? Overall resistance to treatment or cognitive impairment secondary to the depression can each interfere with the patient's ability to be treated in an outpatient setting. Evaluating the basics of self-care sometimes requires the help of significant others, since, as an example, patients may not volunteer that they are eating poorly when depressive apathy, fatigue, and cognitive impairment make it impossible to go to the supermarket.

Similar to treating unipolar depression, using these criteria, only the more severe bipolar depressions need to be treated in a hospital-based setting, and these comprise only a small minority of these episodes. Of course, another nonclinical consideration is medical insurance. Those without insurance have a far more difficult time being hospitalized, even when it is clinically appropriate, compared to those with private insurance or Medicare. Hospitals for the uninsured or for those with Medicaid are available throughout the United States. However, since there are woefully insufficient numbers of available beds in these hospitals compared to the number of patients who need them, the threshold of severity for hospitalizing patients is far higher.

## PRETREATMENT EVALUATION

Similar to the pretreatment evaluation of mania/hypomania as discussed in Chapter 4, the pretreatment evaluation for depression is usually relatively simple. Prior to treating the depression, there are areas that need to be addressed: the use of recently introduced nonpsychiatric medications that may cause depressive symptoms, such as steroids, some antihypertensives or tretinoin (Retin-A); recent drug and alcohol abuse or cessation of substances (including caffeine and nicotine); and, if not recently obtained, a basic chemistry panel and a test of thyroid function, such as TSH measurement. For the latter, hypothyroidism (low thyroid function), characterized by a high TSH, is associated with depressive symptoms. Rarely will there be a need for neuroimaging tests such as a CT scan, MRI, or fMRI. As in other clinical situations, some factors dictate a more aggressive laboratory examination, such as a recent onset of neurological symptoms, a first depressive episode after age 60, or cognitive impairment disproportionate to the depressive symptoms.

## OVERALL CONSIDERATIONS

As noted earlier, there is no agreed-upon treatment approach for bipolar depression. Some central areas of controversy are as follows: What are the relative merits of the different mood stabilizers in acutely treating bipolar depression? What is the place of antidepressants in treating bipolar depression? How great a risk do antidepressants confer for precipitating a manic/hypomanic episode? How frequently should antidepressants be used as part of a long-term maintenance treatment regimen? Which bipolar patients should be in adjunctive psychotherapy? How does one pick a specific form of therapy?

Despite the lack of agreement (and lack of data) on these issues, there are some general treatment principles for bipolar depression, listed in Table 5.1. A first general principle is that, despite the same range of treatment options, it is clinically wise to distinguish bipolar I from bipolar II depression and use a different algorithm/order of treatment. Bipolar I depression and bipolar II depression are clinically indistinguishable in both symptoms and severity. However, since bipolar II patients switch into manic/hypomanic states less frequently compared to bipolar I patients, the risk of using antidepressants diminishes with bipolar II disorder. A second principle is that clinical urgency matters. Some approaches that may be effective—lamotrigine (Lamictal), for example, or psychotherapy—may take longer than other approaches. If the patient is mildly to moderately depressed, the time needed for efficacy may well be justified. With more severe depressions, a quick-acting treatment, such as quetiapine (Seroquel) or even an antidepressant, may need to be started (sometimes along with the slower-acting treatment) to "jump-start" the efficacy.

Third, because there is far greater evidence for the efficacy of psychotherapy in depression than in mania/hypomania, psychotherapy for

---

**TABLE 5.1. General Treatment Principles for Bipolar Depression**

- Distinguish between bipolar I and bipolar depression.
- Clinical urgency matters in treatment choice.
- Consider psychotherapy regardless of whether new pharmacotherapies are instituted.
- Patient preferences for treatment should be taken into account.
- Treat to remission; even mild depressive symptoms have clinical consequences.
- Always consider suicide risk during bipolar depression.
- Persist, and help your depressed patient persist, in different therapeutic approaches until significant clinical improvement is seen.

bipolar depressed patients should always be seriously considered (Chapter 7). Fourth, since there is such a broad range of treatment options with little clear consensus, patient preferences (including but not limited to those related to medication side effects) should and do play a role in treatment choice. A fifth principle is that bipolar depression should be aggressively treated. Even mild depressive symptoms are associated with functional impairment and a greater risk of relapse into another mood episode in the near future. Thus, vigorous clinical efforts should *always* be made in targeting *remission*—the near complete resolution of depressive symptoms—as the only reasonable treatment goal of bipolar depression. Sixth, since suicide in bipolar disorder is overwhelmingly most likely during the depressive phase of the disorder, suicide risk should always be addressed during the treatment of bipolar depression. Finally, since successfully matching specific treatments to individual patients is still not predictable, both patient and professionals need to be both flexible and persistent. If the first treatment (or the first two or three!) does not work, try another.

One other overall consideration is the paucity of FDA-approved treatments for acute bipolar depression. In contrast to mania, for which 10 treatments are approved, or maintenance treatments (see Chapter 6), for which six treatments are approved, only three medication approaches have FDA approval for bipolar depression. They are quetiapine, the combination of olanzapine (Zyprexa) plus fluoxetine (Prozac), marketed as Symbyax, and lurasidone (Latuda) (all three are described below in more detail). However, even though all three medications show clear efficacy, for reasons described below, Symbyax is rarely prescribed, quetiapine is appropriate for only a minority of bipolar depressed patients and lurasidone was just recently FDA approved for bipolar depression (in 2013), resulting in a paucity of clinical experience with it as a treatment for bipolar depression. Thus, most bipolar depressed individuals are treated by off-label medication treatments.

## PHARMACOLOGICAL TREATMENT
## OF BIPOLAR I DEPRESSION

Table 5.2 presents the medication options for treating acute bipolar depression. It is helpful to distinguish between two different clinical scenarios[1]: (1) the currently untreated bipolar patient who presents in a depressive episode versus (2) the bipolar patient on a maintenance regimen who is suffering a "breakthrough" depressive episode.

When a bipolar I depressed patient who comes to treatment is not on any medications, a reasonable approach is to start the patient on a mood stabilizer, with or without other treatments (other medications or psychotherapy). Since acute antidepressant treatment will inevitably evolve into longer-term maintenance treatment, many, but not all, of the factors used to choose an individual mood stabilizer are the same as those discussed in Chapter 6. The key, extra consideration for treating bipolar depression is whether the mood stabilizer itself has acute antidepressant properties (in contrast to preventative efficacy).

**TABLE 5.2. Medication Options for Acute Bipolar Depression**

| Medication[a] | Starting dose | Usual dose range | Efficacy rating | Safety/ tolerability | Comments |
|---|---|---|---|---|---|
| quetiapine (Seroquel) | 50–100 mg | 200–600 mg | +++ | Sedation, weight gain | Side-effect profile limits strong efficacy |
| lurasidone (Latuda) | 20–40 mg | 20–120 mg | ++ | Nausea, restlessness | Preliminary positive data |
| lamotrigine (Lamictal) | 25 mg | 100–400 mg | +–++ | Rare disastrous rash; otherwise, benign | Clinical experience better than published data |
| lithium | 300–600 mg | 900–1,800 mg | +–++ | Polyuria, tremor, weight gain | Infrequently used in the United States |
| valproate (Depakote, Depakene) | 250–500 mg | 1,000–2,000 mg | +–++ | Weight gain, sedation | Infrequently prescribed |
| olanzapine/ fluoxetine (Symbyax) | 6–25 mg | 6/25–5/50 | ++ | Weight gain, sedation | Rarely prescribed |
| olanzapine (Zyprexa) | 5 mg | 5–15 mg | +–++ | Weight gain, sedation | Rarely used |
| aripiprazole (Abilify) | 2.5–5.0 mg | 5–15 mg | + | Restlessness, sedation | Clinically more popular than study data suggest |

*Note.* For antidepressants, see Table 5.4.
[a]Trade names are in parentheses.

## First-Line Medication Treatment Options for Monotherapy

The mood stabilizers most likely to be considered for acute bipolar depression in an untreated patient are quetiapine or lamotrigine, and somewhat less commonly (at least in the United States), lithium or valproate (Depakote). Although it has not been evaluated as a mood stabilizer, lurasidone should also be considered as a first-line treatment for bipolar depression.

Quetiapine's antidepressant properties in bipolar disorder have been well established in five separate large-scale, double-blind, placebo-controlled trials, giving quetiapine far more evidence of antidepressant efficacy than any other bipolar antidepressant treatment.[2] Doses of 300 and 600 mg have been evaluated and found to be identical in efficacy. Given the equivalent efficacy of the two doses, 300 mg should be the usual target dose. The efficacy of lower doses is unknown from these studies, but, anecdotally, at least some patients will respond to daily doses in the range of 150–250 mg.

Lurasidone, the most recently released SGA, has demonstrated efficacy as a monotherapy for bipolar depression in doses ranging from 20 to 120 mg, with no difference in efficacy comparing low dose (20–60 mg) to high dose (80–120 mg).[3] Lurasidone should be prescribed with food in order to optimize its absorption from the GI tract. Nausea, restlessness, and sedation were the most common side effects observed.

Despite its lack of FDA indication for bipolar depression, most clinicians (as reflected by their place in treatment guidelines in different countries) perceive lamotrigine to be effective for bipolar depression and, importantly, very tolerable, leading to high patient acceptance. The lack of an FDA indication for lamotrigine reflects that only one of five double-blind studies for bipolar depression was positive. Adding the results of the five studies together demonstrates some, albeit weak, efficacy.[4] However, the more severely depressed patients across all five studies did respond significantly more to lamotrigine than to placebo.[5] Therefore, it may be that lamotrigine's proper place in bipolar depression is in the subgroup of more severely depressed patients.

Lithium's efficacy in acute bipolar depression has yet to be fully evaluated by large, well-designed studies despite its ongoing use for close to 50 years. Partly, this reflects the fact that lithium, as an essential mineral, is unpatentable. Therefore, no pharmaceutical firm has had the incentive to sponsor a large enough study to test lithium's antidepressant efficacy. More difficult to explain is why no governmental agency has sponsored such a study. Only a handful of small studies has evaluated lithium's antidepressant efficacy.[6] In the only recent, large study, lithium was not more effective than placebo in treating acute bipolar I and II depression.[7] However, the relatively low doses and blood levels (average = 0.61 mEq/liter) make the results of this study anything but definitive. European psychiatrists tend to prescribe lithium for acute bipolar depression far more than do American psychiatrists.

Valproate is rather infrequently prescribed for acute bipolar I depression. Nonetheless, each of four small, placebo-controlled studies demonstrated greater antidepressant efficacy than placebo, which suggest valproate's potential efficacy for this purpose.[8]

The decision as to which mood stabilizer to prescribe first for acute bipolar depression depends, as usual, on the relative efficacy versus side effects. As an example, lamotrigine is the most tolerable of the mood stabilizers, but it takes the longest to work (because of the obligatory slow-dose titration; see Chapter 6 for details) and the studies are not as positive as one would like.[9] On the other hand, quetiapine has the best antidepressant data but is associated with substantial weight gain and sedation, which for some patients is very problematic. Thus, a discussion with the patient about the relative advantages and disadvantages of the mood stabilizer options will help generate the right treatment algorithm *for that patient.*

### Second-Line Medication Options

As noted earlier, the combination of olanzapine plus fluoxetine (Symbyax) is one of only three FDA-approved treatments for bipolar depression,[10] yet it is rarely prescribed. The reasons are as follows:

1. Most physicians are taught to avoid combination treatments such as Symbyax, since the fixed ratio of the two medications limits the ability to alter flexibly the dose of one medication without altering the dose of the other. If both olanzapine and fluoxetine are appropriate treatments, then one could always prescribe them as two separate prescriptions, thereby enhancing dosing flexibility.
2. Olanzapine's deserved reputation as the medication causing the most weight gain in all of psychopharmacology (along with clozapine [Clozaril]) and its marked sedative profile makes its prescription for a group of depressed, often fatigued, hypersomnic, bipolar depressed patients unattractive.

Olanzapine as a solo agent is also infrequently prescribed for acute bipolar depression because of the side effect considerations just mentioned. However, in one double-blind study, olanzapine was somewhat more effective than placebo in treating acute bipolar depression.[10]

Aripiprazole (Abilify) has not been demonstrated as effective for acute bipolar depression in two large placebo controlled trials.[11] Yet because of its clearly demonstrated efficacy as an adjunctive treatment (when added to an ineffective antidepressant) for unipolar depression, a number of clinicians prescribe it for bipolar depression. In the two negative studies, the doses used (average doses of 16 and 18 mg) were much higher than those used in the unipolar depression studies. The most common side effects of aripiprazole are restlessness, sedation, and constipation.

Among the other SGAs, risperidone (Risperdal) has not been evaluated as a solo agent for bipolar depression. Ziprasidone (Geodon) was found to be ineffective for bipolar depression in two studies.[12] Neither risperidone nor ziprasidone is prescribed with any regularity for bipolar depression.

A handful of small studies have found that carbamazepine (Tegretol, Equetro) may have efficacy as an antidepressant in patients with bipolar disorder. Nonetheless, it is rarely used for this purpose due to the same difficulties limiting its use in acute mania, as described in more detail in Chapter 4: side effects, concerns about agranulocytosis, and drug–drug interactions.

The vast majority of clinicians appropriately avoid prescribing antidepressants as solo therapeutic agents for bipolar I depression, in view of both the lack of solid evidence demonstrating their efficacy and for fear of triggering a manic/hypomanic episode in the absence of a mood stabilizer. The addition of an antidepressant to a mood stabilizer is discussed below, as is the place of antidepressants as solo agents in treating bipolar II depression.

## Combining a Mood Stabilizer with an Antidepressant

In some clinical situations, the simultaneous initiation of a mood stabilizer with an antidepressant is warranted for bipolar I depression. The concerns about this practice are not only the usual considerations about antidepressants for bipolar depression (considered in detail below) but also the fact that, with simultaneous initiation, the mood stabilizer has not had sufficient time to reach therapeutic blood levels to diminish the risk of an antidepressant-triggered mania/hypomania. Yet clinicians use this treatment with some regularity in one very specific and urgent situation: when a bipolar I patient who comes to treatment is taking no medications at all, is moderately to severely depressed, and has a history of prior response to an antidepressant. In this circumstance, other treatments may be considered but are of unproven efficacy *for that individual*. Thus, starting the mood stabilizer first, waiting for it to have full effect, then adding the antidepressant is indeed the conservative path for treatment, but it takes many weeks, which is a very long time for a severely depressed individual. Therefore, in this very specific situation, some clinicians start the mood stabilizer and antidepressant simultaneously, assuming (and hoping) that even the gradual dosage increase of the mood stabilizer will still prevent the emergence of an antidepressant-induced mania, while the initiation of the antidepressant will help to improve the patient's mood relatively quickly. No study has examined the efficacy of this approach, but it is commonly utilized by clinicians.

## PSYCHOTHERAPY

As indicated in Chapter 7, psychotherapy can be initiated during a bipolar depressive episode and may decrease the time to stabilization. However, psychotherapy should be initiated in combination with mood stabilizers or atypical antipsychotics, not as a solo treatment. Currently, there is no evidence that psychotherapy alone hastens recovery from bipolar I depression, although there is beginning evidence that it may be a monotherapy choice for some bipolar II patients (see Chapter 7).

## TREATMENT OF BREAKTHROUGH DEPRESSION

The other, more common clinical situation arises when a bipolar patient who has been on a stable regimen of one or more mood stabilizers—lithium, valproate, lamotrigine, carbamazepine, or one of the SGAs—then becomes depressed. Only a handful of studies has systematically examined effective medication strategies in this situation, so recommendations are based primarily on clinical opinion (expert and otherwise) and experience. Figure 5.1 presents the options for treating bipolar depression in patients already on a mood stabilizer regimen.

As is the case when treating mania, a first consideration in treating breakthrough depression is to increase the dose of the mood stabilizer. No study has examined this commonly used strategy, so its efficacy is unknown. But for mood stabilizers or antipsychotics that have at least some acute antidepressant efficacy—quetiapine, lurasidone,

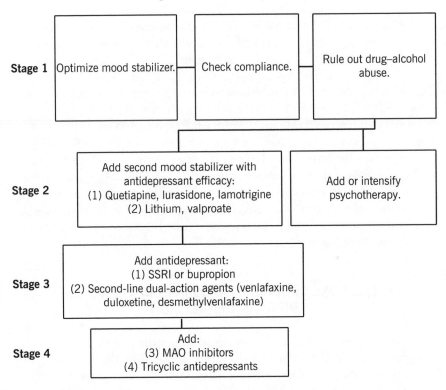

**FIGURE 5.1.** Stages in the treatment of patients with bipolar depression.

lamotrigine, and possibly lithium or valproate—this strategy makes good clinical sense.

Second, as in the treatment of manic episodes, other potential triggers for depression, such as poor adherence to a maintenance medication strategy or drug–alcohol misuse and abuse, should be evaluated and addressed. Interestingly, sleep disruption, which is frequently a trigger for manic symptoms, is less likely to be associated with the emergence of depressive symptoms.

Third, psychotherapy should be considered during breakthrough depressive episodes. Patients whose depression can be related to a series of discrete stressful events (e.g., loss of a loved one) or ongoing chronic stressors (e.g., severe family conflict, financial difficulties) may benefit from an action-oriented, problem-solving therapeutic approach, as described in more detail in Chapter 7.

Core medication approaches for breakthrough depression treatment consist of adding another mood stabilizer or adding an antidepressant. When adding another mood stabilizer, of course, it makes the most sense to prescribe an agent that has some antidepressant properties. Quetiapine and lamotrigine are the most commonly prescribed medications in these situations. Lurasidone would also be an appropriate recent choice in this situation. Although quetiapine has far more empirical support for antidepressant efficacy, lamotrigine is more frequently prescribed due to its greater tolerability. No study has examined the efficacy of quetiapine when added to another mood stabilizer to treat bipolar depression. In the only study examining lamotrigine's efficacy when added to another mood stabilizer (lithium), lamotrigine was indeed more effective than placebo.[13] Lurasidone has clear efficacy for bipolar depression when added to another mood stabilizer, such as lithium or valproate.[14] The efficacy of adding lithium or valproate as an antidepressant has not been evaluated.

## THE ROLE OF ANTIDEPRESSANTS IN TREATING BIPOLAR DEPRESSION

The major controversy in this area surrounds the proper role of antidepressants added to a mood stabilizer regimen in the treatment of bipolar I depression. Opinions are passionate on both sides, with the minimal amount of existing data presented to justify whatever position is being argued. The overall thrust of the competing arguments is presented in Table 5.3. Making this question even more difficult is the dramatic disparity between research findings and "academic" recommendations based on this research, versus clinicians' behavior. As we examine just below, evidence supporting the efficacy of antidepressants for bipolar depression is weak at best, and many scholarly articles, practice guidelines, and textbooks argue against their use except after multiple other approaches have failed. Yet in a study published only 7 years ago, 50% of all initial prescriptions for bipolar disorder were for antidepressant monotherapy.[15] Thus, clinicians, voting with their prescription pads, perceive antidepressants as being effective for bipolar depression despite the barrage of contrary recommendations. Additionally, there are cultural differences, in that European academic psychiatrists seem more accepting of antidepressants for bipolar depression than do their American counterparts.

Part of the problem is the unfortunate dichotomous nature of the question as it is usually posed: Are antidepressants helpful? Are antidepressants harmful? A more nuanced approach assumes that the questions are more complex. First, it is reasonable to assume that a

**TABLE 5.3. Antidepressants for Bipolar Depression: Competing Arguments**

| Against antidepressants | For antidepressants |
| --- | --- |
| There is no consistent evidence of efficacy. | Efficacy is seen at trend level; still insufficiently studied. |
| They may cause manic/hypomanic switches. | There is little evidence of switch with modern antidepressants, especially when added to mood stabilizers. |
| They may cause mood instability. | Most data are derived from old tricyclic studies; little evidence with modern antidepressants. |
| There is little evidence of suicide prevention. | The only evidence for suicide prevention is for lithium, not all mood stabilizers; successfully treating the primary cause of suicide (depression) will inevitably decrease suicide. |

subgroup of bipolar depressed patients may not only respond but also not be harmed by antidepressants, whereas another subgroup may not respond, switch to a manic episode, or both. Therefore, the question should be: *Which* bipolar depressed patients might be effectively and safely treated with antidepressants? Second, antidepressants should not be considered a unitary class of medications. Based on the handful of studies addressing the issue, some antidepressant classes confer a smaller risk of switching to a manic episode compared to the tricyclic antidepressants (see below). Third, there is consistent evidence (although not universal across studies) that adding an antidepressant to a mood stabilizer is associated with a much lower switch rate compared to prescribing the antidepressant as a solo medication.[16] Fourth, short- and long-term risks may differ. As an example, switch rates for antidepressants in an acute antidepressant trial—typically 6–8 weeks—may present a different risk–benefit ratio than the use of the antidepressant over months to years. And finally, when trying to make causal attributions—such as "The patient switched into mania because he was taking an antidepressant"—it is vital to remember that up to 50% of bipolar patients have mood swings characterized by a depression followed by a mania. Thus, emergence of a manic episode in a bipolar patient 6 weeks after the initiation of antidepressant treatment may be related to either the natural history of that individual's bipolar disorder *or* the antidepressant. With any individual patient, we should be wary of ascribing the cause of an event to one specific factor (e.g., the recent prescription of an antidepressant) without other evidence. Our position is that whereas antidepressants can be exceedingly helpful for some bipolar patients, they can be destabilizing for others.

Regarding efficacy, the best summary statement is that the effectiveness of antidepressants for bipolar disorder remains unknown. A well-done meta-analysis of the only six controlled studies for which sufficient information was available (a remarkably small number given the importance of the topic) compared an antidepressant to placebo in bipolar depression and found broad differences in results across studies. [17] Overall, antidepressants showed no benefit compared to placebo. These six studies examined only four different antidepressants—two SSRIs, imipramine (a tricyclic antidepressant) and bupropion (Wellbutrin). Of note, not all subjects in these studies were taking a mood stabilizer, thus making generalizations on the classic situation of adding an antidepressant to a mood stabilizer impossible.

Additionally, there are too few studies comparing one antidepressant to another for treatment of bipolar depression to give recommendations for specific agents. (Table 5.4 lists all the antidepressant classes, as well as the individual agents.) In the largest recent study, neither bupropion nor paroxetine (Paxil, an SSRI) was more effective as monotherapy than placebo, and they were equivalently ineffective.[18] In another recent double-blind study, bupropion, sertraline (an SSRI), and venlafaxine (Effexor) were equivalent in terms of effectiveness, but since no placebo was included in the study, it is not possible to gauge how effective these agents were, only that they were equivalent.[19] In the absence of sufficient data, most clinicians who prescribe antidepressants for bipolar depression assume relatively equivalent efficacy.

The same meta-analysis also focused on the question of antidepressant-induced mania/hypomania.[20] Rates of switching did not differ at all between bipolar patients treated with antidepressants and those treated with placebo (7.7 vs. 7.2%) despite the fact that not all patients were taking mood stabilizers. However, other studies using different research methods have shown a higher rate of switches with antidepressants. As noted earlier, different antidepressant classes may differ in their relative switch rates into mania based on their differing biological mechanisms of action. Although too few systematic studies are available for definitive conclusions, the information available suggests that bupropion and SSRIs have the lowest switch rates, followed by serotonin–norepinephrine reuptake inhibitors (SNRIs) such as venlafaxine (also called *dual-action agents* and described in more detail below); tricyclic antidepressants are associated with the highest switch rates. In the two studies that examined this issue, venlafaxine, a dual-action antidepressant that increases both norepinephrine and serotonin, conferred twice the risk of switching into mania/hypomania compared to either SSRIs (in both studies) or bupropion (in one study).[19,20] Most psychiatrists assume that switch rates with other dual-action agents such as duloxetine (Cymbalta) or desmethylvenlafaxine (Pristiq) are similar to that of venlafaxine. No data are available on either efficacy or switch rates associated with mirtazapine (Remeron) or vilazodone (Viibryd).

An additional concern about antidepressants in bipolar depression, which is much more difficult to measure and for which there is even less research, is whether antidepressants cause greater overall mood instability even if a switch into mania or hypomania does not occur. This greater mood instability may take place over months or even years, making it much more difficult to observe in both research and clinical settings. The terminology of this mood instability varies: It has been described as inducing rapid cycling, acceleration of episode frequency, cycle acceleration, increased mood lability, roughening of the course, and so forth. The core phenomenon being described by these varied terms is an increase in mood shifts per unit time.

Mood instability/cycle acceleration can be expressed in two ways. One example would be a patient who has three mood episodes—including manias, hypomania and depressions—within a 2-year time frame before antidepressants versus six mood episodes in a subsequent 2-year period during which an antidepressant was part of the treatment regimen. A second example would be a patient who, when taking antidepressants (potentially along with a mood stabilizer) had greater day-to-day mood instability, characterized by a day or two of mild depressive symptoms or a few days of feeling "racy," with fewer truly euthymic days compared to when antidepressants were not part of the treatment regimen. Studies from decades ago did demonstrate that some bipolar patients showed cycle acceleration when given antidepressants.[21] However, these studies exclusively evaluated the effects of tricyclic antidepressants in patients who were not taking mood stabilizers. It is a major leap to assume that these early observations are universally relevant to treatment with modern antidepressants such as SSRIs and bupropion in patients also taking mood stabilizers. At this point, then, our best recommendation is that when antidepressants are prescribed for bipolar depression, treating clinicians should simply be alert to the possibilities of both switches into mania/hypomania (which are relatively easier to see) and an overall period of greater mood instability (which is much more difficult to observe).

In summary, antidepressants, especially SSRIs or bupropion, can be prescribed when added to mood stabilizers for bipolar I depression. They are relatively safe in the context of consistent clinical monitoring. The SNRIs and tricyclics appear to have higher switch rates than the SSRIs.

## TREATMENT OF BIPOLAR II DEPRESSION

Compounding the relative paucity of bipolar depression studies is the unfortunate fact that most of these few studies have included only individuals with bipolar I depression as their subjects. Some bipolar depression studies included both bipolar I and bipolar II patients. However, in most of these studies, there were too few bipolar II patients to analyze the results separately from the bipolar I patients, making data-based recommendations for bipolar II depression very difficult. Nonetheless, since bipolar II disorder is dominated by depressive symptoms and episodes, the question of specific treatment strategies for these patients occurs frequently in clinical work. In general, most clinicians think somewhat differently about treating bipolar II (vs. bipolar I) depression—especially the place of antidepressants—for a number of reasons. First, by definition, hypomanias are substantially less destructive than manias, so there is (or should be) less concern about the damage done by an affective switch related to antidepressants. When depressed bipolar II patients switch into hypomanic or manic episodes in association with antidepressants, they develop hypomanias 95% of the time; bipolar II switches into full-blown mania are relatively infrequent. (In contrast, when bipolar I patients switch, they switch into hypomania 55% of the time and into mania 45% of the time.)[22] Although most psychiatrists are deeply concerned about the switch even into hypomania, others suggest that hypomania, especially if it is mild, should not be a major source of concern and does not even need always to be treated.[23]

Second, in contrast to bipolar I patients, those with bipolar II disorder are approximately half as likely to switch when given antidepressants.[22] Because of these considerations, most, but not all, clinicians prescribe antidepressants more liberally to bipolar II patients than to bipolar I individuals.

Of course, the concerns about cycle acceleration we described earlier are relevant to bipolar II disorder, just as they are for bipolar I disorder. Here, too, clinicians need to be conscious of and monitor for evidence of greater mood instability in bipolar II patients treated with antidepressants. As noted, this is a problem typically expressed over longer time frames than acute episodes and is a more central concern during maintenance treatment.

Despite the previous discussion about weighing the relative risks and benefits differently for bipolar II depression and bipolar I depression, many clinicians still adopt the conservative path for treating bipolar II depression, using the same principles as those for bipolar I depression: prescribing mood stabilizers first and foremost, using antidepressants only in limited circumstances. As noted, with the exceptions of quetiapine and lurasidone, no other mood stabilizer or antipsychotic has been demonstrated to be effective in treating bipolar depression. In the only set of studies with sufficient numbers of bipolar II patients to analyze responses to this subgroup separately, quetiapine was effective for bipolar II depression, just as it was for bipolar I depression.[2] Neither lithium nor valproate has been sufficiently evaluated as treatments for bipolar II depression. Additionally, in the only placebo-controlled trial in bipolar II patients, lamotrigine was not more effective than placebo.[24]

Despite this lack of evidence for efficacy from controlled studies, lamotrigine has become a commonly prescribed and very popular agent for treating bipolar II depression. Most clinicians, ourselves included, perceive lamotrigine to be more effective than has been demonstrated in controlled studies. Additionally, and of great clinical importance, lamotrigine is well tolerated, does not cause weight gain or sedation (in contrast to quetiapine), requires no blood monitoring (in contrast to lithium), and is not associated with switches into hypomania (in contrast to antidepressants).

As with bipolar I depression, there is no substantial research evidence of efficacy of the addition of antidepressants to mood stabilizers for acute bipolar II depression. In the largest study, which included both bipolar I and bipolar II patients, antidepressants were not more effective than placebo in either subgroup.[18] A few small studies have demonstrated the efficacy of antidepressants as solo agents (i.e., without mood stabilizers) for bipolar II depression.[25] In these small studies, switch rates into hypomania were low, and in one study, switch rates were comparable between the antidepressant and lithium. Some clinicians therefore prescribe antidepressants as solo treatments for bipolar II depression. We await further data on the efficacy of monotherapy with antidepressants before recommending this option on a broad scale.

## Summary of Treatment Options for Bipolar II Depression

Given the remarkable lack of data in the area of bipolar II depression, clinicians are left with little to guide treatment decisions other than individual clinical experience. Reasonable options include classic mood stabilizers, such as lithium or valproate, and more recently available agents, such as lamotrigine, quetiapine, lurasidone, or antidepressants, with or without concomitant mood stabilizers.

# STRATEGIES FOR PRESCRIBING MEDICATIONS AND FOR MANAGING SIDE EFFECTS

In this section, we discuss those medications described in Chapter 4 (e.g., mood stabilizers, antipsychotics, and antidepressants), underscoring differences in dosing regimens for depressed patients.

## Quetiapine

In studies evaluating quetiapine for bipolar depression, doses were relatively rapidly increased (within a week) to the final dose of 300–600 mg. For many patients, however, this would cause intolerable sedation. Many experienced clinicians prescribe a slower dose increase over a few weeks. An initial dose may be 25–50 mg, with 50-mg dose increases every few days as tolerated, until the target dose is reached. At any dose titration schedule, sedation remains the limiting acute side effect. Weight gain is also frequently problematic, but it is an even greater difficulty in long-term treatment with quetiapine (see Chapter 6).

## Lamotrigine

A difficulty in prescribing lamotrigine for acute bipolar depression is the obligatory, very slow dose increase that is required to avoid a rare but potentially disastrous side effect (see below). Using the required dose schedule, it takes 6 weeks to achieve a typical dose of 200 mg daily. Usual full daily doses are 100–400 mg, with 200 mg being the usual target dose. Therefore, for patients who are moderately to severely depressed, and for whom urgent treatment is required, lamotrigine as the sole therapy would not be a first choice.

Lamotrigine is one of the most benign medications in psychopharmacology, with very few side effects. It is not associated with sedation or weight gain, and no blood tests are required with its use. A mild benign drug rash may be seen in 5–9% of treated patients. If the therapist is seeing the patient frequently, he may be the first to observe a rash in lamotrigine-treated patients.

The major concern with lamotrigine is its capacity to cause an immunological reaction called Stevens–Johnson syndrome, manifested by a severe whole-body rash, along with a flu-like syndrome that includes fever (which often precedes the rash), mucous membrane (mouth, inside of nose) involvement, and liver enzyme abnormalities. In severe cases, this syndrome may even be fatal. The likelihood of Stevens–Johnson syndrome is one in thousands of treated patients. Because it is more likely with rapid dose increases, and the great majority of these cases occur in the first few months of treatment, lamotrigine should be slowly increased over 6 weeks, as noted earlier.

The key issue in lamotrigine therapy is distinguishing between the common benign rash and the rather rare but severe rash. When in doubt, an emergency dermatology consultation, if available, would be appropriate. Of note, however, Stevens–Johnson syndrome typically explodes over hours to a few days at most. Therefore, any patient who describes a rash that has been present for many days is overwhelmingly likely to have a more classical non-life-threatening drug rash.

### Lithium

When prescribed for acute bipolar depression, lithium should be initiated more slowly than when it is prescribed for acute and emergent mania. As with its use in acute mania and maintenance treatment, the lithium dose for bipolar depression is dictated by the serum lithium level, which should be checked after 4–5 days at any dose. A reasonable starting dose would be 300–600 mg, either given all at once or divided into 300 mg twice daily, with dose increases of 300 mg every 3–5 days as tolerated. When lithium is prescribed for acute bipolar depression, typical daily doses are 900–1,500 mg. Optimal lithium levels for acute bipolar depression have not been established; generally, target lithium levels should be 0.6–1.0 mEq/liter, and a full trial should last 6–8 weeks. Common lithium side effects in treatment for depression are the same as those seen in acute mania—nausea, diarrhea, tremor, increased urination, thirst, and cognitive dulling (described in more detail in Chapter 4). Weight gain from lithium typically occurs over longer time frames and is a more important issue in maintenance treatment (see Chapter 6).

## Valproate

As is the case with lithium, when valproate is prescribed for bipolar depression, the speed of dose escalation, as well as the target doses and blood levels, are somewhat lower compared to when it is prescribed for acute mania. Valproate is usually initiated at 250–500 mg for bipolar depression, with increases of 250–500 mg every 4–7 days as tolerated. Usual doses are 1,000–2,000 mg. Optimal valproate levels for treating acute depression are unknown, but a reasonable range would be 50–100 μg/ml. The most common short-term side effects of valproate when prescribed for acute depression are those described in Chapter 4—nausea, diarrhea, sedation, and tremor. Similar to lithium, weight gain properties of valproate are a more central issue in longer-term maintenance treatment.

## Antidepressants

Table 5.4 lists the classes and 30 individual antidepressant agents available in the United States. Medications within the same class typically share similar biological properties, such as which neurotransmitter(s) they affect and a similar (but not necessarily identical) side-effect profile. The novel agents do not define a specific class; these four agents all differ from each other but cannot be classified with other groups. Table 5.4 also lists the typical starting dose and the usual dose range for each agent. It is impossible to recommend specific antidepressant doses in treating bipolar depression from the clinical trials. It is reasonable, however, to use the same doses prescribed for nonbipolar depression. In cases in which there is a history of antidepressant-induced mania, doses are typically increased more slowly (even though it is unclear whether higher doses of antidepressants are associated with higher switch rates). However, if an antidepressant is prescribed at a lower dose and the patient has not responded, the dose should be increased.

SSRIs are the most commonly prescribed class of antidepressants. These six agents share the biological property of increasing the amount of serotonin in the synaptic cleft (the space between neurons). Their popularity reflects their relatively benign side effects and the ease of prescribing them, since the initial dose is very close to the therapeutic dose, making slow dose titrations unnecessary. A third factor in their popularity is that SSRIs demonstrate consistent additional efficacy in treating anxiety and affective reactivity. Common side effects for all

SSRIs include nausea, activation (insomnia, nervousness), occasional sedation, and sexual side effects. The nausea and activation effects are maximal early in treatment and tend to diminish over the first few weeks. Fluoxetine and sertraline are the most stimulating; paroxetine and fluvoxamine (Luvox) are most likely to cause sedation. SSRIs do not cause weight gain in the short term. However, some patients who take SSRIs (especially paroxetine) gain weight after many months to a year into treatment. All SSRIs are currently available in generic form, thereby making cost an irrelevant consideration in drug choice.

Bupropion is a stimulating antidepressant that enhances norepinephrine and dopamine function. Its side-effect profile is similar to most other stimulating medications: anxiety, insomnia, tremulousness, dry mouth, constipation. Of note, it never causes weight gain and is associated with virtually no sexual side effects (in contrast to the SSRIs). Bupropion confers a slightly higher risk of seizures compared to other antidepressants. It should not be prescribed to individuals with seizure disorders or active eating disorders (which may increase the risk of seizures independently). It is very commonly prescribed for bipolar depression because of its relatively low switch rates into mania/hypomania and its stimulating quality, which is particularly attractive to bipolar depressed patients, who are frequently lethargic and psychomotor retarded.

The other novel agents listed in Table 5.4 are prescribed relatively infrequently as antidepressants for bipolar disorder. Trazodone (Desyrel) is commonly prescribed as a sleep aid because at low doses (50–200 mg) it is very sedating. Consistent with this, at its full antidepressant dose of 300–600 mg, trazodone is too sedating for most patients. Similar considerations about sedation apply for nefazodone (Serzone), which is infrequently prescribed due to concerns about its hepatotoxicity (liver inflammation). This does occur, but so rarely that the risk is negligible. Mirtazapine has never been studied in bipolar depression. It is most commonly prescribed for geriatric depression, conferring frequent side effects of sedation and weight gain. Vilazodone (Viibryd) shares biological properties with the SSRIs, increasing serotonin, but it also has properties similar to those of buspirone, a mild antianxiety agent. Early studies suggest that vilazodone is associated with relatively few sexual side effects but can be rather stimulating. Vortioxetine (Brintellix), the most recently released antidepressant, has not been evaluated for treating bipolar depression. The most common side effects of vortioxetine are gastrointestinal disturbances, such as nausea, constipation and vomiting.

**TABLE 5.4. Antidepressant Classes and Specific Agents**

| Class[a] | Typical starting dose (mg) | Usual dose (mg daily) |
|---|---|---|
| Selective serotonin reuptake inhibitors (SSRIs) | | |
| citalopram (Celexa) | 10–20 | 20–60 |
| S-citalopram (Lexapro) | 5–10 | 10–30 |
| fluoxetine (Prozac) | 10–20 | 10–80 |
| fluvoxamine (Luvox) | 25–50 | 100–300 |
| paroxetine (Paxil) | 10–20 | 20–60 |
| sertraline (Zoloft) | 25–50 | 50–200 |
| Novel antidepressants | | |
| bupropion (Wellbutrin) | 100–150 | 300–450 |
| mirtazapine (Remeron) | 15–30 | 15–60 |
| nefazodone (Serzone) | 50 | 400–600 |
| trazodone[b] (Desyrel) | 50 | 150–400 |
| vilazodone (Viibryd) | 10 | 20–40 |
| vortioxetine (Brintellix) | 10 | 20 |
| Dual-action agents | | |
| desmethylvenlafaxine (Pristiq) | 25–50 | 50–100 |
| duloxetine (Symbalta) | 20–30 | 60–120 |
| levomilnacipran (Fetzima) | 20 | 40–120 |
| venlafaxine (Effexor) | 37.5–75.0 | 150–300 |
| Tricyclics + related compounds | | |
| amitriptyline (Elavil, Endep) | 25–50 | 100–300 |
| amoxapine (Asendin) | 50–100 | 150–400 |
| clomipramine (Anafranil) | 25–50 | 100–250 |
| desipramine (Norpramin, Pertofrane) | 25–50 | 100–300 |
| doxepin (Sinequan, Adapin) | 25–50 | 100–300 |
| imipramine (Tofranil) | 25–50 | 100–300 |
| maprotiline (Ludiomil) | 25–50 | 100–225 |
| nortriptyline (Aventyl, Pamelor) | 10–25 | 50–150 |
| protriptyline (Vivactil) | 10 | 15–60 |
| trimipramine (Surmontil) | 25–50 | 100–300 |
| MAO inhibitors | | |
| isocarboxazid (Marplan) | 10–20 | 30–60 |
| phenelzine (Nardil) | 15–30 | 30–90 |
| selegiline (Eldepryl) | 10 | 20–60 |
| selegiline transdermal (Emsam patch) | 6 | 6–12 |
| tranylcypromine (Parnate) | 10–20 | 30–60 |

[a]Trade names are in parentheses.
[b]Rarely used as antidepressant; prescribed more in low dose as a hypnotic.

Dual-action agents—venlafaxine, duloxetine, desmethylvenlafaxine, and levomilnacipran (Fetzima)—increase both norepinephrine and serotonin in the central nervous system. Their side-effect profile is similar to that of the SSRIs, but with more constipation and nausea in the case of duloxetine and more overall gastrointestinal side effects and sweating with levomilnacipran. Venlafaxine and probably desmethylvenlafaxine are associated with new-onset hypertension at medium to high doses. Sexual side effects of duloxetine specifically may be less than is typically seen with the other dual-action agents or the SSRIs.

Monoamine oxidase (MAO) inhibitors have shown efficacy in a few systematic studies of bipolar depression.[26] However, they are not popular among psychiatrists and patients due to (1) their side-effect burden, such as difficult-to-treat insomnia and orthostatic hypotension; (2) the requirements for mandatory dietary restrictions (especially aged cheeses) in order to avoid a hypertensive crisis (sudden increase in blood pressure, with its attendant medical risks); and (3) the contraindication of combining an MAO inhibitor with many other medications, including all strongly serotonergic antidepressants, such as the SSRIs or dual-action agents, because this combination confers a significant risk of serotonin syndrome which, when severe, may be fatal. Because of these concerns, MAO inhibitors are usually considered as options for treatment-resistant bipolar depression. MAO inhibitors are generally thought to be associated with fewer switches into mania/hypomania than tricyclic antidepressants (see below) but more than the modern antidepressants such as SSRIs or bupropion.

---

Jessica is 47 years old and has suffered from severe bipolar I disorder since her early 20s. She has had multiple psychotic manias, each of which required hospitalization and multiple severe suicidal depressions. Her episodes emerge despite reasonably good treatment adherence to many individual and combination regimens of mood stabilizers and psychotherapy. One year ago, she became depressed despite an ongoing regimen of adequate doses of lithium and lamotrigine plus low-dose aripiprazole. Increasing the dose of each of these three agents was unhelpful. The addition of an SSRI, duloxetine, and bupropion were also ineffective. Tranylcypromine (Parnate), an MAO inhibitor was then added to her three mood stabilizers. Jessica showed a partial response to 40 mg daily (low-medium dose). At a daily dose of 80 mg of tranylcypromine, Jessica showed marked improvement. Although she had some residual fatigue and disliked both the insomnia and the dietary restrictions of the MAO inhibitor, she continued the medication due to its unquestionable efficacy for her.

---

## Tricyclic Antidepressants

Tricyclic antidepressants, one of the two oldest classes of antidepressants, are usually close to the bottom of the algorithm of bipolar depression. This reflects the legitimate concern that tricyclics are associated with the highest rate of manic/hypomanic switches among the antidepressants and is the class most associated with causing mood instability.[27] Aside from these concerns, tricyclics are associated with a great number of side effects, which has limited their use in nonbipolar depression, too. The most common side effects, which differ in frequency and intensity across individual tricyclic agents, are sedation, orthostatic hypotension (dizziness on standing up due to decreased blood pressure), constipation, dry mouth, and weight gain. Additionally, tricyclics easily can be lethal when taken in overdose. Therefore, they should be prescribed with great caution to acutely suicidal depressed patients.

## TREATMENT-RESISTANT BIPOLAR DEPRESSION

There is no established definition of treatment resistance in bipolar depression. Thus, it is difficult to assert specifically which treatments are for "usual" bipolar depression and which are for treatment-resistant cases. As a working definition, a bipolar depressed patient who has failed to respond to at least two mood stabilizers (e.g., lithium, an anticonvulsant, or an antipsychotic) plus at least two antidepressants *and* psychotherapy can be considered treatment-resistant. As always, before utilizing other treatments, it is clinically wise to ensure that (1) the patient is adherent to treatment and not missing either all or a substantial percentage of doses; (2) comorbid drug–alcohol use–misuse is not interfering with treatment; (3) if psychotherapy is being used, the patient is appropriately engaged in the process. Assuming that these are not central factors in the patient's lack of response to treatment, options listed in Table 5.5 should be considered. Many of these—such as antidepressant combinations, adjunctive antidepressants, and ECT—are the same options considered for treatment-resistant nonbipolar depression but have never been formally examined in bipolar depression. Others, such as pramipexole (Mirapex), may be more specific to bipolar depression.

Prescribing combinations of mood stabilizers presumes that, for some patients, there would be additive antidepressant effects, especially when the specific mood stabilizers have at least some antidepressant efficacy. Reasonable combinations would include lurasidone, quetiapine, lamotrigine, and lithium and/or valproate. Similarly, combinations

**TABLE 5.5. Treatment Options for Treatment-Resistant Bipolar Depression**

- Mood stabilizer combinations
- Antidepressant combinations
- Adjunctive antidepressant treatments
  - T3 (Cytomel)
  - Stimulants such as methylphenidate (Ritalin), amphetamines (Dexedrine), Adderall, Vyvanse, modafinil (Provigil), and armodafinil (Nuvigil)
- ECT
- Omega-3 fatty acids
- Pramipexole (Mirapex)

of antidepressants from different classes—such as an SSRI plus bupropion, or venlafaxine plus mirtazapine—should also be considered. However, special caution should be taken when using multiple antidepressants for patients who are mania-prone or have a past history of antidepressant-induced mania.

Adjunctive treatments for depression are medications that, by themselves, are not antidepressants but augment the efficacy of antidepressants when added to them. Lithium and low doses of some antipsychotics, such as aripiprazole or quetiapine, are well established but may already have been considered, since they are also mood stabilizers or have primary antidepressant effects. T3 (Cytomel) is a thyroid hormone that has been used with some efficacy to augment antidepressants in nonbipolar depression.[28] Two different types of stimulants may be considered:

1. Modafinil/armodafinil (Provigil/Nuvigil) have been demonstrated to be effective in at least one controlled study with each agent in bipolar depression and seems not to increase the risk of inducing mania.[29,30]
2. The older class of stimulants—methylphenidate (Ritalin, Concerta, and others) or amphetamines (Dexedrine, Adderall, Vyvanse)—have not been systematically tested in bipolar depression, but anecdotal experience has been positive.[31] These medications *may* confer a greater risk of inducing manic/hypomanic states (there are few data on this issue) compared to modafinil/armodafinil and may be abused by those with a history of stimulant use; therefore, they should be prescribed cautiously.

ECT is the oldest (available for more than 50 years) antidepressant treatment and is assuredly underutilized in bipolar depression. ECT is as effective a treatment for bipolar depression as it is for nonbipolar depression.[32] However, because of its inherent disruptiveness (treatment three times per week with anesthesia, whether the patient is in the hospital or an outpatient), side effects associated with its use (e.g., transient memory problems), and its dreadful image and reputation derived from its use–abuse and other side effects decades ago (when it was regulated quite differently than it is today), ECT is an infrequent choice. Nonetheless, for severely depressed and/or very treatment-resistant patients, it is the most rapid and effective treatment.

---

Stephen's bipolar I disorder was dominated by his prolonged and difficult-to-treat depressions. Although he had had three manias, two of which required hospitalizations, he spent far more of his life depressed, sometimes mildly and at other times severely enough to keep him out of work and cause him to lose relationships. He was completely adherent to treatment, and life stressors seemed to play no role in triggering his depressive episodes. Most recently, he had become markedly depressed, despite taking two mood stabilizers at adequate dosage. Trials of quetiapine, two antidepressants, and an antidepressant combination were ineffective. At this point, 9 months into this depressive episode, Steven had become progressively more discouraged that he would ever feel better, and his low-grade suicidal thinking was intensifying. Although he was terrified of the potential cognitive side effects (when he was well, he worked as a programmer in the computer industry), Steven agreed to a trial of outpatient ECT. His mood began to improve after the fourth treatment and by nine treatments, his mood was essentially normal. His memory was, as expected, a bit fuzzy for the weeks of ECT treatment, but his longer-term memory was minimally affected and improved to its pretreatment levels after the end of ECT treatment. Following ECT, he was restarted on his mood stabilizer regimen with an antidepressant. One year after ECT, Steven continued to feel relatively well and was back at work.

---

Omega-3 fatty acids, especially ethyl-eicosapentaenoate (EPA), are available without a prescription in health food stores at typical doses of 1-2 grams daily, and are sometimes prescribed at higher dose. Omega-3 fatty acids has been shown to be effective in some but not all studies of bipolar depression, and then only as an add-on to standard mood stabilizers or SGAs.[33] Omega-3 fatty acids are associated with minimal side effects. Many patients are positively inclined to take "natural" substances in preference to prescribed medications, but they should be aware of the efficacy limitations of these substances.

Pramipexole, which increases the neurotransmitter dopamine and is more commonly prescribed for Parkinson's disease or restless legs syndrome, was effective in two small studies of bipolar depression. It is infrequently prescribed for this purpose.[34,35]Most recently, ketamine, with a unique mechanism of action relative to classic antidepressants, has demonstrated rapid efficacy (typically after a single intravenous dose and sustained for many days) in bipolar depression when added to a mood stabilizer.[36] However, ketamine cannot be administered orally; in addition, its potential side effects of psychosis and dissociative symptoms, and its use as a street drug (called K or Special K) make it unlikely to be used with any frequency.

## CONTINUATION TREATMENT OF BIPOLAR DEPRESSION

Analogous to treatment principles for acute mania, it is generally assumed that all effective treatments—both pharmacological and psychotherapeutic—for bipolar depression should be continued for some time after the patient improves. Following clinical improvement, continuation sessions of psychotherapy should focus on the gains made, on practicing and strengthening the types of life changes that may have contributed to improvement (e.g., regular sleep–wake habits), and on delineating the early warning signs of a potential depression in the future. If the medications prescribed are also mood stabilizers and part of a long-term treatment plan, then continuation and maintenance treatment merge into each other. However, when a specific medication, such as an antidepressant, has been added to the treatment regimen to target depressive symptoms, it may not need to be continued for an extended time period. Unfortunately, no study has examined the proper length of continuation treatment for antidepressants in bipolar depression. A reasonable time frame is 2 to 6 months, which is shorter than the usual continuation period for nonbipolar depression. As with almost any psychotropic medication, when antidepressants are discontinued, they should be tapered gradually over at least 1 month, unless the discontinuation is triggered by an emerging manic episode. We discuss the longer-term use of antidepressants as part of a maintenance treatment in bipolar disorder in Chapter 6.

## SUMMARY

Treatment of an acute depressive episode of bipolar disorder requires a careful balance between maximization of treatment efficacy and speed of response, and, conversely, minimization of side effects, including the possibility of causing a switch into mania/hypomania. Effectively

# CHAPTER 6

## Pharmacological
## Maintenance Treatment

The goal of maintenance treatment is to prevent mood recurrences, both (hypo)manias and depressions. Arguably, the maintenance phase of bipolar disorder is the most important phase. When episodes break through, as they often do, there is usually impairment in psychosocial functioning, which, of course, can have a pervasive negative effect on the patient's life. The occurrence of acute episodes beyond the first episode reflects the imperfections of our maintenance treatments. Nonetheless, well-planned pharmacotherapy can be powerful in preventing mood episodes (this chapter), especially when combined with psychoeducational forms of psychotherapy (Chapter 7).

Given that bipolar disorder is inherently a recurrent disorder, the question for maintenance/preventative treatment is not *if* there will be a next episode but rather *when*. Many patients are resistant to this idea, especially when they are in the beginning stages of the disorder. Regrettably, they often reject the idea that they must take complex combinations of medications to prevent future episodes (see Chapter 8).

It is ironic that even though depression is the dominant and most impairing pole of bipolar disorder, the focus of research has been the prevention of manias. This is analogous to our far greater knowledge base about the acute treatment of mania compared to the acute treatment of depression, as discussed in Chapter 5.

Maintenance treatment naturally follows continuation treatment for either mania/hypomania or depression. Unfortunately, there is no clear definition as to when continuation treatment evolves into maintenance treatment. In general, once a patient has been stable for 3–6 months after either (hypo)mania or depression, further treatment can be considered to be maintenance therapy.

The mainstays of maintenance pharmacotherapy are the mood stabilizers. Here, too, there is no consensus as to the precise definition of the term *mood stabilizer*.[1] Since the goal of maintenance treatment is to prevent mood episodes, at the very least, the expectation is that the mood stabilizer would prevent an episode at both poles of the disorder. The optimal definition of a *mood stabilizer* would also include effective treatment of acute depression and acute mania.

## GOALS OF MAINTENANCE TREATMENT

At the simplest level, the primary goal of maintenance treatment is the complete prevention of future episodes (see Table 6.1). However, as noted in Chapter 2, virtually all studies over the last 20 years in both the United States and Europe have shown that even patients in ongoing treatment have high relapse rates, with 1- to 2-year relapse rates of 40–60% and 4- to 5-year relapse rates of 60–85%.[3-5] Therefore, clinicians and patients need to consider goals of maintenance treatment other than a complete cessation of episodes. Moreover, intermediate treatment goals need their own measures of efficacy.

In order to show that a maintenance treatment is working, clinicians need literally to count the episodes in a certain time period before a treatment is instituted, then compare it with the number of episodes the patient has while being treated (a "mirror image" comparison). For example, if a patient has had two mood episodes per year in each of the last 2 years (equaling four episodes in 2 years), then after the initiation of maintenance treatment experiences one episode over the next 2 years, the treatment yielded a 75% improvement (one episode vs. an expected four episodes). This treatment is therefore very effective but not perfect, since the patient still experienced one breakthrough episode. (All these considerations presume treatment adherence, an assumption that

---

**TABLE 6.1. Goals of Maintenance Treatment**

- Abolish mood episodes and reduce mood swings.
- Decrease the number, intensity, and length of episodes.
- Achieve greater mood stability (less subsyndromal symptoms) between episodes.
- Enhance functioning.

---

*Note.* From Gitlin and Frye.[2]

frequently may be incorrect). Patients and clinicians alike tend to focus on the one breakthrough episode and conclude that the preventative treatment was ineffective, ignoring the evidence of *partial efficacy*.

Similarly, decreasing the intensity or amplitude of episodes may be very therapeutic even though the patient still experiences mood cycles. If the episodes during treatment are mild depressions, during which the patient neither gets fired nor becomes suicidal, and during the manias/hypomanias the patient does not get hospitalized or become psychotic, then the treatment has been effective, again, albeit imperfectly. Of note, reducing episode intensity (from mania to hypomania and severe incapacitating depression to mild depression) will also significantly reduce work and social impairment.

---

Jonathan, a 27-year-old man with bipolar I disorder since age 18, had severe manias and severe depressions. His manic episodes were characterized by frenzied hyperactivity, irritability, increased use of drugs and alcohol, and psychotic thinking. When depressed, he hibernated, sleeping hours on end and rarely leaving the house. He also reported contemplating suicide, although he had never made an attempt. Not surprisingly, he had been hospitalized numerous times for both types of episodes, had lost a number of jobs, and had been unable to sustain any long-term romantic relationships. Over the previous 3 years, he had experienced five mood episodes and three hospitalizations, two for mania and one for depression. After multiple ineffective maintenance trials of individual mood stabilizers, he was placed on a combination of lithium and valproate (Depakote). Over the next 3 years, Jonathan had three episodes (two depressions and one hypomania). Although his thoughts raced and he was expansive, irritable, and somewhat hyperactive during hypomania, he was neither psychotic nor as belligerent as in previous episodes. He had begun to try to attend college classes and was able (barely) to finish the semester. His depressions during treatment were still characterized by hypersomnia and fatigue, but he was able to go to classes and study to some degree. He was not suicidal. Because of the lower intensity of his depressions, Jonathan was not hospitalized for any of these episodes. Thus, he had a positive reaction to maintenance treatment with lithium and valproate.

---

Similarly, a positive effect of maintenance treatment may be simply to shorten the length of mood episodes. A 1-month episode would certainly be less detrimental to a patient's life than a 6-month episode, regardless of whether the episode is manic or depressive. Finally, amelioration of subsyndromal symptoms, which are consistently associated with functional impairment and earlier manic and depressive relapses, also demonstrates maintenance therapy efficacy.[5,6]

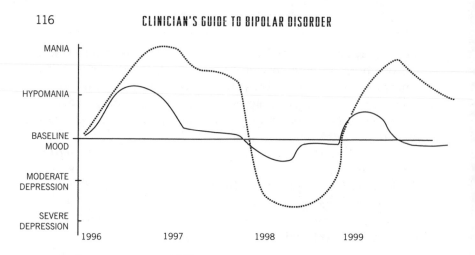

**FIGURE 6.1.** Albert's long-term cycling on and off medications. Solid line, on appropriate medications; dotted line, off medications. From D. J. Miklowitz. *The Bipolar Disorder Survival Guide.* 2nd ed. New York: Guilford Press; 2011. Copyright 2011 by The Guilford Press. Reprinted by permission.

Figure 6.1 illustrates the way in which long-term illness course—in this case, the duration and severity of episodes—can improve during maintenance treatment, even if episodes cannot be fully prevented. The patient, Albert, had severe episodes before taking maintenance medications (dotted lines). Once stabilized on maintenance treatment, his breakthrough episodes became less frequent, shorter and less severe.

## GENERAL GUIDELINES FOR MAINTENANCE TREATMENT

Almost always, the first question about maintenance treatment is: When should this long-term, potentially lifelong treatment commence? Most practice guidelines recommend that maintenance treatment start after the first manic episode. This recommendation sounds very clear in principle, but it is surprisingly difficult to implement in real-world practice. Since bipolar disorder typically emerges in the person's late teens or early 20s, we often are discussing long-term treatment with young people still working on separation from their parents. Many of these young people still harbor grandiose notions of the control they have in shaping their lives. They have yet to internalize the challenges everyone faces in achieving life goals. Suggesting to a 23-year-old male, who has had one manic episode characterized by expansive thinking, that he needs to be on preventative treatment for a lifetime is usually ineffective. Even those who initially agree to such a treatment goal frequently stop their medications within a few months, once they feel some sustained relief from their symptoms and the traumatic memories of prior manic episodes recede into the past, and they forget or deny the consequences of untreated bipolar disorder.

---

Bart had no psychiatric history until age 19, when, as a sophomore in college, he had a classic manic episode during the spring semester. He was eventually hospitalized. Although initially ambivalent about taking medications while overtly manic, he ultimately agreed to take medication and improved rather rapidly on valproate and olanzapine (Zyprexa). Bart withdrew from school for the semester. In the early summer, olanzapine was tapered slowly and without problem. By August, in discussing his return to school, Bart wanted to discontinue the valproate, too, insisting that the manic episode was an aberration. He had long discussions with his psychiatrist, who not only educated him about the recurrent nature of bipolar disorder and the risks of another manic episode but also empathized with Bart's desire to discontinue treatment. Bart's disappointment that he could not control his own brain and that he was "marked" by taking medications were central issues in the discussion. Bart agreed to continue the valproate when he returned to school. By December, however, he had gradually tapered and stopped the valproate, which his psychiatrist found out after the fact. They again discussed the risks of being off medication, but this time the psychiatrist helped Bart to clarify the early symptoms of his prior manic episodes, in the hope that Bart would recognize them if they recurred. Bart did well until the next spring, when his manic symptoms reemerged. However, he recognized the symptoms and returned to treatment quickly enough that it was effective and he was able to continue the semester.

---

In constructing a maintenance treatment regimen with a patient, sophisticated clinicians know that one size does not fit all. The two major criteria that should always be considered in developing an individualized maintenance pharmacotherapy regimen are (1) the ratio of manic to depressive dominance, and (2) side-effect sensitivity *for that individual patient*. Bipolar disorder can be described as *mania-dominant, depression-dominant* (most bipolar II patients), or *pole-nondominant* (episodes of equal frequency and severity across the two poles). Because some mood stabilizers have greater efficacy in preventing manias/hypomanias and others are better at preventing depressions, one can thoughtfully match medications to patients based on these criteria.[7] Of course, to do this effectively, the treating clinician must take a careful enough history to know about relative frequency and severity of past mood episodes. Similarly, all mood stabilizers have side effects, but these side effects differ from each other across agents. For some patients, weight gain would be a paramount concern; for others, sedation would be intolerable. Another patient who depends on motor control for his livelihood (e.g., a violinist, surgeon, or artist) might find tremors most problematic.

Because most patients have breakthrough episodes, it is critical that patients and significant others—parents, children, spouses, lovers— know the initial or prodromal signs of an emerging mood episode. Educating patients and family members about early warning signs is discussed in detail in Chapter 7.

## MAINTENANCE PHARMACOTHERAPY

Typically, the initiation of a maintenance treatment follows treatment of an acute episode, either mania/hypomania or depression. In this circumstance, the pretreatment evaluation described in Chapters 4 and 5 would suffice. In the less common situation in which a new, asymptomatic patient presents for maintenance treatment and is not taking medications, the psychiatrist should conduct a pretreatment evaluation, including a thorough review of currently prescribed medications (for nonpsychiatric and other psychiatric disorders) and standard screening tests (basic chemistry panel and TSH measurement for thyroid function). Depending on which mood stabilizer is prescribed (see below), other blood tests might also be ordered. If conducting psychotherapy as well, the clinician should evaluate the history of prior episodes in the context of psychosocial triggers (e.g., loss events, changes in daily routines and sleep–wake cycles, marital separations/conflicts).

Maintenance medication treatments for bipolar disorder, their general dose ranges, and most common side effects are listed in Table 6.2. In contrast to the dosing of these medications for acute mania, doses of mood stabilizers in maintenance treatment may remain stable or even be reduced. If they need to be increased, this will occur slowly, for two reasons:

1. There is typically little clinical urgency when starting a long-term preventative treatment.
2. A slower and more gradual dose escalation results in less burdensome side effects, making treatment adherence more likely.

**TABLE 6.2. Maintenance Medications for Bipolar Disorder**

| Medication[a] | Starting dose (mg) | Maintenance dose range (mg) | Common side effects |
|---|---|---|---|
| lithium | 300–600 | 900–1,800; levels = 0.6–1.0 mEq/liter | Increased urination, thirst, tremor, weight gain |
| lamotrigine (Lamictal) | 25 | 100–400 | Rash, nausea |
| valproate (Depakene, Depakote, Depakote ER) | 250–500 | 750–3,000 | Nausea, tremor, weight gain, sedation |
| olanzapine (Zyprexa) | 5 | 10–15 | Sedation, weight gain |
| aripiprazole (Abilify) | 5 | 10–30 | Akathisia/stimulation effects, sedation |
| quetiapine (Seroquel) | 25–50 | 200–800 | Sedation, weight gain |
| ziprasidone (Geodon) | 40 | 80–160 | Sedation, akathisia/ stimulation |
| risperidone long-acting injection (Risperdal Consta) | 25 | 25–50 (intramuscular, every 2 weeks) | Sedation, weight gain, akinesia, tremor, akathisia |
| carbamazepine (Tegretol, Equetro) | 100–200 | 400–1,200 | Dizziness, poor balance, double vision, fatigue |
| oxcarbazepine (Trileptal) | 300 | 600–800 | Dizziness, poor balance, double vision, fatigue |

[a]Trade names are in parentheses.

## Lithium

### Efficacy and Techniques of Administration

Lithium was the first treatment that was available and for many decades was the only medication with any demonstrated efficacy in preventing both manias and depressions. Although still a first-line treatment, many patients, especially in the United States, are treated with other agents first, due partly to the marketing blitzes from pharmaceutical firms promoting more recently released medications and partly to the perception (somewhat accurate) of lithium as a burdensome drug in terms of side effects, organ toxicities, and the requirement for regular blood tests. Nonetheless, lithium is still thought of as the "gold standard" for maintenance treatments; new medications are often tested in comparison to lithium in order to demonstrate efficacy.

Across many studies, lithium consistently appears to prevent mood episodes better than placebo.[8] The most recent studies, although still demonstrating lithium's efficacy, seem to indicate less robust preventative effects. This change in effect size almost assuredly reflects differences in how these studies were designed and the types of subjects/patients who enter these studies. Moreover, lithium prevents manias/hypomanias more effectively than it prevents depressions.[9] Not surprisingly, this has long been a major complaint of people with bipolar disorder, who typically dread depressions more than manias.

Patients who do best on lithium are those who fit the classic profile of bipolar disorder.[10] These classic features include discrete episodes with typical symptoms, a family history of bipolar disorder (as well as a family history of lithium response), a mania–depression interval (MDI) pattern of episodes (in contrast to biphasic episodes that begin with a depression followed by a mania [DMI pattern]), an intermediate age of onset (not pediatric and not geriatric), and full remission between episodes. In contrast, mixed features and a rapid-cycling pattern of episodes predict a poorer response to prophylactic lithium treatment, although rapid cycling probably predicts a poorer response to any mood stabilizer, not just lithium.

As noted in Chapter 4, prior to starting lithium, blood tests measuring renal (kidney) function (serum creatinine), thyroid function (TSH), and possibly serum calcium should be obtained. An EKG for those older than age 40 and a pregnancy test for women of childbearing age are also advisable.

When prescribed as a maintenance treatment, lithium is typically started at 300–600 mg daily, with increases of 300 mg every 4–5 days. Usual daily doses of lithium range between 900 and 1,800 mg but may be higher for some individuals. As with its use in treating acute mania, the extended release form of lithium should be reserved for those patients who develop prominent nausea with lithium capsules. Additionally, lithium can be prescribed once daily. The daily dose can be given twice daily in a divided dose if nausea is excessive with a once-daily regimen.

Target blood levels for maintenance lithium treatment are 0.6–1.0 mEq/liter, lower than the levels targeted for acute mania. Higher maintenance serum levels of lithium, 0.8–1.0 mEq/liter, may result in better preventative efficacy but are associated with greater side-effect burden and more nonadherence compared to lower serum levels.[11] Consistent with its use in acute mania, lithium levels of 0.4–0.6 mEq/liter may be sufficient for older patients.

## Side Effects and Their Management

As noted in Chapters 4 and 5, the most common acute side effects of lithium are nausea, diarrhea, tremor, increased urination, thirst, and cognitive dulling.[12] With the exception of nausea, which tends to diminish and/or remit with time, these other side effects may also occur during long-term lithium treatment. Long-term side effects are weight gain and negative effects on both the thyroid and the kidneys. It is relevant to distinguish between the most common side effects and those that are most distressing, since the latter are more associated with medication discontinuation. The most distressing side effects associated with lithium are the weight gain and the cognitive effects. Chapter 8 discusses the relationship between side effects and treatment adherence.

Tremor, classically of the hands, is a common side effect of lithium. Lithium-induced tremor is described as postural and intentional; it is increased with effort such as holding a coffee cup or writing (sometimes leading to a change in handwriting). This type of tremor is distinct from the tremor seen in Parkinson's disease or in association with antipsychotics, with which the tremor is worst at rest, not with effort. Lithium-induced tremor is worsened by anxiety or stimulation effects from caffeine or other stimulants. The tremor can be effectively treated with low doses of beta blockers such as propranolol (Inderal).

## Lithium and Cognition/Creativity

Cognitive side effects are of more concern during maintenance treatment than in the treatment of acute mania. Patients on lithium complain of poor concentration, impaired memory, and a sense of dullness or diminished creativity. Certainly, some of these complaints are not due to lithium but are secondary to the loss of the heightened senses associated with the hypomanias, which are diminished with lithium. However, cognitive problems due specifically to lithium clearly occur with some patients. Cognitive side effects from lithium are dose-related; thus, lowering the dose may decrease this problem.

The subtle decrease in creativity is more difficult to measure but unquestionably occurs with some musicians, artists, writers, and actors.[13] For most artists who have bipolar I disorder, the generally increased productivity on lithium—due in large part to spending less time depressed, dysfunctional, psychotic, or hospitalized—makes up for the potential loss of short-term creative bursts. This is a rather sensitive issue, however, and often requires a more extensive discussion between the physician and patient of risk–benefit ratios of medication treatment. One might point out the risks and benefits more concretely by examining the actual creative output of the patient when she is having more mood symptoms or episodes compared to euthymic times. Unless they have blessedly mild to moderate hypomanias and can stay self-disciplined while symptomatic, most patients realize that even though they *feel* more creative with mood swings, their careers have suffered because of the decreased productivity associated with depressions. It is also helpful to point out that side effects are dose-related. It is usually possible to find a dose of lithium that is effective but still allows creative output.

## Lithium-Induced Weight Gain

Significant weight gain (usually defined as gaining 7% of baseline body weight, which translates to 10 pounds in a 150-pound person) occurs in up to 25% of lithium-treated patients.[14] Of course, weight gain may be due to myriad reasons, including the weight gain effect of other prescribed medications, increased appetite and decreased exercise associated with depression, hypothyroidism (from lithium; see discussion below), edema (water retention infrequently caused by lithium), and increased ingestion of high-calorie soft drinks in response to lithium-induced thirst. As would be expected, the management of the weight gain depends on the cause. Treating the depression, increasing exercise (always a right answer!), switching to noncaloric drinks, and treating hypothyroidism, if present, are all reasonable clinical strategies. For classic lithium-induced weight gain, the best treatment strategies are (1) prevention, with early education and attention to diet and exercise patterns *before* weight gain occurs, and (2) diet and exercise. Patients can lose weight on lithium via the usual means but it takes more work. As an example, a diet and exercise program that would typically result in a 2-pound weight loss per week may be associated with a 1-pound weekly weight loss in patients taking lithium.

To keep dieting patients from growing discouraged, it is helpful to educate patients on lithium about weight management. For example, one might inform patients that weight loss may be slow on lithium, but it is entirely possible and probable. It may also be helpful to point out that the key to maintaining a healthy body weight is to develop better habits toward diet and exercise, which will be effective whether one takes lithium or not.

A number of agents may be utilized to combat weight gain when caused by any medication, including lithium. Agents with stimulating properties, such as phentermine (Adipex-P) or *d*-amphetamine (Dexedrine) are generally avoided in bipolar disorder because of concern about mood destabilization and/or abuse. However, these medications may be safely prescribed for some bipolar patients. Topiramate (Topamax) or zonisamide (Zonergran), two anticonvulsants with clearly demonstrated weight-loss properties may be prescribed without concern about destabilizing mood.[15] However, every medication is associated with at least some side effects. As an example, topiramate is frequently associated with sedation and/or cognitive side effects. Therefore, adjunctive weight-loss medications should be prescribed only when other therapeutic strategies have failed.

## Lithium Organ Toxicity: Thyroid and Kidneys

It has been known for decades that lithium has negative effects on thyroid and kidney function. Lithium's effect on thyroid function may result in a low thyroid state.[16] Before any symptoms emerge, blood tests may indicate an increase in TSH levels, indicating that the thyroid gland needs more than the usual stimulation by the pituitary to make sufficient amounts of circulating thyroid hormone. Later, the patient may exhibit typical overt hypothyroid symptoms such as fatigue, anergia, weight gain, poor concentration, depression, cold intolerance, and brittle hair. (All except the last two symptoms are also completely consistent with bipolar depression. Only the TSH measurement will help to distinguish between the two disorders.) Women are at higher risk for lithium-induced hypothyroidism, since they are more vulnerable to hypothyroidism from any cause.

When the TSH is clearly high (>10) and/or the patient has any symptoms consistent with a low thyroid state, it is appropriate to treat the hypothyroidism. Luckily, lithium-induced hypothyroidism is easily treated by L-thyroxine, prescribed by either the treating psychiatrist or a primary care physician. Lithium-induced hypothyroidism is *not* a reason to stop lithium treatment, if it has been effective. What is more controversial, and what different competent psychiatrists handle in different ways is whether thyroid treatment should be instituted if the TSH measurement is only slightly high (e.g., 4–10) and the patient has no symptoms consistent with hypothyroidism. Our position is that if a patient has a TSH in the range of 4–10 and complains of lethargy/lassitude or fatigue, a trial of L-thyroxine is warranted.

It has also been clear for many decades that lithium can have negative effects on renal (kidney) function.[17] Symptomatically, the most common manifestation of this is *polyuria* (frequent urination caused by a greater urine volume, not obstruction, as would be seen with enlarged prostates in older men) and thirst. Early in lithium treatment, these negative renal effects are functional and reversible, and reflect lithium's effect on the tubular system in the kidneys that regulates salt and water balance. With ongoing lithium use over years and decades, this effect becomes irreversible, with clear evidence of structural damage to the tubular system and then the glomerular system (primarily associated with the filtering function of the kidneys). If the filtering function of the kidneys is only minimally affected, the symptoms of increased urination and thirst are annoying but not dangerous (as long as the patient continues to stay well hydrated given the increased urine volume). In approximately 20+% of lithium-treated individuals, the serum creatinine, which is a measure of filtering function, starts to rise, a phenomenon colloquially described as "creeping creatinine," indicating damage to the glomeruli/filtering system of the kidney.[18] When the serum creatinine rises above a certain level (around 1.5 ng/ml), consultation with a nephrologist, lithium discontinuation, and switching to another mood stabilizer should all be seriously considered. If lithium is continued despite the rising creatinine, renal damage may in a small number of cases progress to renal failure and the need for renal dialysis or transplantation.[19]

Symptomatic treatment of lithium-induced polyuria by some diuretics is frequently helpful, with hydrochlorothiazide (Microzide) being most commonly prescribed for this purpose. There is some evidence that once-daily lithium dosing if started early in treatment (in contrast to dividing the daily dose into two or three doses) may be associated with less polyuria and fewer negative effects on the kidneys.[20]

## Lithium Toxicity

Finally, there is only a small difference between therapeutic and toxic doses of lithium. Therefore, lithium toxicity is always a concern in long-term lithium therapy. The causes of lithium toxicity are all related to changes in hydration or salt balance, since lithium is not metabolized at all by the liver but is excreted unchanged by the kidneys (which regulate salt and water balance). Common causes of lithium toxicity include change in diet (especially if salt intake is decreased), viral illness with dehydration, some anti-inflammatory drugs or diuretics, and less commonly, a change in renal function.[21] The early symptoms of lithium toxicity are ataxia (poor balance), diarrhea, and worsening hand tremor. When lithium toxicity is suspected, lithium treatment should be suspended until a lithium level can be drawn and the patient is medically evaluated.

Given the need to keep lithium levels within a narrow therapeutic range, as well as concerns about lithium's effects on kidneys and thyroid disease, lithium levels, TSH levels for monitoring thyroid function, and creatinine levels for monitoring renal function are mandatory components of lithium therapy. For stable patients, lithium levels may be measured every 4 months (or 6 months in very stable individuals). TSH and creatinine levels should be monitored every 6–12 months. More frequent measurements are required if either TSH or creatinine levels begin to rise.

## Lamotrigine

### Efficacy and Techniques of Administration

Lamotrigine (Lamictal) has become a very commonly prescribed maintenance treatment regimen in bipolar disorder, reflecting both its efficacy and relative lack of side effects. It received an FDA indication as a bipolar maintenance treatment in 2003, only the second medication to be so designated (lithium was the first). Given its greater efficacy in preventing depressions than manias/hypomanias, lamotrigine should be more strongly considered in depression-dominant bipolar patients. These patients experience depressions that are more frequent, longer lasting, more intense and, in general, more problematic compared to the manias. Most bipolar II patients are depression-predominant since, by definition, the hypomanias are not that intense. (If they were, the proper diagnosis would be bipolar I disorder.) Depression may also be the dominant feature of bipolar I disorder. Thus, even with bipolar I patients, lamotrigine should still be considered as a potential first-line therapy. Patients for whom lamotrigine would typically be considered either second-line or prescribed in conjunction with another mood stabilizer would be mania-dominant bipolar I patients: those who have had multiple destructive manic episodes with more infrequent and/or milder depressions.

In the head-to-head studies comparing lamotrigine to lithium, two of which included a placebo treatment, the two medications were equivalently effective in preventing mood episodes overall.[22] Lamotrigine was somewhat better at preventing depressions, while lithium was superior in preventing manias. In another study, lamotrigine was better than placebo in preventing episodes in bipolar II rapid-cycling patients, but not in bipolar I patients.[23]

As noted earlier, lamotrigine treatment must be started very slowly in order to avoid a severe rash (see Chapter 5, pages 102–103, for details). The typical initial dose schedule is 25 mg weekly for 2 weeks, then 50 mg weekly for 2 weeks, then 100 mg in week 5 and 200 mg daily starting in week 6. Most patients show optimal response to lamotrigine as a maintenance treatment in the 100–200 mg range. Doses may be increased to 400 mg daily if needed and, occasionally higher. Lamotrigine may be prescribed on a once-daily regimen, typically in the morning.

### Side Effects and Their Management

Aside from the severe rash that occurs in one in thousands of treated patients (described in detail in Chapter 5), lamotrigine has a rather benign side-effect profile and is associated with neither sedation nor weight gain. It can cause a more typical, nondangerous drug rash (unrelated to severe rash, referred to as Stevens–Johnson syndrome) in 5–9% of patients, and occasionally, nausea, insomnia, or headache. No laboratory monitoring is necessary during long term lamotrigine therapy. Lamotrigine blood levels can be measured but, since it is not known whether these levels correlate with efficacy in bipolar disorder, they are not a standard part of long-term treatment.

### Valproate

### Efficacy and Techniques of Administration

Valproate has been a mainstay as a maintenance treatment of bipolar disorder for close to 20 years. Unlike lithium and many of the other medications reviewed below, it does not now nor will it ever have an FDA indication for this purpose. This lack of an FDA indication as a maintenance treatment (it does have the indication for acute mania) reflects the failure of the one large-scale controlled study to demonstrate efficacy for this purpose.[24] Almost assuredly, the failure of valproate (in the form of divalproex) to prevent mood episodes better than placebo was due to certain methodological features of the study that made it less likely that any medication would have been effective. In fact, lithium, used in the study as a comparison medication, was also not more effective than placebo, in contrast to its positive effects in most other studies. Nonetheless, as demonstrated by its recommendations in most treatment guidelines, most psychiatrists (M. J. G. included) consider valproate to be an effective mood stabilizer and prescribe it regularly for this purpose.

Predictors of a good response to maintenance valproate are not well established. But since many patients who are unresponsive to lithium respond to preventative valproate (and vice versa), valproate should routinely be considered for those patients who have failed to respond to another mood stabilizer.

The results of the two head-to-head studies comparing valproate to lithium as maintenance treatments in bipolar disorder showed discrepant results (which is surprisingly common in psychiatric treatment studies). In the first study (Bowden et al.[24]), neither agent was more effective than placebo, but valproate was slightly more effective than lithium in preventing depressive episodes. In the second study, the BALANCE study, lithium was superior to valproate on a number of (but not all) measures, including prevention of depression.[25]

Similar to its use in acute mania, prior to starting valproate maintenance treatment, blood for a standard set of laboratory tests, such as a chemistry panel and CBC, should be drawn. When prescribed as a maintenance treatment, valproate is started far more slowly than when it is prescribed for acute mania. Usual starting doses of valproate when used as a maintenance treatment are 250–500 mg, with increases of 250 mg every few days as tolerated. An average dose of valproate is 1,500 mg daily, with a range of 750–3,000 mg. Valproate may be given once daily, typically at night, since sedation is a common side effect. Dividing the dose should be considered if there is significant nausea, or if daytime sedation is used for calming purposes. All available forms of valproate (see Table 6.1) are equally effective.

Valproate has significant drug–drug (pharmacokinetic) interactions with other medications by inhibiting their metabolism, thereby increasing their levels. The most important of these interactions are with lamotrigine and carbamazepine (Tegretol), both of which are also used to treat bipolar disorder. Valproate doubles lamotrigine blood levels; therefore, if lamotrigine is added to valproate, the usual dose increases should be half the usual rate. Therefore, the usual lamotrigine target dose of 200 mg should be 100 mg when valproate is also prescribed. Similarly, valproate increases carbamazepine levels, requiring a slower dose titration. Conversely, carbamazepine decreases valproate levels, often requiring an upward dose adjustment of the latter.

## Side Effects and Their Management

In the beginning of treatment, the most common side effects seen with valproate are nausea, vomiting, diarrhea, sedation, and tremor.[26] Nausea may be less with the more extended release forms of valproate. Thus, Depakote ER is associated with less nausea than is Depakote, which is associated with less nausea than Depakene (valproic acid). Nighttime dosing of valproate helps to diminish the sedation. Valproate-induced tremor may be treated in the same manner as lithium tremor—with a beta blocker such as propranolol, but possibly with less consistent positive results.

The most important side effects associated with long-term maintenance treatment are weight gain, alopecia (diffuse hair loss) and polycystic ovarian syndrome. Weight gain is somewhat more common with valproate than with lithium but less problematic compared to olanzapine. Strategies for combating weight gain from valproate are identical to those described earlier for lithium-induced weight gain. Alopecia is, not surprisingly, more problematic and distressing (although not more common) for women patients treated with valproate. Anecdotally, selenium and zinc supplements are reported to counteract valproate-induced hair loss, although one of us (M. J. G.) has never seen it work. If valproate is discontinued, hair gradually resumes its normal thickness over months, not weeks.

Polycystic ovarian (PCO) disease is caused more often by valproate (in the range of 6–10% of treated women) than by other anticonvulsant mood stabilizers or lithium.[27] Symptoms of PCO disease include irregular menses, hirsuitism (abnormal facial or body hair), and acne. Because of this concern and the relationship of PCO disease to decreased fertility, many psychiatrists are wary of prescribing valproate to young women of childbearing age.

Infrequently, valproate may cause pancreatitis and even, more rarely, hepatitis. When valproate is prescribed in combination with other anticonvulsants, the rate of hepatitis increases from rare to infrequent. Additionally, a mild increase in liver enzymes can be seen. Generally, as long as the liver enzymes are less than 2.5 to 3 times the upper limit of normal, valproate therapy can be continued.

Finally, valproate confers a significant risk of fetal malformations when the fetus is exposed to the medication during the first trimester. This is discussed in more detail in Chapter 9.

## Laboratory Monitoring during Valproate Treatment

Valproate blood levels are frequently monitored. Unfortunately, in contrast to lithium levels, no studies have shown a relationship between valproate levels and preventative efficacy in bipolar disorder. Most clinicians target valproate levels of 50–100 µg/ml during maintenance treatment, borrowing this range from valproate studies in epilepsy. Other laboratory monitoring during valproate treatment should include occasional blood counts (since a low platelet count—thrombocytopenia—can be seen with valproate), and measurement of liver enzymes every 6–12 months.

## Second-Generation Antipsychotics

Possibly the most remarkable evolution in the maintenance pharmacological treatment of bipolar disorder has been the emergence of antipsychotics as important options. As discussed in more detail in Chapter 4, antipsychotics—both the older agents and the more recently released ones—have been mainstays of treatment of acute mania for many decades. From the 1960s through the 1990s, anecdotal experience and a few small studies gave clinicians no reason to believe that antipsychotics (during that time, the first-generation agents, e.g., haloperidol [Haldol]) should play any central role in the maintenance treatment of bipolar disorder. They did not seem to prevent mania very well, they did not prevent depression at all (and may have even made depression more likely) and, with long-term treatment, they conferred the risk of tardive dyskinesia, a potentially irreversible movement disorder (discussed in detail below). However, studies of the SGAs over the last decade have demonstrated that these newer medications do indeed have a place in long-term treatment of bipolar disorder. Five of these medications (see Table 6.3) have FDA approval as maintenance treatments in bipolar disorder. Overall, they consistently prevent mania. With the exception of quetiapine (Seroquel), however, prevention of depression with SGAs is less clear. Yet, appropriately, side-effect considerations—primarily weight gain and its attendant health risks, sedation, and tardive dyskinesia—continue to concern both clinicians and patients, and have prevented the SGAs from being prescribed more frequently despite clear evidence of their efficacy.

Evidence for the efficacy of SGAs as mood stabilizers derives from two types of studies, both of which utilize the usual double-blind design. The classic studies are drug versus placebo, in which patients, typically stabilized after an acute episode, are treated with either the SGA or placebo for between 6 months and 2 years, and relapse rates in the two treatments are compared. Partly due to the ethical concerns of having patients on maintenance placebo for long time periods, the second type of study is described as an *adjunctive design*. In these studies, all patients take lithium or valproate prescribed openly (i.e., not blinded), and either the SGA or placebo is prescribed in a blinded manner, combined with the openly prescribed medication for the 6-month to 2-year time period. Thus, these studies evaluate the *additive* efficacy of the SGA. The distinction between these two types of studies is relevant, since the FDA approves some SGAs specifically for adjunctive use, others for solo agent treatment, and still others for both. Table 6.3 lists these FDA indications.

Among the most important concerns surrounding the SGAs are their side-effect profiles and health risks. The individual SGAs differ sufficiently from each other to warrant separate discussions below on side effects. However, the one important side effect that is common to all agents of this class is the liability for causing tardive dyskinesia (TD). The most common forms of TD are (1) facial movements such as tongue thrusting, chewing movements, lip smacking, or tongue writhing, and (2) movements of the fingers (and, less commonly, the toes) that are "snake-like," described as *choreoathetoid* (which, technically, means "dancing without position or place"). Of course, both types of movements may be seen in one individual. The greatest concern about TD is its potential irreversibility. With virtually any other side effect, if the medication is discontinued, the side effect dissipates. The potential irreversibility of TD, however, changes the risk–benefit ratio. TD is, by definition, tardive (or late); these movements are seen after months or, more typically, years of antipsychotic exposure. The longer the length of exposure to the antipsychotic, the higher the risk of TD.

**TABLE 6.3. Second-Generation Antipsychotics as Maintenance Treatments for Bipolar Disorder**

| Medication[a] | Solo agent | Adjunctive agent | Efficacy for preventing mania | Efficacy for preventing depression |
|---|---|---|---|---|
| olanzapine (Zyprexa) | X | | Yes | Yes, but less than for depression |
| aripiprazole (Abilify) | X | X | Yes | No |
| quetiapine (Seroquel) | | X | Yes | Yes |
| ziprasidone (Geodon) | | X | Yes | No |
| risperidone long-acting injection (Risperdal Consta) | X | X | Yes | No |

[a]Trade names are in parentheses.

One of the few indisputable advantages of the SGAs compared to the first-generation agents is that they are associated with lower rates of TD. With the exception of clozapine (Clozaril), used only in treatment-resistant patients (see below), rates of TD are approximately equal among SGAs. The best estimate is that the SGAs cause TD at approximately one-seventh the frequency of that seen with the first-generation agents, which translates to a rate of 0.8% after 1 year.[28] This is a dramatic improvement, but the TD rate with the SGAs is *not* zero. Therefore, any consideration of using an antipsychotic as a maintenance treatment of bipolar disorder must include the risks of TD.

### Olanzapine: Efficacy and Side Effects

Olanzapine was the first SGA to show efficacy as a maintenance treatment in bipolar disorder.[29] Its efficacy is greater at preventing manias than depressions; therefore, it is more strongly considered in mania-prone bipolar individuals. Olanzapine is usually started at 5 mg, with typical daily doses of 10–15 mg. In one controlled study, olanzapine was more effective than lithium in preventing manias.[30]

Olanzapine's major drawback is its side-effect profile. Although sedation is the dominant early side effect of olanzapine, the most important long-term side effects associated with its use are weight gain, new-onset diabetes mellitus, and metabolic syndrome, a complex of signs and symptoms, including increased cholesterol, increased triglycerides, increased blood sugar, and truncal obesity (in which fat is deposited selectively at the waist), that together increase the risk for cardiovascular disease.[31] With the possible exception of clozapine (which is only used for patients with very treatment-resistant bipolar disorder), olanzapine causes the most weight gain of all the antipsychotics and confers the greatest risk for these health-related negative outcomes.

### Aripiprazole (Abilify): Efficacy and Side Effects

Aripiprazole has received FDA indications as both a solo-agent maintenance treatment and an adjunctive medication.[32,33] According to published studies, its efficacy is in preventing manias, not depressions. Many clinicians (including us) believe that aripiprazole also prevents depression (despite the lack of data supporting this idea). The usual starting dose of aripiprazole is 5 mg. Doses used in controlled studies are 15–30 mg daily; because of the design of these studies, higher doses were more likely to be used. Here too, many expert clinicians believe that aripiprazole doses between 10 and 20 mg are often sufficient for maintenance treatment.

Paradoxically, aripiprazole is associated with either sedation *or* activation (manifested as insomnia, general feelings of being wired, or akathisia, characterized by physical restlessness). When the restlessness is prominent and does not diminish with time (as commonly happens), it can be treated by benzodiazepines (e.g., lorazepam [Ativan] or clonazepam [Klonopin]) and/or beta blockers such as propranolol. Weight gain is seen in only a small subset of aripiprazole-treated patients, but it can be problematic for this small group. It is not associated with increased risk of new-onset diabetes or metabolic syndrome.

### Quetiapine: Efficacy and Side Effects

Alone among the SGAs, quetiapine shows equal efficacy in preventing manias and depressions. It has demonstrated effectiveness as both a solo-agent treatment and as adjunctive therapy, although its FDA approval is only for adjunctive therapy.[34–36] Usual starting doses are 25–50 mg, with daily doses in the maintenance studies in the range of 400–800 mg, although many clinicians believe that efficacy also may be seen in the 200- to 400-mg range. Quetiapine was as effective as lithium in one controlled study.

Quetiapine's side-effect profile as a maintenance treatment stands midway between olanzapine and aripiprazole in its propensity to cause weight gain and sedation (somewhat less than the former and significantly more than the latter).[37] It can increase blood glucose and blood lipids (e.g., cholesterol), but less than is seen with olanzapine.

### Ziprasidone: Efficacy and Side Effects

Ziprasidone (Geodon) decreases manic relapses (but not depressive relapses) when prescribed as an adjunctive agent.[38] Usual maintenance daily doses are in the 80- to 160-mg range. Unlike other mood stabilizing medications, ziprasidone should be taken with food to increase absorption.

Like aripiprazole, ziprasidone can be either sedating or activating; insomnia, restlessness, and sedation are the most common side effects. It is seemingly weight-neutral. Consistent with this, ziprasidone is not associated with increases in cholesterol, triglycerides, or other metabolic syndrome parameters. Earlier concerns regarding ziprasidone's effect on cardiac conduction (specifically, the QTc interval) have appropriately diminished and should no longer be considered a major concern.[39]

## Risperidone Long-Acting Injection (Risperdal Consta): Efficacy and Side Effects

Risperidone long-acting injection (RLAI), marketed as Risperdal Consta, is a version of risperidone (Risperdal), given as an intramuscular 25- to 50-mg shot every 2 weeks. The advantage of a long-acting, injectable mood stabilizer is obvious: Patients do not need to struggle with treatment adherence on a daily basis. The disadvantage is equally obvious: Patients struggle with needing to go to the doctor's office to get a shot every 2 weeks. Because of the latter considerations, RLAI is infrequently prescribed as a mood stabilizer. Ironically, given the paucity of its use in the community for bipolar disorder, RLAI has FDA indications as both a solo-agent therapy and an adjunctive maintenance treatment for bipolar disorder in the prevention of mania but not depression.[40,41] It is reasonable to presume that the efficacy of oral risperidone is similar or even identical to that of RLAI. Of course, oral risperidone has neither the advantages nor disadvantages of being administered as an injection every 2 weeks.

Not surprisingly, side effects of RLAI are the same as those seen with oral risperidone. Its propensity for causing sedation, hyperglycemia, and weight gain is moderate: less than with olanzapine and quetiapine, but more than with aripiprazole and ziprasidone. RLAI causes more classic extrapyramidal side effects, such as akinesia (motor slowing) stiffness, muscle rigidity, tremor, and akathisia (motor restlessness), than all other SGAs. These side effects can be effectively treated by a class of medications called anticholinergics, such as benztropine (Cogentin) or trihexyphenidyl (Artane). RLAI (and risperidone) can also increase prolactin levels, which manifests as galactorrhea (inappropriate breast milk production) and menstrual irregularities in women, and erectile dysfunction in men.

### Carbamazepine/Oxcarbazepine

#### Efficacy and Techniques of Administration

Although carbamazepine was the first anticonvulsant evaluated as a treatment for bipolar disorder, it is rarely prescribed now as a first-line maintenance treatment. Asssuredly, this reflects a number of factors, including (1) the relative lack of studies demonstrating its efficacy, (2) its side effect profile, and (3) its prominent drug–drug interactions, which makes combining carbamazepine with other medications rather difficult (see below).

Most maintenance treatment studies on carbamazepine have compared its efficacy to lithium, not placebo, thereby precluding clear conclusions as to its ability to prevent mood episodes.[42,43] Overall, the studies comparing lithium and carbamazepine found that lithium was somewhat more effective than carbamazepine as a maintenance treatment. However, in contrast to lithium, for which atypical bipolar features predicted a *poorer* response, carbamazepine seemed to be effective in these very patients.[42,44] Thus, carbamazepine should be considered as a maintenance treatment for those patients with mixed states, rapid cycling, incomplete remission, and so forth.

Carbamazepine treatment is typically started at 100–200 mg daily, with dose increases of 200 mg daily every 4–7 days. An average dose of carbamazepine is 900 mg, with the usual range extending from 400 to 1,200 mg daily (but occasionally higher). Initially, carbamazepine is prescribed twice daily in order to minimize side effects associated with ingesting a large dose at once.

Oxcarbazepine (Trileptal), an analogue of carbamazepine, is very similar in chemical structure and shares a number of properties but is sufficiently different to be evaluated separately. Many psychiatrists think of prescribing oxcarbazepine as a mood stabilizer, since it has fewer side effects than carbamazepine (see below). Unfortunately, as modest as the evidence is for the efficacy of carbamazepine as a mood stabilizer, oxcarbazepine's database is even weaker. In the only small, controlled study that has evaluated its efficacy as a bipolar maintenance treatment, oxcarbazepine was weakly helpful in preventing mood episodes when added to lithium.[45] Thus, when it is prescribed for bipolar disorder, it is on the hope and assumption that it will be as effective as carbamazepine, which may or may not be true.

Oxcarbazepine should be started at 300 mg daily, typically in divided dose, with dose increases of 300 mg every 4–7 days. An average dose is 1,200 mg, with the range of 600 to 2,100 mg daily.

## Side Effects and Their Management

Long-term side effects with carbamazepine are similar to those seen when the drug is used acutely, described in Chapter 4. Neurological side effects predominate—dizziness, ataxia (poor balance), a general feeling of being unwell, diplopia (double vision), and blurred vision, along with fatigue and nausea. Hyponatremia (low sodium), which is more common in older adults, a mild increase in liver enzymes, or thrombocytopenia (low platelet count) may also be seen. Of note, carbamazepine is associated with less weight gain than many other mood stabilizers and is sometimes recommended as a mood stabilizer because of this. As with its use in acute mania, another concern with carbamazepine is its capacity to cause the very rare but potentially life-threatening side effect of agranulocytosis, in which the bone marrow stops making blood cells.

A very important complication that makes carbamazepine a difficult maintenance medication in bipolar disorder is its ability to lower the blood levels of many other medications by increasing their hepatic (liver) metabolism (including oral contraceptives, potentially making the latter ineffective if the dose is not adjusted). Since most patients with bipolar disorder are taking multiple medications, this makes monitoring of doses far more difficult.[46,47] Like valproate, carbamazepine is associated with relatively high rates of fetal malformations when used in the first trimester of pregnancy (see Chapter 9).

Oxcarbazapine shares the same general side-effect profile as carbamazepine but in much milder form.[48] Additionally, agranulocytosis seems not to occur with oxcarbazepine. Drug–drug interactions appear to be less common; however, oral contraceptives may be less effective when combined with oxcarbazepine. The only side effect that is seen more commonly with oxcarbazepine than with carbamazepine is hyponatremia (low sodium).

## Laboratory Monitoring with Carbamazepine/Oxcarbazepine

Monitoring of the blood count, especially in the first year of carbamazepine treatment, is typical, although given the rarity of agranulocytosis, it is unlikely that these blood counts are either helpful or cost-effective. The optimal frequency of these measurements is unclear. Some treatment guidelines recommend measurements every other week during the first 2 months, followed by once-monthly then monitoring every 3 months. Others recommend less frequent monitoring, such as two or three measurements in the first few months and less frequently thereafter. Regardless of how frequently blood counts are monitored, it is prudent to tell patients that a blood count should be obtained immediately, especially within the first year of treatment with carbamazepine, if they have any sort of infection and/or fever (since these would be a potential clinical sign of agranulocytosis). Other blood tests to monitor during long-term carbamazepine treatment include occasional measurement of platelet count (which would typically be included in a blood count), liver enzymes, and serum sodium.

Carbamazepine levels can be obtained, but there is no evidence that these levels correlate with clinical outcome. Thus, the typically quoted range of carbamazepine levels of 4–12 µg/ml should be considered a very crude estimate of *usual* levels, not therapeutic levels. Routine blood monitoring with oxcarbazepine is not needed, since it is not associated with agranulocytosis.

### Antidepressants as Part of Maintenance Treatment Regimens

As discussed in Chapter 5, there is great controversy as to the proper place of antidepressants in treating bipolar depression. Just as controversial is whether (or how frequently) bipolar patients should be treated with antidepressants as part of a maintenance treatment regimen. The concerns described in Chapter 5 about antidepressants—precipitating switches into mania/hypomania, inducing a period of greater mood instability—are, if anything, of greater concern in maintenance treatment because of longer-term exposure to these medications. Yet clinicians frequently prescribe antidepressants as part of maintenance treatment in bipolar disorder—and patients just as frequently are reluctant to stop their antidepressant for fear of relapsing into depression.

Systematic studies in this area, of course, show conflicting results. Some studies seem to demonstrate that the use of long-term antidepressants confers a greater risk of switching into mania and shows only a small benefit in preventing depressions. However, a number of these studies—those published prior to the 1990s—evaluated the efficacy of tricyclic antidepressants, which are known to have the highest rate of pharmacological switches into mania and are rarely used today. Additionally, other studies compared the efficacy and switch rates of antidepressants when used as solo-agent treatments in bipolar I patients and not as part of a treatment regimen with a mood stabilizer. The results of both types of studies are not necessarily relevant to the question of whether modern antidepressants—SSRIs, bupropion (Wellbutrin), and so forth—can be safely prescribed as maintenance treatments, typically in addition to mood stabilizers.

Over the last decade, a number of studies have shown that for a subset of patients with bipolar disorder, antidepressants may play a vital role as part of a maintenance treatment regimen. In these studies, patients who had responded to antidepressants (in combination with mood stabilizers) during acute or continuation treatment were maintained on antidepressants over the long term.[49,50] These patients had fewer depressive relapses compared to those whose antidepressants were discontinued, with no increase in manic relapses. In one study, there were *fewer* manic relapses in those who continued antidepressants.[50] This seemingly paradoxical result can potentially be explained by the overarching positive effect of mood stability (and, conversely, the negative effect of mood instability) on the likelihood of staying well. Those patients who relapse into depression may be at higher risk for any mood episode, including mania.

There are no data to guide the choice of a specific antidepressant when prescribed as part of maintenance treatment regimen. Given that SSRIs and bupropion are generally associated with the lowest switch rates in acute treatment studies, it is reasonable to assume that they are safest in maintenance treatment, too.

Of course, these studies should not be interpreted as meaning that any and all bipolar patients can be treated with long-term antidepressants without risk. Rather, they suggest that a subset of patients will do best on the combination of mood stabilizers plus antidepressants. Patients for whom antidepressants may most likely be associated with mood instability are those with rapid-cycling bipolar disorder.

---

Now 31 years old, Bertha has had bipolar I disorder since she was a teenager. She has had two full-blown manic episodes, the first at age 19, when she was hospitalized, and a milder manic episode at age 25, when she was treated as an outpatient. However, she has struggled with low-grade depressive symptoms most of the time and has had four major depressive episodes. After much early ambivalence about taking medications preventatively, over the last 5 years, Bertha has been impressively adherent to treatment. Treated with an ongoing regimen of lithium plus lamotrigine, she has had no manias but has continued to struggle with depressive symptoms. Therefore, after an extensive discussion of the potential risks of antidepressants, bupropion, increasing to 300 mg daily, was added to her medication regimen with excellent antidepressant efficacy. Bupropion was continued for 4 months, after which an attempt was made to discontinue it. Bertha quickly became more depressed. After a second attempt to discontinue bupropion again resulted in greater depression, Bertha and her psychiatrist decided that she should continue on lithium plus lamotrigine plus bupropion. Over the next 3 years, Bertha had no manic episodes and her depressive symptoms were markedly diminished. Like many patients, Bertha's optimal treatment regimen appeared to include an antidepressant as adjunct to mood stabilizers.

---

Just as some bipolar II patients can be treated in acute phases of depression with antidepressant monotherapy (without a mood stabilizer), a subset of bipolar II patients may be safely and effectively treated with a maintenance regimen of antidepressants alone. In one study, bipolar II depressed patients who responded acutely to fluoxetine (Prozac) showed the fewest depressive relapses over 1 year compared to those switched to either placebo or lithium, with no increase in hypomanic relapses (but with a slight increase in more subtle measures of mood instability).[51] This practice should be considered controversial for now and is appropriately considered only for highly selected patients.

## MEDICATION COMBINATIONS AS MAINTENANCE TREATMENTS IN BIPOLAR DISORDER

As noted, mood stabilizer combinations are the rule rather than the exception in the maintenance treatment of bipolar disorder. Many naturalistic studies have demonstrated the frequency of multiple medication treatment in the maintenance phase of bipolar disorder. As one of many examples, a recent multicenter study found that the *average* bipolar patient was taking three medications.[52] Another study found that almost 20% of bipolar patients were taking four *or more* medications at baseline.[53] To be sure, not all of these medications are mood stabilizers; some may be sleeping pills or tranquilizers or antidepressants. Of course, this reflects the less than optimal results with solo-agent treatment.

The individual medications reviewed earlier are unquestionably more effective than placebo in preventing mood episodes, but the relapse rate on medication is still unacceptably high. Using the first maintenance treatment study of an antipsychotic as an example, mood episode relapse rates for patients with bipolar disorder over 1 year on placebo was 80 versus 47% for those on olanzapine.[29] This difference is both statistically and clinically significant, but almost half of the patients on olanzapine still relapsed within 1 year. Patients and mental health professionals alike would consider a 1-year relapse rate of 50% unacceptably high.

As noted earlier, four SGAs have received FDA indications as adjunctive therapies, in which the SGA plus lithium or valproate was more effective in preventing mood episodes than lithium or valproate alone, demonstrating that combination treatment may be more effective than monotherapy for many patients. Additionally, the BALANCE study showed that lithium plus valproate was generally more effective than either medication alone in preventing bipolar mood episodes over 2 years.[9]

Thus, when a bipolar patient has breakthrough episodes to a solo-agent maintenance therapy, adding a second medication (vs. switching to a different medication) is a typical therapeutic approach. This allows the prescriber to preserve the partial response of the first medication, while seeking to prevent future episodes more effectively. Switching from one mood stabilizer to another, especially in the circumstance of a partial response, confers the risk of losing the partial response of the first treatment. However, when multiple medications are prescribed, care must be taken to repeatedly evaluate the efficacy of each treatment. It is too easy to add a second, then a third or a fourth medication, hoping that the latest addition will augment the prior treatments, all the while missing the fact that the patient is no better with four (or five or six) treatments than with one.

On the surface, it sounds as if a medication regimen of four (or more) treatments is the mark of an unobservant and sloppy psychiatrist. However, when a patient has recurrent episodes, psychiatrist and patient alike will try desperately to prevent these destructive relapses. Physicians treating younger patients sometimes add agents in response to multiple requests from patients' family members to augment the regimen. The key is to be conscious of the burden of multiple medications and to review medication regimens on a regular basis to ensure that patients are being prescribed only those agents that have shown some benefit.

---

Samantha, age 26, has had bipolar II disorder for 8 years. Although initially she stopped her mood stabilizers when she was feeling well, over the last 3 years she had taken her prescribed medications regularly. Unfortunately, despite her treatment adherence, she continued to have mood episodes. She spent almost half her time in one mood episode or another, mostly depressions with occasional hypomanias. Lamotrigine seemed to help diminish the intensity of her depressions, but it did little to prevent depressive episodes and did not change the frequency or intensity of her hypomanias. The effect of lithium added to lamotrigine was less clear. Samantha's hypomanias seemed less frequent, but this was a weak effect at best. In discussing the next step, Samantha was reluctant to stop either the lamotrigine or the lithium, afraid that her mood episodes would worsen, despite the weak evidence of their efficacy. Therefore, valproate was added to the lamotrigine/lithium regimen (necessitating a dosage change of her lamotrigine), with the plan to use all three medications as a maintenance treatment in an effort to prevent future mood episodes, especially depression. Although she continues to cycle, she now spends less than 20% of her time in a mood episode, which is a significant improvement.

---

One last general consideration about combination treatment concerns rapid-cycling bipolar disorder. As discussed in Chapter 2, rapid cycling may be a difficult phase of the disorder that may simply resolve over time or it may represent a longer-term pattern of mood episodes for an individual. Most important to remember in treating this subgroup is that maintenance preventative treatments simply work less well than they do for patients without rapid cycling. Initially, it was thought that rapid-cycling patients responded poorly to lithium alone. However, at this point, it is clear that the poor response to maintenance treatment is probably generalizable to all mood stabilizers. Inevitably, patients who are rapid cyclers are treated with multiple mood stabilizers; a regimen of two, three, or four mood stabilizers prescribed simultaneously is not unusual. There is some evidence (albeit small) that combination treatment is more effective than monotherapy in rapid cyclers.[54] In most cases, polypharmacy with rapid-cycling patients is based more on the clinician's wish to help rather than what the research (albeit limited) recommends.

## MAINTENANCE APPROACHES TO TREATMENT-RESISTANT BIPOLAR DISORDER

When a patient has continued mood cycling despite reasonable preventative treatments, a number of other, less commonly prescribed treatments are considered. Although no formal consensus definition of *treatment resistance* is available, a reasonable working definition would be "repeated mood episodes despite ongoing maintenance treatment." The question of how many breakthrough episodes and how many different maintenance treatments should be prescribed before the term *treatment resistant* is used is left vague in this definition. Certainly, a pattern of two or more mood episodes per year is unacceptable. (Implied in this definition is that a patient in treatment with rapid-cycling bipolar disorder should in most cases be considered treatment resistant—if she is adherent to her medication regimen.) Equally, at least two different mood stabilizers and at least one combination treatment should be considered standard treatment. Beyond these crude guidelines, the definition depends on the nuances of each patient's clinical course. Before considering these less commonly used treatments, however, four basic questions, listed in Table 6.4, should be addressed.

The first issue is treatment adherence. It is foolish to switch medication regimens when a patient is not taking medications or is taking an inappropriate dose. The exception to this, of course, is when nonadherence is due to unacceptable side effects. In this situation, switching to another treatment may be appropriate. Chapter 8 provides an in-depth review of adherence issues and strategies to enhance adherence.

Second, as in evaluating breakthrough episodes, the possibility that substance abuse may be interfering with the efficacy of maintenance treatment should always be considered. Substance abuse can not only interfere directly with medication efficacy but it can also create cognitive difficulties that undermine treatment adherence and increase the likelihood of emerging mood episodes.

Third, psychiatrists should also take stock of patients' life stresses and their coping strategies. Stressful life events often precede mood episodes. Identifying episodic or chronic stressors in a patient's life allows a focus on coping strategies—cognitive, interpersonal, and/or environmental—for dealing with these stressors.

Fourth, if the patient is taking an antidepressant, presumably due to multiple depressive episodes, consideration should be given to discontinuing it. As we discussed earlier in this chapter, although a subset of bipolar patients may be optimally treated with a combination of mood stabilizers and antidepressants, another subset of unknown size may show mood instability or increased cycling when treated with antidepressants, especially if these are being taken without a mood stabilizer or SGA. Therefore, any patient with continued cycling on antidepressants should have that part of their treatment reevaluated. Optimally, one would systematically compare the cycling pattern in the period before the antidepressant was started to the cycling pattern after the antidepressant was started. Frequently, however, prior history information is less than precise and other variables (life stresses, etc.) interfere with making a definitive statement regarding the relationship between antidepressant use and cycling patterns. In these situations,

**TABLE 6.4. Maintenance Strategies for Treatment Resistant Bipolar Disorder**

Overall considerations

- Evaluation of treatment adherence
- Reconsider potential substance abuse
- Reevaluation of life stresses
- Reconsideration of antidepressants if currently prescribed

Treatment choices

- More aggressive mood stabilizer combinations
- Clozapine
- High-dose T4 (thyroid hormone)
- Calcium channel blockers
- Omega-3 fatty acids
- ECT

psychiatrist and patient must have an open discussion regarding the risks and benefits of antidepressant discontinuation.

Assuming that these four areas have been evaluated and do not appear to explain the failure of maintenance treatment to prevent mood episodes, other treatment options should be considered. As described earlier, the usual first step for continued cycling is a more aggressive combination of mood stabilizers. Different combinations of two medications—usually lithium plus an anticonvulsant mood stabilizer (lamotrigine, valproate, carbamazepine or oxcarbazepine) or an antipsychotic—make more sense than combining two antipsychotics. Two anticonvulsants, however, may make sense, since they have such different biological effects. Three or more mood stabilizers, such as lithium, an anticonvulsant, and an antipsychotic, are also commonly considered in treatment-resistant cases.

Clozapine, the most effective—and the most dangerous—antipsychotic available is an appropriate consideration for very treatment-resistant patients. Multiple case series and one controlled study demonstrate that, as with treatment-resistant schizophrenia, clozapine can be effective when other treatments have failed.[55,56] Clozapine is usually added to an ongoing mood stabilizer regimen, but it may also be used as a solo agent. Usual daily doses of clozapine are 300–600 mg, with occasional patients needing up to 900 mg, using a slow dose titration beginning with 25 mg. Clozapine blood levels in schizophrenia correlate with better outcome when the level is more than 350 ng/ml.[57] No studies of this kind for bipolar disorder are available, but clozapine levels are easily obtained, and most psychopharmacologists use the schizophrenia guidelines.

Unfortunately, clozapine treatment presents two enormous difficulties. First, clozapine is a dangerous drug, with a small percentage of treated patients suffering agranulocytosis (the same potential side effect seen more rarely with carbamazepine, discussed above). Without white blood cells, patients become vulnerable to overwhelming infections. Because of this complication, regular blood tests to monitor white blood cell counts are a mandatory part of clozapine treatment. In the United States, the requirement is for weekly blood tests for 6 months, every other week for another 6 months, then, assuming the white blood cell counts have been within normal limits, once monthly for the duration of clozapine therapy. Because these blood tests are mandatory, there are no involuntary clozapine-treated patients. If a patient refuses the blood test, the clozapine is immediately discontinued.

Clozapine-induced agranulocytosis is generally estimated to occur in just under 1% of treated patients. Almost 80% of agranulocytosis cases occur in the first 5 months of clozapine treatment, justifying the more frequent blood monitoring during this time period.[58] However, a number of cases have been reported even after years of treatment. With proper monitoring (and with discontinuing the medication if the white count drops below a certain threshold), the fatality rate from clozapine-induced agranulocytosis is 3%.

The second set of difficulties with clozapine reflects its general side-effect profile. Similar to olanzapine, clozapine causes sedation, substantial weight gain, risk of new-onset diabetes, and increased risk for metabolic syndrome (high cholesterol and triglycerides, etc.) described earlier. It can also cause drooling (primarily at night), seizures at high dose, and rare cases of myocarditis (inflammation of the heart muscle).[59] Given this side-effect profile, clozapine represents a distinctly high-risk/high-gain strategy to be considered only in clearly treatment-resistant patients who will be adherent to the mandatory blood monitoring. Nonetheless, virtually all psychiatrists with experience in treatment-resistant bipolar disorder (including M. J. G.) have treated patients for whom clozapine was lifesaving.

Typically, adding high-dose T4 (a thyroid hormone, usually prescribed as L-thyroxine [Synthroid, as a proprietary brand]) to a mood stabilizer regimen has been shown to diminish mood cycling in a few very small studies.[60,61] The concern with high-dose T4 is that the doses used are three to four times the usual dose of L-thyroxine prescribed to treat hypothyroidism. At these high doses (300–500 µg daily, in contrast to the usual thyroid replacement daily dose of 100–125 µg), there is the infrequent risk of atrial fibrillation and the long-term risk of osteoporosis (since high levels of thyroid hormone leach calcium from bones, thereby making them softer). Thus, high-dose T4 should only be considered in relatively young, healthy patients who understand the potential risks.

Calcium channel blockers (CCBs), a class of medications used for hypertension, migraine headaches, and other medical disorders, have been effective as maintenance treatments in a few small studies.[62] In the few studies published, the most commonly used medications of this class were verapamil (Calan) and nimodipine (Nimotop). Given the relative weakness of the evidence in support of the efficacy of these medications in bipolar disorder, CCBs are usually only added to the regimen when classic mood stabilizers and SGAs have not proven adequate in prophylaxis.

Omega-3 fatty acids, a class of compounds available without a prescription, are occasionally used as (primarily) adjunctive maintenance treatments in bipolar disorder. However, so far, no controlled studies have demonstrated the efficacy of omega-3 fatty acids as a maintenance treatment.[63] The evidence for omega-3 fatty acids in bipolar depression (briefly discussed in Chapter 5) is somewhat stronger.

Finally, ECT is sometimes recommended as a maintenance treatment for those bipolar patients whose rapid cycling cannot be controlled. When used in this way, the goal is to give ECT much less frequently than when it is used for acute depression. Typically, a once-monthly treatment is the target frequency. Only small case series attest to ECT's efficacy in this area.[64] If ECT is used as a maintenance treatment, it should not be combined with lithium, since that combination is associated with marked cognitive impairment. Lamotrigine, valproate, and carbamazepine interfere with ECT's efficacy because they are anticonvulsants and prevent the electrical seizure that is a necessary component of ECT treatment. Sometimes, the anticonvulsant can be temporarily withheld for 1 to 2 days prior to maintenance ECT treatments.

## SUMMARY

This chapter has focused on pharmacological decision making in the maintenance phase of bipolar disorder. The choices among agents are many, and different treatment plans are usually needed for patients who are mania-dominant versus depression-dominant, rapid cycling, or otherwise treatment resistant. Psychotherapy—especially treatment models that emphasize symptom management and relapse prevention—should always be considered during the maintenance phase if it has not already been introduced during acute treatment. Some patients who cannot be stabilized with complex combinations of mood stabilizers and antipsychotics or who have been nonadherent with medications, will have a better course of illness when psychotherapy rather than simply another pharmacological agent is added. We address these topics in the next chapter.

# CHAPTER 7

## Psychosocial Treatment
## for Recovery and Maintenance

Psychotherapy is often begun with bipolar patients during an acute
episode of mania or depression, sometimes in an inpatient setting. It
can be difficult to make significant progress in the acute phase beyond
developing a therapeutic alliance with the patient or encouraging him
to follow a medication regimen. Yet the therapeutic relationship will
be substantially strengthened by these initial contacts. The real work
of psychotherapy usually begins after the patient has been discharged
from the hospital and returned home, and even then, the patient may
not be in shape to address major life issues or learn significant skills
to help prevent future episodes. Patients are often most motivated to
receive help just after an acute mood episode, when they discover the
difficulties of returning to prior work and relationships.

Clinicians who work psychotherapeutically should keep the different illness phases in mind; the goals during the acute, recovery, and
maintenance phases may be quite different. Moreover, one may plan
psychotherapy differently if the patient is still manic or hypomanic versus depressed, or if comorbid disorders complicate the picture (see also
Chapter 11). Some psychotherapy programs (e.g., group psychoeducation, mindfulness-based cognitive therapy) require that the patient has
been stable for some months, which may limit their utility in acute care
services.

Practitioners usually feel most competent to treat patients if they
have a "tool chest"—a set of therapeutic objectives and associated techniques on which to draw for different kinds of patients in different
phases of illness. This chapter describes some of these tools. Even if the
clinician cannot be trained in any of the full manualized treatments

described here, adapting these principles and integrating them into an eclectic model will be of significant help to most patients.

There are controlled studies supporting the efficacy of protocol-driven intervention programs (as reviewed here), but few data guide our choices for individual patients at different illness stages, or patients who do and do not have certain comorbid disorders. We also know surprisingly little about what interventions to prioritize if one only has a short time to work with the patient. Therefore, in this chapter we present treatment strategies as options in the same way that pharmacotherapy options were considered—what works for one patient may not work for another, and what works at one phase of the illness may be less effective with the same or a different patient at another phase.

As we discuss in more detail in Chapter 11, psychosocial treatments are usually most effective if there is an ongoing dialogue between the therapist and psychiatrist (assuming they are not the same person), especially when patients change states quickly. Clinics are usually set up to make this kind of communication possible, but in private practice settings, clinicians may need to go to some effort to share information. Furthermore, it is important to give psychosocial treatments an adequate chance to work. As was true for medications, switching modalities too quickly can reduce the chances of seeing a therapeutic effect.

## PSYCHOTHERAPY WITH WHOM?

The research literature describes four ways of structuring therapy for bipolar disorder: individual therapy, family/marital treatment, psychoeducational groups (with or without a mental health professional), or caregiver/patient ("multifamily") groups. The choice of one structure over the other is usually driven by what practitioners feel competent to recommend in a given setting, but patient preferences should also play a role. For example, some patients dread the idea of meeting with strangers and sharing stories, thereby limiting the role of group therapy, whereas others prefer this format.

As explained in prior chapters, it is almost always useful to bring in family caregivers (i.e., parents, spouse, siblings, grandparents, or other persons who have a role in the patient's care) for one or more treatment sessions, even if family or marital therapy is not the practitioner's goal. In the best-case scenario, caregivers help patients to recognize early warning signs of recurrence, remember to take medicines, stay on regular sleep cycles, and limit drinking habits. Of course, family sessions can also deteriorate into angry, mudslinging back-and-forths that appear to do more harm than good. In either case, involving family members is informative to the clinician in understanding the milieu in which the patient is recovering. In the sections that follow, we discuss ways to develop an alliance with family members so that session time is used productively.

## TARGETS OF PSYCHOTHERAPY DURING THE POST-ACUTE CONTINUATION PHASE

As discussed in earlier chapters, the continuation treatment phase is the period after resolution of acute symptoms when the goal is to produce a sustained recovery. The length of the continuation phase—the time it takes to achieve a minimum of 8 symptom-free weeks (*recovery*)—may last anywhere from 2 months to 1 year or more; the average is 3–4 months for a manic episode and 6–9 months for a depressive episode.[1] The overall goal of psychotherapy during this phase is to increase the speed of recovery, using the subsidiary aims listed in Table 7.1. Note that enhancing quality of life is not listed as a goal of the continuation phase, although it is the central goal of the maintenance phase. Nonetheless, psychosocial treatment during the continuation phase usually eases the patient's reentry into work, student, or parenting roles.

There is one large-scale, randomized trial—the Systematic Treatment Enhancement Program for Bipolar Disorder (STEP-BD) trial—that tested the effectiveness of psychosocial treatment when added to a stable medication regimen during the continuation phase following a bipolar (I or II) depressive episode.[2] Participants were randomly assigned to up to 30 sessions of intensive therapy (family-focused therapy [FFT], interpersonal and social rhythm therapy [IPSRT], or

**TABLE 7.1. Objectives of Psychotherapy during the Continuation Phase**

- Develop a working alliance with the patient and caregiver(s).
- Educate patients and family members about early warning signs of recurrence.
- Develop a relapse prevention plan.
- Encourage patients to track their moods daily.
- Stabilize sleep–wake rhythms.
- Use behavioral activation (i.e., pleasant events scheduling) for depression.
- Minimize the role of drug or alcohol abuse.
- Maintain consistency with medication regimens.

cognitive-behavioral therapy [CBT], all described below) or to three sessions of individual psychoeducation ("collaborative care"). Over a 1-year period, patients who received the intensive therapy recovered more quickly (110 days on average) from their depressive episode than patients in collaborative care (269 days). Also, in any study month, patients in intensive therapy were 1.6 times more likely to be clinically well than patients in brief treatment. The three intensive psychotherapies did not differ in time to recovery, but all were more effective than the briefer collaborative care treatment.[2] In all, adding intensive therapy to a mood stabilizer regimen appeared to be more effective in STEP-BD than adding an antidepressant to the regimen.[3]

What do the results of STEP-BD mean for practitioners? First, patients who are recovering from an acute depressive episode benefit from *psychoeducation*. Clinicians in all three treatments worked with patients to use daily mood-monitoring strategies and to recognize early warning signs of recurrence, develop relapse prevention strategies, regulate their lifestyles and sleep habits, and adhere to medication regimens. Educating family members about the disorder and learning communication and problem-solving strategies to manage stress in relationships (e.g., learning how to talk and listen during arguments) may have played a role in recovery given that the numerical effect sizes for FFT exceeded that of at least one of the other individual therapies, CBT.

We do not know whether the same results would have been observed had patients been recovering from manic instead of depressive episodes. Nonetheless, the therapy strategies recommended for hastening recovery from mania have many similarities to those for depression. Below, we discuss some of the strategies that were used in STEP-BD and other studies of psychotherapy for bipolar disorder. Later chapters address the role of psychotherapy in addressing pharmacological nonadherence (Chapter 8) and comorbid disorders (Chapter 11) during continuation or maintenance treatment.

### Educate the Patient and Family about Early Warning Signs of Recurrence

There is considerable evidence that FFT, when administered alongside medications in the post-episode period, can delay recurrences, reduce symptom severity, and improve medication adherence (for review, see Geddes & Miklowitz[4] and Miklowitz & Scott[5]). In research trials, FFT is given in up to 21 weekly and biweekly sessions that include the patient and caregivers (spouse or romantic partner, parents, siblings, or close friends). The critical criterion for including a caregiver is that this person consider it part of her role to help the patient manage the disorder.

Early on in the continuation phase, while the patient is being medically stabilized, a clinician can invite the patient to bring in one or more family members to assist in illness management and relapse prevention planning. As indicated in earlier chapters, caregivers are often the first to recognize when a patient is becoming ill (e.g., "He gets that look in his eyes"), or when medications are producing adverse reactions. When inviting the family members in for the first family session, the clinician can introduce the treatment plan as follows:

> "An episode of illness can be quite traumatic to members of the family. Just like with any illness, you may be worrying about the future. These sessions may help all of you to learn more about bipolar disorder: what it is, what causes it, and what you can do to help _____ control it. What do you think?"

At this point, the patient may voice objection to the characterization of his behavior as "recovery" or even the bipolar diagnosis. If that is the case, the clinician can encourage him to clarify how he sees his recent experiences, keeping in mind that residual mania or depression may be coloring his perceptions. It is best not to encourage a confrontation between the patient and caregivers at this point. Instead, the clinician can redirect the issue:

> "It's understandable that you'd have these questions at this point. I know each of you may be in very different places about this. But let me give you a sense of how some family sessions might help."

The clinician then asks the patient to describe to the caregiver(s) what he just went through: how the most recent episode began, what stress factors may have contributed to it, and what symptoms or behaviors he remembers having. Likewise, the clinician poses the same questions to the caregiver(s): "What made you think he was getting ill— what was different? Had you seen this before? How did you try to manage it?"

A handout such as that in Figure 7.1 may make the material more salient for the patient and family members. Describe the patient as the "expert" in the disorder:

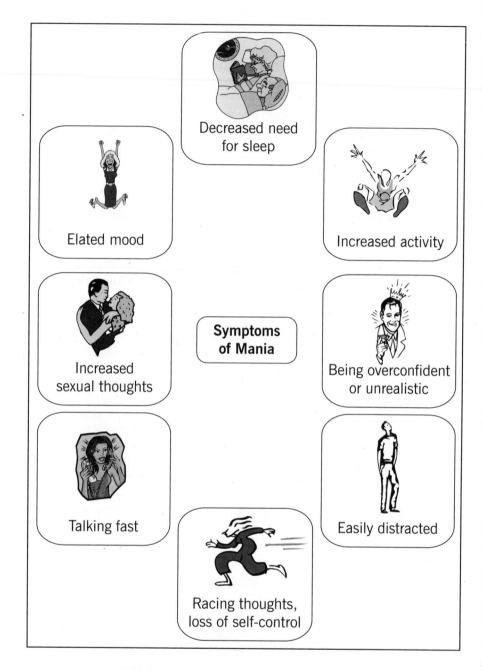

**FIGURE 7.1.** Handout on symptoms of mania.

From *Clinician's Guide to Bipolar Disorder* by David J. Miklowitz and Michael J. Gitlin. Copyright 2014 by The Guilford Press. Permission to photocopy this figure is granted to purchasers of this book for personal use only (see copyright page for details). Purchasers can download a larger version of this figure from *www.guilford.com/miklowitz5-forms*.

"You're the one who's had these experiences—we're going to depend on you to help us understand what you've gone through. Which of these symptoms on the handout do you remember having right before you went in the hospital?"

After the patient has been given time to describe the episode in his own words, the clinician encourages the caregiver(s) to review the handout and discuss what symptoms they remember best.

The goal of this discussion is to help the patient and caregiver to clarify the *prodromal signature* of the most recent manic or depressive episode. It is likely that future episodes will be preceded by similar sets of symptoms. For example, Phil, age 25, described his manic episodes as beginning with "creative thoughts," which then turned into long verbal diatribes when he felt "I have to get all of my thoughts out before they disappear." His mother experienced his irritability and impatience as being similar to the early phases of prior episodes, along with his "strange bedtime habits." His creative thoughts, she felt, only appeared after nearly a week of highly driven, irritable, sleep-deprived behavior. Moreover, they didn't sound all that creative to her; she described them as "unrealistic scenarios of what he might accomplish if we gave him unlimited resources."

If caregivers are available for ongoing sessions, a relapse plan can be developed in which prodromal signs are paired with specific actions that can be taken by patients, family members, or doctors to prevent the full escalation of mania or the worsening of depression. Figure 7.2 illustrates the relapse plan that Phil, age 25, developed with his parents and older brother. Note that the family decided to label the plan "version 1.0"; in fact, the plan was revised many times before it became useful as a preventative device.

### Patients with Multigenerational Histories of Bipolar Disorder

As the clinician introduces patients and family members to the psychoeducational material, she may run across resistances, particularly among young people in families with multigenerational histories of bipolar illness. As mentioned in Chapter 2, knowledge that bipolar disorder runs in one's family can lead to outright rejection of the diagnosis. For example, a teenager or young adult with suspected bipolar disorder may fear that the diagnosis and its treatments mean living like Dad, who has a long history of psychiatric hospitalizations, drug abuse, and poor functioning. Addressing these issues may require seeing the young person individually and discussing his fears about the future—some of which may be warranted and some not.

**Early Warning Signs**
Sleeps less, gets up more during night
Gets irritable and cranky
Obsessed with video games and pornography websites
Talks loudly about elaborate money-making schemes

**Recent Stressful Events**
Arguments with Mom
Fired from job
Pet [dog, expensive fish] died

**Coping Strategies**
Contact Dr. Benson for medication check or adjustment
Try to have the same bedtime as the rest of the family
Talk about my problems with my brother Pete
Stay away from friends who make me want to smoke weed

**FIGURE 7.2.** Phil's relapse prevention plan (Version 1.0).

If the bipolar parent is not attending sessions because of ongoing illness, the clinician may wish to draw distinctions between the young adult and the parent, such as differences in personality, social supports, age at first treatment, family relationships, knowledge of the disorder, or even the availability of better treatment options than in the past; these are all variables that can affect long-term illness course. In these cases, the goal is to encourage the young person to see his life trajectory as different from the parent's. In contrast, if the bipolar parent is stable, she may be able to explain to the offspring how she achieved stability; the different phases she went though in coming to accept her disorder; what medications or therapies she found helpful; and how she used social or familial supports. In this case, the goal is to encourage the young person to use the parent's current approach to the illness as a model for achieving stability.

### Tracking Symptoms with a Mood Chart

Whether one chooses to see the individual alone or with her family, one of the most useful between-session assignments is a daily mood and sleep chart, such as the one pictured in Figure 7.3. The purpose is to teach the patient to observe even minor fluctuations in mood and

Week of _____

## Mood Chart

| | Monday | Tuesday | Wednesday | Thursday | Friday | Saturday | Sunday |
|---|---|---|---|---|---|---|---|

**Moods**

Elevated

Energized

Balanced

Mildly
depressed

Very
depressed

Woke up at:  _____  _____  _____  _____  _____  _____

Went to bed at:  _____  _____  _____  _____  _____  _____  _____

Additional  _____  _____  _____  _____  _____  _____  _____
symptoms

Stressful events  _____  _____  _____  _____  _____  _____  _____
(yes/no)

Additional symptoms: I = irritability; A = anxiety; S = substance use; R = rumination;
P = paranoia/suspiciousness

Use single words or phrases to describe each mood state (e.g., "can't get going," "stay in bed," "on top of the world"):

| Elevated | Energized | Balanced | Mildly depressed | Very depressed |
|---|---|---|---|---|
| | | | | |
| | | | | |
| | | | | |
| | | | | |
| | | | | |

**FIGURE 7.3.** Mood chart. From D. J. Miklowitz and E. L. George. *The Bipolar Teen.* New York: Guilford Press; 2008. Copyright 2008 by The Guilford Press. Reprinted by permission.

activity levels that may herald the development of more serious episodes, or may become a focus of intervention in themselves. Patients who track their day-to-day environmental stressors or "hassles" (e.g., a job interview, relationship conflicts, their child's academic problems) may be able to clarify further the nature of the stress–symptom relationship. The psychopharmacologist will also find mood charts useful because they often reveal a developing episode that the patient has trouble describing, or suggest that a specific medication may be causing unexpected mood changes. Mood charting will have more impact during the continuation/recovery phase, when there is likely to be more mood upheaval, than during the maintenance phase, in which more stability can be expected.

Mood charts have proliferated recently, and, in addition to those distributed by drug companies, include online web forms and smartphone apps (e.g., *www.sleepcycle.com*). In our experience, the format is less important than that the patient buy into the idea of a mood chart and agree to fill it out on a daily or at least weekly basis. The chart in Figure 7.3 has been used successfully by both adolescents and adults, and can be adapted using the patient's own language (e.g., rating oneself as *elevated, excited, amped, energetic, racing*, or another term).

The components of a mood and sleep chart are (1) a 1-week or 1-month timeline in which the patient makes a daily depression and mania rating; and (2) spaces to record bedtimes, wake times, and daily events. Mixed moods are typically indicated by simultaneously rating depression and elevation on the same day.

When giving the patient the mood chart, explain that "this is one of the things you can do other than take medicines to stabilize your moods. . . .It puts you in the driver's seat if you can see what's setting off your highs and lows." Ask her to make at least one mood rating each day below the day of the week (or if she prefers, a "best" and "worst" rating), and record what time she went to bed each night and woke up the next day. If the patient says that the mood descriptors are irrelevant to her (e.g., "I don't really get elevated"), ask her to substitute terms that describe her experience (e.g., angry, irritable, "chaotic," "tired but wired"). If the patient complains that she has several mood changes per day, ask her to rate the morning and evening separately. Some patients obtain input from their spouse or roommates when they have trouble gauging their own moods.

Patients can list stressful events or daily hassles in a separate section of the chart. No stressor should be considered too trivial to be a trigger for mood swings: Traffic jams, unpleasant interactions with strangers, or problems with pets have all been listed by patients. The patient can pose questions to herself, such as "What happened before I started feeling irritable?" The actual timing or specifics of the event may be less important than the patient's realization that mood fluctuations are nonrandom and often the joint product of a poor night's sleep and an accompanying stressor.

The next session should begin with a review of the mood chart, along with praise for the patient's efforts to complete one. If she has not completed it, the clinician should explore the reasons and, if appropriate, further indicate the importance of the task by producing another blank copy and saying, "Let's fill it out together now." It can help to encourage the patient to fill out the chart at the same time each day. When a week's data have been recorded, assist the patient in drawing conclusions for that week, even if the conclusions are as simple as "My mood didn't change" or "I get more depressed every time I talk to my dad." The role of sleep disturbance in these mood fluctuations can often be highlighted with summary statements, such as "You seem to have a tougher time moodwise on weekends than during the week— any idea why that would be?" or "What jumps out at you about your sleep and how it tracks with your mood?"

Patients who are successful in this task can be encouraged to keep a similar record of anxiety, irritability, or target behaviors, such as rumination, drinking, or compulsions. Some patients find it useful to track the onset–offset of their menstrual periods in relation to mood changes. Ideally, the patient should keep a mood chart throughout therapy, although its role in sessions may vary over time. For example, mood monitoring may be central when one is recovering from an episode or changing medications, and less important when the patient's moods, medications, and sleep regimens have been stable for many weeks. Nonetheless, mood charting can anchor the treatment and give a visual and numerical index of progress.

Of course, not every patient will agree to chart his moods. Although the clinician can explore the nature of the patient's resistances (e.g., not liking being reminded of one's moods; disliking therapy homework; misunderstanding the purposes of the task), in our experience some patients will not follow through no matter what strategies are undertaken. Furthermore, some patients may not be cognitively able to carry out this task. In these cases, online mood chart applications that come with text or e-mail reminders can be used, making the task less cognitively challenging (see recommendations at *www.healthline.com/health-slideshow/top-iphone-android-apps-bipolar-disorder#2*).

## Tracking Substance Abuse on the Mood Chart

Patients who have ongoing problems with drug or alcohol abuse, as well as mood instability, should be involved in chemical dependency treatment in addition to treatments for their bipolar disorder (see Chapter 11). Nonetheless, it is useful for the patient to track his daily use of substances on the mood chart. The chart can be adapted so that number of drinks, joints ("blunts"), or pills is recorded at the end of each day, and mood and sleep shifts are recorded as well. The clinician can frame this as an experiment: "Let's see how much your mood and sleep change on days after you've drunk more than two beers the night before, and how that compares to days when you haven't had anything to drink." The patient may be surprised to learn how intertwined substance abuse, sleep, and mood have become. One patient assumed that drinking was a means of self-medicating her anxiety, but was surprised to find that her anxiety levels were not very high when she reached for a drink. In fact, her anxiety ratings reached their maximum the day after she had been drinking heavily.

## Stabilizing Sleep–Wake Rhythms

Identifying and maintaining regular daily and nightly routines are essential to recovery from a manic or depressive episode. Behavioral treatments for insomnia have recently been applied to bipolar disorder, with preliminary data suggesting that regulating bedtime and wake times leads to overall improvements in sleep.[6] The effects of these behavioral strategies on stabilizing mania or depression symptoms, however, have not been demonstrated.

IPSRT,[7] an individual therapy that emphasizes regular daily and nightly routines, and the events that disrupt them, has been shown to be effective in preventing recurrences of bipolar I disorder. IPSRT combines social rhythm stabilization with exploration and resolution of key interpersonal problems that contribute to mood instability. In a study of 175 bipolar patients who began treatment in an acute episode, patients were randomized at the beginning of the continuation period to weekly IPSRT or an equally intensive individual clinical management approach, along with mood stabilizing medications. Patients were randomized a second time once they recovered and entered a 2-year maintenance phase, during which their therapy sessions were tapered to monthly intervals. Patients who received IPSRT in the continuation phase had longer periods of wellness before their next recurrence than those who received clinical management. Relapse prevention was contingent on whether patients were successful in regulating their sleep–wake patterns, which was more likely to occur in IPSRT than in clinical management. Patients who received IPSRT also recovered their vocational functioning earlier than those who received clinical management.[8]

IPSRT makes use of a more expanded mood chart called the Social Rhythm Metric,[9] which helps patients track when they wake, eat, drink coffee, exercise, and go to bed, along with levels of social stimulation. These more detailed records show patients that their irregular bed and wake times are often due to the erratic timing of events earlier in the day or evening. Generally, the clinician should emphasize the *regularity* of the sleep pattern rather than the *number* of hours slept (a common confusion). For example, some individuals do fine with only 6 hours of sleep but become unstable when this 6-hour block changes from night to night.

Many patients who believe that they should exercise right before bed to tire themselves in fact become overstimulated by the exercise. Some patients eat dinner right before bed, or drink caffeinated drinks late in the afternoon and then cannot fall asleep. Daily records may also assist in spotting minor changes to routines that affect sleep and mood. For example, Rosslyn, a 38-year-old biology professor who was on the East Coast of the United States on an academic sabbatical, communicated with her graduate students through Skype. Her students, however, were in a time zone that was 3 hours earlier, often requiring Rosslyn to stay up 1–2 hours beyond her ordinary bedtime. Her mood became more elevated after this fairly ordinary change in routines, which became clear from her social rhythm charting.

Not surprisingly, the assignment to regulate routines is usually met by some degree of resistance. First, some people seem to be "larks" and others, "owls." Most patients feel encumbered by having to adhere to a strict bedtime and wake time; younger patients feel oppressed by it. College students may report that their social life depends on a later bedtime, yet they also have no choice but to schedule morning classes. People who have worked hard all week may resent the idea that they cannot "sleep binge" on the weekends (which tends to disrupt their sleep during the week). Therefore, regular sleep–wake rhythms must be negotiated in steps with the patient, sometimes over several months.

The clinician can empathize with the difficulty of having regular routines (e.g., "I can see that going to bed regularly means giving up a lot, maybe more than I realized") and encourage the patient to try an experiment for 1 week (e.g., "For this next week, try going to bed between 12:00 and 1:00 every night week and getting up between 8:00 and 9:00, and record your mood each day") or to change one aspect of the routine that seems to interfere with sleep stability ("How about moving your workout to 5:00 P.M. instead of 8:00 . . . is that doable for 1 week?"). Finally, frame the need for regularity as being tied to recovery: "I think this plan will be very important in speeding up your recovery from your depression, so for the next 2–3 months let's try to stick with it closely. After you've recovered maybe you'll be able to experiment with more variability."

### Behavioral Activation

If the patient's most recent episode was a depression, and depressive symptoms persist, a behavioral activation or "pleasant events" schedule will almost certainly be helpful. Research on major depressive disorder has shown that the behavioral activation component of CBT is as powerful or even more powerful than the cognitive restructuring component in stabilizing major depressive episodes.[10] The premises of behavioral activation are simple. First, because its primary characteristic is withdrawal, depression makes it less likely that the person will do those things that would be reinforced by others (e.g., initiating a conversation). Second, lack of social reinforcement worsens a person's depression and makes her withdraw even more. Combined with the biological predispositions inherent to depression, social withdrawal can create a negative spiral.

During the continuation phase, patients may go in and out of phases of activity as their mood varies up or down. If their most recent episode was manic or hypomanic, they may be doing too many things. Their hyperactivity may have driven friends away, so that they have little positive input from others to guide their choices. If the most recent episode was depressed or mixed, they may be active on some days and not others; reject others' attempts to connect; or sleep all day, then become active when others are unavailable. In any of these scenarios, patients cannot take full advantage of their social support systems, and their mood worsens.

---

Danielle, age 41, was recovering from a mixed episode that had evolved into a lengthy state of depression. Despite lamotrigine (Lamictal) and bupropion (Wellbutrin), she complained of lethargy and anhedonia. Her friends had encouraged her to come out with them, usually to go hiking or biking, as they had done many times in the past. She complained that she did not have any interest in these activities, and that her friends seemed boring. Worse yet, she felt they were tolerating her or seeing her only out of a sense of duty. Her recent relationship breakup had caused some of her friends to side with her previous boyfriend, leaving her with a smaller social network than before. Her limited social input contributed to her worsening state of depression, which in turn made her less likely to accept her friends' invitations.

---

The key task of the therapist is to introduce to the patient a slate of rewarding and pleasurable (or at least stimulating) activities. Start by explaining the vicious cycle of depression and social withdrawal (usually endorsed by the patient). Then, the patient generates a list of activities that are potentially pleasurable and do not seem onerous. The patient should choose activities that can be done each day (or every other day) during the next week. Using a calendar, she marks days and times in which she believes she can accomplish these activities. If the patient has not been keeping a mood chart, encourage her to record her mood before each activity and again after the activity.

The first week's assignments should be relatively minor (e.g., walking to a coffee shop and greeting at least one other person; calling one friend about plans for the following week). The patient should reward herself for accomplishing these objectives with relaxing and pleasing activities, even if they do not involve others (e.g., cooking a favorite meal, taking a bath, watching a humorous movie). If the patient's initial attempts at behavioral activation have gone well, she should be encouraged to plan more activities each day, such that previously long stretches of empty time are punctuated by activities that bring her into contact with others.

Often, behavioral activation plans fail because the patient chooses too many activities too soon, or cannot balance pleasant activities and "must-do" activities. So, for example, Danielle's plan originally included gardening and painting. In fact, these activities had "shoulds" attached to them (e.g., "The garden looks awful. I'd better get the weeding done before it's too late"; "I should go buy some brushes and an easel to get back into my painting, to make myself feel better"). Pleasurable activities should be those that (1) keep the patient engaged with others so that she feels liked or respected, (2) provide a feeling of competence, or (3) present an opportunity to experience emotions other than depression. If the patient has been unable to follow through on her plans, and it is clear that she tried to do too much, then the bar should be set lower. She might be encouraged, for example, to spend 5 minutes each day outside doing some mild exercise, such as walking the dog while listening to music that evokes positive memories, and then to increase the length of time outdoors by 5 minutes each day. Sometimes, behavioral activation can be combined with mindfulness meditation exercises (see Chapter 9).

In a minority of cases, the clinician may feel that the patient's social calendar is chaotic and has become dominated by hypomanic behavior. The patient may be constantly planning events with different people in a way that seems overly forced or driven. In these cases, the goal of behavioral activation may change to regulating the timing and frequency of activities. So, for example, the patient who plans to exercise, have dinner with a friend, go to a movie, and then catch up on work all in the same evening can be encouraged to scale back the plan to only one of these activities. Once again, the patient should make a mood rating on any day of the week that she has completed her activity plans.

## PSYCHOTHERAPY DURING THE MAINTENANCE PHASE

As is true of pharmacotherapy, the main objective of psychotherapy during the maintenance phase is to help the patient stay relapse-free. This is done through continual monitoring of early warning signs and implementation of stress management skills. As patients enter a period of *recovery*—arbitrarily defined in the literature as an 8-week period of minimally symptomatic functioning—the clinician can experiment with more insight-oriented approaches that the patient may not have been able to tolerate earlier. Although all of the strategies introduced during the continuation phase will continue to be relevant (e.g., mood charting, sleep–wake cycle regulation, and behavioral activation), the focus can move toward prevention of recurrence, improved quality of life, acceptance of the disorder, and illness-related issues that often accompany higher levels of functioning (e.g., stigma, job discrimination, relationship problems). Enhancing quality of life usually means facilitating the patient's reentry into new or preexisting work, educational, and social roles. It may also involve educating family members on how to help the patient manage new mood cycles or interpersonal challenges.

We have already discussed one form of prevention—the introduction of behavioral management strategies when the patient has a worsening depression or is becoming hypomanic. One can also explore how to prevent the social–environmental circumstances that led to a relapse in the first place. For example, if the patient has had a succession of difficult romantic relationships, the focus may change to adapting one's behavior toward the partner when one's moods change. If the patient clearly has a conflictual relationship with one or both parents, the focus of family sessions can change to learning conflict resolution skills.

## Enhancing Interpersonal Relationships

When patients have symptomatically recovered, they may be motivated to repair relationships that were damaged during the latest mood episode, or to improve relationships at home or at work that are conflict-ridden and stressful. In the IPSRT approach, these issues are broadly summarized as grief reactions (depression regarding a previous loss), interpersonal disputes (e.g., marital conflicts), role transitions (e.g., having to find new work or a new place to live), and interpersonal deficits (i.e., ongoing problems with social skills).[7]

Consider Frank's[7] example of IPSRT in a young woman with family relationship problems. In contrast to FFT, the IPSRT approach would proceed individually and focus on how this patient could negotiate differently with her parents.

> Lisa came to IPSRT treatment at age 19. She had had several manic and depressed episodes, all of which had seriously interfered with her family and social relationships. . . . Her parents had divorced when she was 6 years old. Although both parents were individually quite devoted to their daughter's welfare, they had only recently been able to work together to help cope with Lisa's mood disorder and interpersonal problems. Perhaps as a result, Lisa typically had had little respect for authority, which was reflected in feelings of moral or professional superiority, especially to teachers, school administrators, coworkers, and her father, whose demands she perceived as evidence of not caring for her or obstacles to her freedom. This stance . . . brought her into frequent conflict with others. . . . Her boss had already told her that unless she became more consistent in her attendance and more respectful of others in the office, he would need to look for a replacement.
>
> Lisa had long had a pattern of making her needs known to her parents only when she was acutely depressed. At those times, the neediness that was underlying her declarations of independence became quite pronounced and she would tend to pull them in to support her, only to push them away when she felt better. . . .As she progressed in therapy, she became increasingly cognizant of this interpersonal pattern and more aware of how the way she had managed her neediness had left her unfulfilled and even angry with her parents, while also keeping her enmeshed with them in an unnecessarily dependent way. She began to question her view of others' inferiority and to consider her own feelings of inferiority. . . . Over the last several months

of treatment, the level of conflict with both of her parents diminished, as she was able to define a set of reciprocal expectations with them. . . .At the time of therapy termination, she was doing well in her job and had formed a long-term relationship.[7] (pp. 109–110)

In many ways, interpersonal therapy with bipolar patients proceeds much like therapy with any patient. The unique elements of IPSRT, however, should not be overlooked: The emphasis is on regulating inconsistent daily routines that can contribute to problems such as inconsistent work attendance, and identifying and exploring the effects of manic or depressive symptoms on social relatedness. Also, the timing of these interventions can be critically important: It is unlikely that the progress made in this case would have occurred in the immediate aftermath of a depressive or manic episode.

The emphasis in this case on separation–individuation from parents versus the need for structure and support, although not unusual in Lisa's age group, is a key issue for young adult bipolar patients that can be addressed during the maintenance phase. Patients strongly value independence, and their manic phases sometimes seem like excessive attempts at autonomy. Yet, in the depressive episodes, they may become very vulnerable, dependent, and passive. As discussed in Chapter 8, interpersonal problems during the continuation or maintenance phases—including attitudes toward parents and other authority figures—can contribute to medication nonadherence and later recurrences.

### Family-Focused Treatment during the Maintenance Phase

A different approach during the maintenance phase is to build on the work the patient and family may have begun during the continuation phase. The relapse prevention plan can now be made more salient for the family as they evaluate strategies to undertake when the patient shows early warning signs. For example, Robert, age 45, who lived with his girlfriend, Jessie, had a manic episode that was preceded by multiple warning signs, most of which Jessie could describe after the fact. He had become more irritable with his children and coworkers, and his thoughts had raced as he became preoccupied with new ideas about expanding his landscaping business. According to Jessie, he had been unusually irritable toward her, yelled and screamed inappropriately during his younger daughter's basketball game, and had angrily confronted his adult son in a public setting. Robert added that as his mania had increased in severity, he became preoccupied with becoming a professional guitarist, buying and selling expensive guitars on impulse. He was finally picked up by the police after threatening suicide.

During his continuation treatment and for several weeks after he recovered, Robert and Jessie went back through the episode step-by-step and developed a prevention contract listing his early warning signs, stressors (increase in business obligations, conflict with his children and ex-wife, conflict with coworkers), and potential early interventions. These included (1) learning to talk as a couple about his emerging symptoms, without allowing the discussion to degenerate into arguments or blame cycles; (2) consulting his psychiatrist to have his lithium level checked and, possibly, his dosage increased or augmented with another agent; (3) avoiding having access to large sums of money; (4) Robert taking a few days off work when he became overly goal-focused; (5) setting a regular bedtime and wake time for the two of them; and (6) Robert avoiding confrontations with his children when Jessie or others noticed his increasing irritability, or when he (or they) recognized other signs of emergent mania.

Robert and Jessie revisited the plan every 3 months during their family treatment. After 1 year of medication and FFT, Robert was continuing to have mood cycles, but his episodes had begun to resemble hypomanias and his periods of depression became shorter. He and Jessie had been able to have productive (albeit tense) discussions about his hypomanic symptoms when they emerged. He was gradually rebuilding his relationships with his children and had ceded some of the financial control of his business to a partner.

The clinician can further assist the patient and family members by focusing on their communication styles. Not surprisingly, patients in families that show greater use of positive communication strategies, such as active listening, praise, problem solving, or nonverbal signs of acknowledgment (e.g., head nodding), have better symptomatic recoveries than patients whose families are negative across time.[11]

In their couple treatment, Robert and Jessie were taught the steps of active listening and positive requests for change (Table 7.2). *Active listening* requires that one partner role-play speaking about a topic of importance while the other listens, reflects, validates, and offers nonverbal signs of attention. When first attempting to train patients and relatives in these skills, it is best to encourage the speaker to pick a nonthreatening topic (e.g., something that happened on the way to work; an interaction with a coworker) rather than one that involves family conflict. Otherwise, the role-play exercises may devolve into shouting matches and accusatory diatribes. The clinician must stop these interactions before they become too heated, ask the members to pause, then start the role play over again, giving the listener instructions to paraphrase, ask clarifying questions, and avoid being judgmental. Sometimes a third try is necessary as well. Between these practice attempts, the clinician can ask, "What did you like about the way she listened just now? What steps did she do on this sheet? What else might she have done?" It is important to praise the listener for even minor attempts to use the skills.

Next, the roles of listener and speaker are reversed. If there are more than two people in the family, the previous speaker can volunteer to hear out another family member, so that everyone participates and dyadic discussions do not become dominated by one person. The family member observing the role play can be asked to comment on what components of the skill the new listener has used.

A related skill, *positive requests for change* (Table 7.2), teaches participants an alternative to criticism or other negative statements that are common during the recovery period. Instead of criticizing another family member, the speaker requests that some activity be done in a more collaborative manner. For example, Robert practiced with Jessie, "When I get like that [irritable, hypomanic], I want you to tell me that you love me, and in a more tender way tell me that you think I need help and why, even if I'm not receptive." Jessie followed up with

---

**TABLE 7.2. Communication Skills**

Active listening

- Look at your family member.
- Attend to what is said.
- Nod your head or say "uh-huh."
- Ask clarifying questions.
- Check out what you heard (paraphrase).

Making positive requests for change

- Look at your family member.
- Say exactly what you would like him or her to do.
- Tell him or her how it would make you feel.
- Use phrases such as:
    "I would like you to _____. That would make me feel _____."
    "I would really appreciate it if you would _____."
    "It's very important that you help me with _____."

*Note.* From D. J. Miklowitz. *Bipolar Disorder: A Family-Focused Treatment Approach.* 2nd ed. New York: Guilford Press; 2010. Copyright by The Guilford Press. Adapted by permission.

"I would appreciate your telling me before you go off of your medications, so that we can talk about it as a couple and I'll know my feelings matter to you."

These strategies are dependent on families being willing to practice on their own. The clinician can assign them the task of choosing 3 days in the week to practice listening skills (without necessarily telling others in the family they are doing so), writing down the "whens" and "wheres" of each conversation, and listing what skill components they used. At the beginning of the next session, the couple or family can be asked to replay the conversation to gain further practice. Even if they do not adopt the skills right away, patients and caregivers benefit from knowing that their parent, spouse, or sibling is working to be more collaborative.

## Group Psychoeducation in the Maintenance Phase

Many patients do not interact regularly with family members or are not partnered. Individual approaches such as IPSRT or CBT may be choices for these patients. Alternatively, some patients (and some clinics) prefer group therapy approaches, in which several patients with bipolar disorder meet with each other.

Several studies of group psychoeducation have been done. These have been large-scale, well-controlled trials (one study[12] had 441 patients enrolled in a health maintenance organization; another[13] included 306 patients from multiple Veterans Administration settings). It appears from these studies that not all group treatments are equally effective: The groups must be structured, educational, and involve skills training and homework assignments. They involve more than just talking about the disorder in front of others, although the "anti-stigma" effects of groups cannot be underemphasized. In one study,[14] patients who were being maintained on mood stabilizers were randomly assigned to 21 structured group sessions or 21 unstructured support group sessions, in which patients could talk about anything they wanted. Those patients in the structured groups had fewer recurrences and hospitalizations, and better social functioning over a 5-year follow-up than those in the unstructured groups.

A typical group agenda might include breaking into pairs and developing a list of prodomal symptoms, discussing the role of substance and alcohol abuse in mood cycles, learning to identify and restructure one's pessimistic beliefs, or troubleshooting disruptions to daily and nightly routines. The groups generally work best when the participants are in clinical remission, even if they have functional impairments. They are usually conducted by a psychologist who edu-cates using Socratic, "give-and-take" methods.

Group psychoeducation appears to be cost-effective. In the study just cited,[14] patients in structured group psychoeducation were signifi-cantly more likely to attend their other treatment appointments and less likely to need emergency consultations. Over 5 years, there was a saving of about 5,000€ (about $6,500) per patient, which was attribut-able to fewer hospital admissions in these patients than in patients who attended support groups without psychoeducation.[15]

### Mutual Support Groups

Many patients and family members feel that only others who cope with bipolar disorder can truly understand their challenges and offer viable solutions. Much like the Alcoholics Anonymous (AA) models, mutual support groups, such as those offered by the National Alliance on Men-tal Illness (NAMI) or the Depression and Bipolar Support Alliance (DBSA), involve talking about one's experiences with medicines and other treatments; how one has dealt with work, family or social prob-lems; and what has or has not been effective in preventing episodes (see resources in Appendix A). Sometimes these groups involve educational lectures by specialists as a supplement to group meetings. Although no controlled studies of mutual support groups have been done in bipo-lar disorder, large surveys of the NAMI and DBSA memberships have consistently shown that mutual support groups make patients more willing to take medications, communicate with members of their treat-ment team, and cope with side effects.

There are also support groups available for family members. For example, NAMI offers a 12-week course called "Family to Family," taught by trained members who have coped with their own or a fam-ily member's illness. Most attendees report that these groups helped them feel less isolated and more effective in coping with their relative's disorder.

Patients are usually reluctant to attend mutual support groups at first, fearing that they will be asked to stand and say, "I'm Fred, and I'm bipolar." In fact, the groups do not pressure patients or caregivers to contribute beyond their comfort level. A good strategy is to suggest that the patient or caregiver attend a single session to see whether the group is a good fit given the stage of the illness and cohort characteris-tics of the group (i.e., other patients of similar diagnosis, age, and func-tioning). Support groups are not a replacement for one's own therapy, but they can be a helpful supplement.

## SUMMARY

Psychotherapy is an important component of the outpatient treatment of bipolar disorder during the continuation and maintenance phases. In addition to assisting the patient in managing symptoms, it may enhance quality of life and offer hope for the future. It may also improve family relationships and the patient's ability to function in the social or occupational milieu.

We have emphasized the importance of matching therapeutic goals to different phases of the illness. Equally important is the structure and setting of treatment, such as whether the family is included or patients prefer a group setting. The patient's financial situation, as well as what treatments are ordinarily provided in the clinical setting, also influence treatment choice.

Most individuals with bipolar disorder benefit from an ongoing therapeutic contract, whether it is occasional check-ins with their psychopharmacologist, weekly appointments with a mental health professional in the same or a different setting, or a clinician-directed or mutual support group. As we discuss more in Chapter 11, cross-disciplinary communication is essential to making a treatment contract effective. We have devoted the next chapter to the ways in which psychotherapy can enhance the goals of the pharmacological plan, through addressing difficulties with medication adherence.

# ─── CHAPTER 8 ───

## Dealing with Medication Nonadherence

Refusing to follow a recommended medication regimen—called *nonadherence* or sometimes *noncompliance*—is a problem in all areas of medicine. Pervasive problems of adherence in bipolar patients have been well-documented.[1] Nonadherence can occur at any stage of bipolar illness, but it is a particular problem during maintenance treatment, when the patient may begin to feel better or, alternatively, experience frustration that residual depressive symptoms have not lifted. When patients discontinue their medications abruptly, their chances of relapsing or committing suicide go up considerably.[2,3]

Any clinician—physician, psychologist, social worker, or nurse practitioner—needs to be aware of the potential for relatively stable patients to discontinue their medications. Clinicians should consider an instance of possible nonadherence to occur when the patient worsens symptomatically (e.g., gets more and more hypomanic) despite a seemingly optimal medication regimen, when she alludes to discomfort or resentment regarding the treatment plan (e.g., "I'm looking forward to the day when I don't have to take these anymore"; "Taking lithium makes me feel like I'm ill"), or when she confidently asserts her ability to control the illness on her own.

This chapter is divided into four sections. We first discuss the relevant research on nonadherence in bipolar disorder to help frame our approach to preventing it. Second, we discuss how to detect nonadherence in a patient who is in ongoing care. Third, we describe practical approaches to nonadherence, such as adjusting dosing frequencies to help patients who forget to take their pills. Finally, we discuss exploratory treatment approaches to address underlying (often unstated) issues. Many patients who become nonadherent report that they (1) enjoy being

168

high, (2) view medications as interfering with their creativity, (3) battle with family members who insist on adherence, (4) struggle with feeling different and stigmatized, or (5) equate medications with a loss of goals and aspirations. Treating psychiatrists may have data that therapists do not have (e.g., the frequency with which prescriptions are being filled). Nonetheless, therapists can aid the physician in promoting adherence by addressing the underlying reasons—some of which may be obvious, and some not—for discontinuing medications.

## REASONS FOR NONADHERENCE

Researchers have been examining medication nonadherence in bipolar disorder for as long as there have been mood-stabilizing medications. As a harbinger of things to come, the first patient treated with lithium, by John Cade in the 1940s, responded quite well but within 6 months went off of lithium against Cade's advice and was rehospitalized.[4] Researchers estimate that up to 60% of patients with bipolar disorder discontinue their medications at some point in the lifetimes, with between 40 and 60% being partially or fully nonadherent in the year after their first hospitalized manic episode.[5,6] Rates of adherence with valproate (Depakote) and the atypical antipsychotics tend to be higher than those with lithium because of milder side-effect profiles.[7,8] More important for our purposes are the reasons for nonadherence, which are summarized in Table 8.1.

Consider the following quote from Kate Millet's account of her bipolar disorder:

> Accusing me of mania, my elder sister's voice has an odd manic quality. "Are you taking your medicine?" The kind of control in furious questions addressed to children, such as "Will you get down from there?" As if by going off lithium I could erase the past, could prove it had never happened . . . of course, I had only to take lithium in order to be accepted back . . . on lithium I would be "all right." But I am never all right, just in remission. If I could win this gamble. . . .[9 (p. 32)]

In this example, one sees several reasons for stopping: the stigma of the disorder, anger over attempts at control by family members and the strong desire to regain autonomy, and the sense of being infantilized. The emotional tug of these conflicts can be a significant cause of nonadherence.

Nonadherence can also revolve around more practical problems. For example, many patients stop taking antipsychotics when they gain

**TABLE 8.1. Reasons That Patients with Bipolar Disorder Discontinue Their Medications**

- Side effects (e.g., weight gain, memory impairment)
- Forgetting
- Being young, male, and dealing with a recent-onset episode (first or second)
- Negative feelings about having one's moods controlled by medications
- Missing high periods and perceived loss of creativity
- Financial/insurance issues
- Substance/alcohol abuse
- Lack of acceptance of illness
- Lack of understanding of the purposes of medications
- Feeling better
- Stigma of bipolar illness
- Rebelling against parents or spouses
- Discomfort with blood tests

too much weight, or lithium when their hands shake. When a patient loses his job, he may no longer be able to afford medication refills. Some of these problems have solutions and others do not.

In the sections that follow, we discuss ways to address each of these problems with patients. Some may be addressed by adjusting dosages or changing from one agent to another (e.g., changing olanzapine [Zyprexa] to aripiprazole [Abilify] to manage weight gain). Others may require more extensive problem solving (e.g., introducing reminders for when to take what pills or enlisting the help of family members in filling prescriptions). Other issues may require mediating conflicts between the patient and family members that may be contributing to the patient's inconsistent use of medications. Before intervening, however, it is important to assess whether a patient has indeed become nonadherent.

## ASSESSING NONADHERENCE

### Blood Levels

Determining whether a patient is consistently taking his medications has challenges. One of the advantages of some of the older antimanic and mood stabilizing medications—lithium, valproate, and carbamazepine (Tegretol)—is that the psychiatrist can measure blood levels on a regular basis (for lithium usually once every 4–6 months during the maintenance phase, unless levels have been irregular; carbamazepine and valproate levels are less useful). Therapeutic levels during maintenance treatment (e.g., 0.6–1.0 mEq/liter for lithium; 50–100 µg/ml for valproate; 4–12 µg/ml for carbamazepine) that vary from one test to another are often a sign of inconsistent adherence. The absolute level is less relevant in this context than the variation in the levels over time.

Some patients "game the system" by taking an extra dosage of their mood stabilizer in the hours before the level is to be taken, leading to an inflated serum level. This strategy is more common when the patient is hypomanic and wants to be on a lower dosage than initially agreed upon. Patients do not come in for blood levels at all when they have stopped taking their medications. As a result, therapeutic levels from blood tests are not always informative about the patient's true medication habits.

### Asking the Patient

Inquiring about the patient's medication habits is often the best way to determine adherence (see Table 8.2). In a longitudinal study, we found that patients' self-reports about lithium usage were more reliable than physician reports, reports from caregivers, or blood levels.[10] However, obtaining accurate information hinges on the therapeutic alliance and how the question is asked. When asked, "Are you taking your medicine?" many patients will respond defensively ("Of course") and lie by omission. It is often better to use an inquisitive but nonjudgmental approach, with an emphasis on normalizing the patient's

---

**TABLE 8.2. Ways to Inquire about Medication Adherence**

- "Do you have any difficulty taking *all* of your medications?"
- "Do you ever try to cope on your own without lithium (or Depakote or Abilify)?"
- "Many people miss taking their medications from time to time; how has it been for you?"
- "It's easy to forget to take your pills when you have to take them at different times of the day; do you ever forget to take your afternoon or evening dose?"
- "Most people have trouble remembering when they travel; how has it been for you?"
- Medication Adherence Rating Scale (Self-Administered) (see below)

doubts about taking medicines. The patient may still dodge the subject, but at least you will have opened the door to further discussion about these issues.

### Pill Counts and Prescription Checks

An obvious and highly reliable method of identifying nonadherence is to know how many pills a patient should have taken in a given interval, and compare that number to how many the patient has actually taken. Some physicians, and even some psychotherapists, ask the patient to bring in the bottles or bubble packs periodically so that pills can be counted, especially if the patient has been previously nonadherent.

If you are the treating physician, you can check when the last prescription was written, and whether the patient called for a refill within the expected time frame. Consider the following interchange between a psychiatrist and a 52-year-old man with bipolar I disorder and a history of alcohol dependence.

> DOCTOR: How has it been with taking the lithium and the Lamictal [lamotrigine]? Any problems?
>
> PATIENT: The Lamictal is pretty good. It's a good drug, it's definitely helping.
>
> DOCTOR: Glad to hear it. How is it helping?
>
> PATIENT: Well, you know, less depressed, sleeping better.
>
> DOCTOR: Good news. And the lithium?
>
> PATIENT: (*Pauses.*) OK. You know, lithium is lithium. (*Smiles.*)
>
> DOCTOR: I'm a bit puzzled by something. I gave you a 3-month supply on June 12. It's now October. You should have run out by now, yes?
>
> PATIENT: Oh, yeah, I thought I'd just ask you to refill both of them when I saw you today. I didn't want to bug you back in September.
>
> DOCTOR: I see. When did you fill that last prescription, do you remember?
>
> PATIENT: Oh, I always fill them in your pharmacy on the way out.
>
> DOCTOR: So, I'm still confused. You must have run out of lithium in September.
>
> PATIENT: (*pausing, somewhat defensive*) No, I had enough left from an old prescription.

DOCTOR: I guess that's possible. But maybe you're having a hard time telling me that you stopped taking it.

PATIENT: (*still defensive*) Yeah, I stopped it back in July. I thought since I had the Lamictal and it was working I'd be OK.

DOCTOR: OK, I know this can be hard to talk about. Can you say a little more about what made you decide to stop the lithium?

In this exchange, the physician has been able to elicit an important piece of information. He learned later in the session that the patient had resumed drinking as well. The patient expressed his belief that lithium was not adequately controlling his symptoms, and that he could better control his depression and anxiety through alcohol and the occasional tablet of lamotrigine.

Note that this method of inquiry is similar to what the physician might do if the patient has been abusing benzodiazepines or sleep or pain medicines. Patients who are taking excessive quantities of alprazolam (Xanax), clonazepam (Klonopin), zolpidem (Ambien), or hydrocodone (Vicodin) often call two or three times more often for refills of these medications as for their mood stabilizer or second-generation antipsychotic (SGA). Keeping clear records of the frequency of refills is an essential method of tracking medication use, especially during the maintenance phase, when appointments may be scheduled far apart.

### Asking the Caregivers

As we discuss more below, nonadherence can become intertwined with family dynamics, particularly in younger patients living at home or married/cohabiting patients who have conflicts with their spouses over dependency. Although patients who are nonadherent may resent the practitioner's questioning of their parents or spouses about medication use, these caregivers can be important sources of information. Parents and spouses are often the first to know when the patient has stopped his medications and is becoming symptomatic.

With the married patient, the clinician can soften the impact of this line of inquiry by telling the patient, "I often find that husbands [wives, partners] provide important information about their spouses' health habits. I'll bet that if she were the one taking medicines, you would be equally helpful about her care." A young adult patient can be told, "Just because I ask your mom doesn't mean that I believe her and don't believe you. It's important for me to get everyone's perspective. But in the end it's really your decision what you want to do."

Be particularly attuned to situations in which patients claim they are being consistent with their prescriptions but caregivers raise doubts. Parents and spouses are usually right when they say that the patient has missed dosages, filled prescriptions late, or canceled treatment or lab appointments to avoid being "discovered."

### Do Any Questionnaires Identify Nonadherence?

Some clinicians use self-report instruments to identify when patients are being inconsistent with medicines. We can see the value of these instruments, especially in the earliest stages of treatment, when you may not know the patient very well. Neither of the two scales below was specifically developed for bipolar disorder, but both have acceptable reliability and validity data in patients with schizophrenia or schizoaffective disorder. We recommend considering these scales and following up with questions to ascertain when nonadherence or discontinuation has occurred, or to clarify assumptions such as "It is unnatural for my mind and body to be controlled by medication."

The Medication Adherence Rating Scale[11] may help determine the source of nonadherence (Figure 8.1). It contains three subscales: Adherence Behavior (items 1–4), Attitudes toward Medications (items 5–8), and Psychotropic Side Effects (items 9 and 10). Those patients who only endorse nonadherent behavior (items 1–4) but not negative attitudes may benefit from reminders; those with significant side effects (items 9 and 10) may benefit from changing medications or doses. Patients with negative attitudes about psychotropic medications (items 5–8) may benefit from psychoeducation about what it does and doesn't mean to take these agents. The Brief Adherence Rating Scale,[12] consisting of three interview questions regarding the number of days or dosages missed in the past month, is also a useful assessment. For example, this scale may reveal that the patient does not know how many pills to take.

## MANAGING NONADHERENCE

Addressing nonadherence requires at least three steps: (1) assessing whether and how often the patient has been inconsistent with mood stabilizers or SGAs, (2) exploring the reasons for nonadherence, and (3) collaborating with the patient and available caregivers to increase consistency. In the sections that follow, we emphasize the importance of clarifying and, whenever possible, validating the patient's point of view

**Medication Adherence Rating Scale (Self-Administered)**

For the following questions, please circle Y ("Yes") or N ("No") based on the last week.

1. Do you ever forget to take your medication?      Y   N

2. Are you careless at times about taking your medication?    Y   N

3. When you feel better, do you sometimes stop taking your medication?      Y   N

4. Sometimes if you feel worse when you take the medication, do you stop taking it?      Y   N

5. I take my medication only when I am sick.      Y   N

6. It is unnatural for my mind and body to be controlled by medication.      Y   N

7. My thoughts are clearer on medication.      Y   N

8. By staying on medication, I can prevent getting sick.      Y   N

9. I feel weird, like a "zombie" on medication.      Y   N

10. Medication makes me feel tired and sluggish.      Y   N


**Brief Adherence Rating Scale (Clinician-Administered)**

Pose the following three questions to patients about their knowledge of the medication regimen.

1. What is the number of doses of each medication you're supposed to take each day?
2. How many days in the past month did you not take the prescribed doses?
3. How many days in the past month did you take less than the prescribed dose?

If patients have trouble recalling the number of days, ask them to give you an estimate of the percentage of days in the last month, where 0 = *none of the days* and 100% = *all of the days.*

**FIGURE 8.1.** Self-report instruments for identifying nonadherence. The Medication Adherence Rating Scale is from K. Thompson et al.[11] *Schizophrenia Research.* 2000;42(3):241–247. Copyright 2000 by Elsevier. Reprinted by permission. The Brief Adherence Rating Scale is from M. J. Byerly et al.[12] *Schizophrenia Research.* 2008; 100(1–3): 60–69. Copyright 2008 by Elsevier. Reprinted by permission.

From *Clinician's Guide to Bipolar Disorder* by David J. Miklowitz and Michael J. Gitlin. Copyright 2014 by The Guilford Press. Permission to photocopy this figure is granted to purchasers of this book for personal use only (see copyright page for details). Purchasers can download a larger version of this figure from *www.guilford.com/miklowitz5-forms.*

about medications. This can be challenging when treating a patient who has been nonadherent on multiple occasions and has relapsed each time, or who seems to have forgotten major periods of illness and blames illness-related events (e.g., car accidents) or poor functioning on the behavior of others. Nonetheless, the key to reestablishing the patient's consistency with the medication regimen is to consider the validity of her viewpoint and collaborate with her in finding a way forward. Altering the treatment regimen, helping to adjust aspects of the immediate environment, and offering the patient didactic information may all contribute to this effort.

### Practical Approaches to Nonadherence

Once nonadherence has been identified, it can often be addressed in a practical way. By practical, we mean (1) giving the patient information about each medication, the expected side effects, dosing options, and risks of discontinuation; (2) adjusting dosages or switching agents to manage side effects; and (3) strategizing with the patient as to how to remember to take medicines at the proper times. These "tricks" to enhance adherence may seem simplistic and obvious—especially to the prescribing psychiatrist—but they may be genuinely new ideas for patients. In the section that follows, we discuss exploratory approaches that address emotional reactions to medications that are often associated with nonadherence.

### The Therapeutic Stance

Many physicians and therapists provide patients with statistics about the risk of relapse when going off recommended medications. Indeed, having data at your fingertips on rates of relapse in patients who discontinue medications may be quite helpful: 60–70% relapse within 1 year, and an even greater number of patients relapse if they stop suddenly; rates of relapse when taking mood stabilizers regularly are 30–40%.[5,13] Suicide risk increases considerably among patients who discontinue medications quickly.[14] However, data from research studies are usually not enough to convince patients, especially if they are hypomanic or grandiose. They may counter that they are part of the 30% that will not relapse.

The clinician's stance on medication nonadherence should not be an argumentative one. Rather, encourage the patient to think about temporal sequences of events and the balance of risk and protective factors in recurrences, so that the patient generates her own conclusions about future risk. In most cases, recurrences are a product of multiple factors, including life events, drug or alcohol abuse, and sleep–wake disruptions. All of these factors, however, will have a greater impact if the patient is not protected by medicines.

The dialogue with the patient can begin with the following:

> "Let's talk about what happened in the past when you've gone off your Depakote. That may tell us something about what's likely to happen this time. How has this worked out in the past? Why would things be different this time?"

The patient may deny the link between prior relapses and nonadherence. For example, he may recall that he became hypomanic, felt powerful and invulnerable, and wanted to accentuate this state by going off his mood stabilizers or SGAs. He may not recall instances in the past that were associated with relapse, or may have a different (and equally viable) explanation for why a relapse occurred (e.g., "I was doing cocaine then"). You can assist him in recalling the last episode if you have information such as the following in the medical chart:

> "According to my records, you stopped taking valproate on April 12, and then stopped risperidone on May 1. Your last hospitalization started on May 6. What do you remember happening at that time?"

### Lack of Understanding about Medicines

You may learn that the patient misunderstands what specific medications are designed to do. For example, he may believe that the mood stabilizer or SGA is only meant to control mania and has no effects on depression. Then, when he feels depressed, he may conclude that mood stabilizers are not necessary or are even the cause of the depression.

---

Ethan, age 48, had bipolar I disorder, and was being treated with valproate, risperidone, and citalopram (Celexa). He complained of sluggishness at work, which he felt was due to the valproate. His psychiatrist did not believe that the citalopram was alleviating his depression. When Ethan complained about his inattentiveness problems, his doctor switched him from citalopram to methylphenidate–extended release (Concerta, a relatively long-acting stimulant), one 30-mg tablet in the morning. Ethan liked the feelings he got from methylphenidate but did not understand that it was long-acting. He began taking a second tablet at noon, and eventually, a third tablet late in the afternoon. Because he now felt wired and energetic, he decided that he did not need his valproate or risperidone and discontinued both. But a few days later, he developed sleep problems and became increasingly aggressive and disinhibited. He was hospitalized a week later with a full-blown manic episode.

Ethan's hospitalization might have been averted had he been given more information about each of his medications. He did not understand what "long-acting" meant, the potential risks of exceeding the recommended dosage of his methylphenidate, or the risks of discontinuing the mood stabilizer. Upon further exploration, the physician found that Ethan also had little understanding of why he was taking risperidone. He had a history of delusional thinking, and believed that antipsychotics should only be taken when he felt paranoid. Because he felt elevated and expansive on methylphenidate, he saw no reason to continue the antipsychotic agent.

### Managing Side Effects

During the maintenance phase, you may learn that the patient no longer believes that tolerating the side effects of her medications is balanced by the protective value of medications on relapse risk. When in remission, patients often consider resuming work or school, which may increase their concerns about how they appear to others. Understandably, they may be particularly concerned about medicines that make them look or feel physically uncoordinated or ungainly (e.g., trembling hands), unattractive (e.g., weight gain), or cognitively impaired.

Take a collaborative approach to managing side effects. The patient should provide information about which side effects are most important to her (e.g., a 27-year-old who is trying to get acting roles may be more bothered by weight gain than by headaches or gastrointestinal distress). Are the side effects dosage-related? Were they present when she was taking a lower dose? As the clinician, you can provide information about the expected side effects of the current medications and the alternatives that should be considered.

There are a number of modifications that can be made for side effects, as elaborated in Table 8.3 (see also Chapter 6). Once a change in regimen has been agreed upon, the patient should keep a daily journal of symptoms and side effects. The mood chart (Chapter 7) can be adapted for this purpose.

**TABLE 8.3. Modifications to Medication Regimens That May Increase Adherence**

| Medication class | Side effects | Potential modifications |
|---|---|---|
| SGAs | Weight gain | Switch to different agent that is more weight-neutral (e.g., lamotrigine, aripiprazole, carbamazepine).<br><br>Add metformin (Glucophage) or topiramate (Topamax). |
| | Sedation | Use nighttime dosing.<br><br>Add modafanil (Provigil) or armodafanil (Nuvigil). |
| | Akathisia (restlessness) | Add:<br>• Beta blocker<br>• Benzodiazepine<br>• Anticholinergic |
| Lithium | Mental sluggishness | Lower dosage. |
| | Memory problems | Switch to valproate (Depakote). |
| | Frequent urination | Thiazide diuretics. |
| | Hand tremor | Add propanolol (Inderal). |
| Valproate | Gastrointestinal distress | Take after eating.<br><br>Switch to extended-release valproate. |
| Lamotrigine | Rash | Switch to different mood stabilizer. |

## Forgetting

Forgetting is a problem with all maintenance medications, but it can become acute when the patient is highly symptomatic, cognitively impaired, or abusing substances. Patients may miss whole days of a medication and take double doses at other times. If family members are not embroiled in conflict with the patient over medications, you may be able to enlist their help in a reminder campaign.

A patient who frequently forgets to take medications may benefit from a brief *problem-solving* exercise. A basic component of most psychoeducational therapies, problem solving involves helping the patient to identify a specific area of difficulty, brainstorm solutions, choose one or more possible solutions, and develop an implementation plan (Table 8.4). In this case, you can help the patient define the problem as "not remembering when to take my medications" or "being confused as to what to take and when." Solutions may include obtaining a pillbox, using the alarm on her watch or cell phone, accepting text reminders from relatives, pairing pill-taking with meals, and other options. When patients or caregivers are generating solutions, it is important that no one interrupt the idea flow by raising doubts about the viability of any one solution. For example, the younger sister of a 17-year-old suggested that they "stick a Post-it note on her head." Although the older sister was not thrilled with this solution, it did generate the alternative that she tape a reminder to the mirror of her medicine cabinet.

Next, encourage the patient (and caregivers, if they are present) to make a list of the advantages and disadvantages of each proposed solution. Implementing solutions may be simple, such as buying pillboxes or stickers, deciding where and how often to leave reminders, or noting the date that refills are due using an online calendar; or more complex, such as evaluating when reminders from others feels intrusive.

**TABLE 8.4. Steps for the Implementation of Family Problem Solving**

1. Define the problem. Get everyone's input.

2. List all possible solutions. Do not evaluate any solutions at this point.

3. Discuss and list the advantages and disadvantages of each possible solution.

4. Choose the best solution or combination of solutions.

5. Plan how to carry out the chosen solutions.
   a. Decide who will do what.
   b. Decide what resources will be needed; list and obtain them.
   c. Anticipate what can go wrong during implementation and decide how to overcome these problems.

6. Rehearse the implementation of the solution(s).

7. Give positive feedback to all participants for their help in solving the problem.

8. If the implemented solution did not work, go back to step 1 and try again.

*Note.* From D. J. Miklowitz.[16] *Bipolar Disorder: A Family-Focused Treatment Approach.* 2nd Ed. New York: Guilford Press; 2008. Copyright 2008 by The Guilford Press. Reprinted by permission.

The physician may be able to alter the regimen to reduce the likelihood of forgetting. One option is once-daily dosing. All mood stabilizers may be given once daily with full efficacy, but dividing the dose can minimize certain side effects. If the patient is taking antipsychotics, he can be switched to depot (injectable) preparations. Patients may be resistant to the idea of getting an injection, but there is increasing evidence that injectable antipsychotics are associated with better adherence and, possibly, cognitive functioning compared to the same agents in pill form.[15]

## EXPLORATORY APPROACHES
## TO MEDICATION NONADHERENCE

Most people with bipolar disorder—or with any medical illness, for that matter—have emotional reactions to the diagnosis and its treatments. We represent these in the sections below with quotes we have heard from patients who have decided to discontinue their medicines. In most cases, a patient will feel safe in exploring her conflicts over medicines if the clinician *validates* her beliefs and *normalizes* them before attempting to intervene. You will see several examples of this stance in the examples that follow.

### *"I feel fine now, so why do I need medicine?"*

Patients often stop taking mood stabilizers when their mood switches from depressed to normal or hypomanic. They may say, "I feel fine. . . . I'll just start taking them if I feel sick again."

The major role of the clinician in these circumstances is to challenge these assumptions. For example, explain that drugs such as lithium, valproate, or SGAs do not work when they are taken intermittently, at the first sign of symptoms. When people are becoming manic, they feel better than usual and may believe that taking medicines is what made them ill in the first place. We have been surprised at how frequently the effects of medications become confounded in the patient's mind with a worsening of the illness.

It may help to acquaint or reacquaint the patient with the notion of *prophylaxis*. When patients are in maintenance treatment and have not had significant mood symptoms in some time, they may start to think of their mood stabilizers as they might think of antibiotics or antihistamines: "I'll take the pills when I'm ill and stop them once I feel better." It is best to remind them that people with bipolar disorder have underlying biological vulnerabilities that require them to take mood stabilizers for preventative purposes. Revisit the notion of a recurrence: a return of symptoms in someone who is biologically vulnerable but has been remitted from the illness for some time.

Acquaint the patient with the nature of biphasic fluctuation. High periods can indeed be enjoyable, but they are usually followed by a depression; in fact, at least 25% of manic or hypomanic episodes are followed *immediately* by a depressive episode.[17] For that reason alone, patients need to be protected by mood-stabilizing agents when well or hypomanic. Of course, many patients—especially those who are currently hypomanic—deny that they will ever relapse again. They may say, "I've got a handle on it now" or "If you want, I'll call you if I think I'm getting worse." Engaging caregivers in the oversight of patients who have discontinued their medications is usually essential in these cases.

### "I miss my high periods and my creativity."

Does a fish know when it's wet? Hypomania felt good to me. It didn't feel at all like there was anything wrong to me, it felt great, and I'd been feeling bad for so long. So I went off my medication, and then I started getting higher and higher. People told me to go back on, but it felt patronizing. I resented their lack of recognition that I was accomplishing things. . . . But then I cycled into a depression and got suicidal.
—38-year-old man with bipolar I disorder[18] (p. 138)

Many patients with bipolar disorder say that mood stabilizers make them feel flat, unemotional, or mildly depressed. They miss the excitement and vitality that often come with (hypo)manic periods. Even if they do not experience mania as a happy state, they may resent the idea that their moods are being controlled by medicines. Many have a love–hate relationship with their own moods. Although they may hate the fact that their emotions and energy levels swing so widely and cause such damage, they may believe that the highs and lows are central to who they are. Acknowledge to the patient that you comprehend these internal conflicts. To be told that you need pills to bring your emotions under control can be extraordinarily humiliating and invalidating. Moreover, missing out on the high periods can feel like a tremendous loss.

If the patient is artistically inclined, she may feel that mood variability is essential to her creativity. As we discussed in Chapter 2, the association between bipolar illness and creativity has been well documented, with many writers or poets (e.g., Ernest Hemingway, Robert

Lowell, Virginia Woolf), artists (Vincent van Gogh, Eduard Munch, Jackson Pollock), and musicians (Ludwig van Beethoven, Robert Schumann) having had periods of (hypo)mania and depression.[19] The mechanisms linking bipolar illness and creativity are not well understood, although high energy, goal directedness and being able to "think outside the box" are often characteristic of highly creative periods.[20]

Start this discussion with a statement of validation, such as "You're absolutely right. Mood stabilizers can make you feel flat. Taking them can mean giving up on the emotional roller coaster, which can be very intoxicating." If the patient is an artist, you can also add, "I don't doubt that mood stabilizers can make it harder to write [paint, play music]. It can be harder to be creative when you feel like you're being kept in this very narrow emotional bandwidth."

Follow up this statement with a discussion of the patient's short- and longer-term goals. An artist may have a commission that must be completed by a certain date. A writer may have a publishing deadline. Remind her that she wants to get back to work, make money, finish her degree, have a romantic relationship, or have a better connection with her children. A good question is, "What do you want to see happen in the next 3 or 6 months? Will medications help you get there? If not, help me understand why not."

If you are the treating psychiatrist, this may be an opportunity to review the patient's dosing plan. During the maintenance phase, some patients function well on a lower dose of lithium or may no longer need their SGA. If the patient is complaining of the negative effects of medications on her creativity or productivity, it may make sense to compromise on lower doses with more frequent monitoring during maintenance care. Although this is far from a fail-safe solution, it may avoid outright medication discontinuation.

## "My medications don't work."

Many patients go through numerous medication adjustments for their disorder but still have residual symptoms of depression or anxiety, or breakthrough episodes of varying levels of severity. Understandably, some come to the conclusion that their medications are ineffective. The reality is that the mood symptoms of bipolar disorder, and particularly the depressive symptoms, are only partially controlled by medications. Therefore, the role of the psychiatrist and other clinical team members is to determine whether the patient's regimen has been optimized. It may be that the patient would respond better to one mood stabilizer over another, that dosages are inadequate, or that there are too many agents in the regimen. However, none of these changes will be effective if the patient is resistant to taking medicines at all.

Ask the patient to keep a mood chart, so that the effects of any recent medication adjustments or instances of nonadherence/inconsistency can at least be recorded. After keeping a record for 1 month or more, the patient may come to recognize that there has been some improvement on the current regimen. If she is married or lives with a parent with whom she has a positive relationship, consider asking her to involve the spouse or parent in tracking her mood or sleep patterns, especially after a change in medications. Relatives may report changes of which the patient is unaware, such as smiling more often, being more energetic in doing housework or cooking, being less irritated at little things, or being more like her old self. The patient may still believe that none of the medications have been helpful, but these observations from relatives may make her reconsider stopping all her treatments.

### "Taking medications means giving up control to my family."

Many individuals, and especially younger patients, complain bitterly about the child-like role in which bipolar illness has placed them. Whereas they may have been quite competent and independent before their first period of illness, one or more episodes may have left them dependent on their parents at financial, emotional, and pragmatic levels. Married or cohabiting patients may complain that their spouses watch them carefully to see whether they are overreacting to people or events, and are quick to call the physician to ask about a higher medication dosage whenever the patient argues with them. This dynamic leads some patients to believe that their caregivers are using medication as a weapon to keep them in their place. Then, they think about discontinuing medicines as a way of fighting back.

An 18-year-old patient hid lithium tablets all over his house, so that his mother would find them—on the kitchen counter, next to the toilet, under her pillow. When she confronted him, he told her, "You're the one who needs them, so I left them for you to take." A 45-year-old man expressed annoyance that his wife would repeatedly ask him, "How is it with the pills today?" even if they were in the company of others. He taunted her by picking up the pills, pretending he was going to take them, then approaching her, saying, "Open your mouth, here comes the airplane!" In such scenarios, it is easy for clinicians to find themselves unwittingly supporting the efforts of the caregiver, and alienating the patient in the process.

We have also seen the reverse, in which parents or spouses actively discourage patients from taking their medications. A 17-year-old who had previously excelled at sports, and who had developed hand tremors from valproate, was told by his father, "You look like a 'spaz,'" when he played basketball with his team. The husband of a 36-year-old woman told her that she was "getting pudgy and unsexy" now that she was taking valproate and quetiapine (Seroquel).

The best way of dealing with these issues is to bring in the patient's parents or spouse and have a family session in which medications—their potential role in the patient's recovery, side effects and dosing, and the patient's need to feel some degree of control in taking them—are discussed openly. The objective is for the patient to feel that the decision to take medicines has been mainly hers, and for the parents or spouse to feel confident that she is making good choices, such that careful monitoring is no longer necessary. Consider the following segment from a family therapy session with a 25-year-old male and his parents:

CLINICIAN: So, I guess you're saying that if you go back on your lithium, it's got to be your decision.

PATIENT: Absolutely correct. My decision only.

CLINICIAN: And, it being your decision, you also want to be able to decide what dosage to take.

PATIENT: How much I want to take, when I take it, how often I get blood tests, and who will be my doctor.

CLINICIAN: Well, I'll certainly go along with that because the reality is that no one can force you to take lithium. What do you think about this, Mrs. Perez [mother]?

MOTHER: We realize that. We never said we were going to make him take it or choose his doctor for him.

PATIENT: (*pausing*) It sure seemed like that's what you were saying.

CLINICIAN: Mr. Perez, can you tell Rich more about what your position is on this?

FATHER: He's 25. He can do what he wants. I don't see any reason for us to treat him like a little kid. (*to the patient*) But that's the way you act sometimes.

PATIENT: Well, that's how I end up feeling. Like a little kid who hasn't eaten his vegetables.

MOTHER: But when we ask you if you've taken it, you get all resentful and huffy, and then you start acting like a kid. And then we start acting like the parents of a little kid. It's not like anybody *wants* to be doing this.

From here, the clinician addressed the larger issue of the patient's struggles with independence, which had become derailed by his illness. He bitterly resented living at home, but at the same time was ill-prepared for full autonomy. His parents made clear that they got no satisfaction from monitoring his medications, and that it made them feel like the family was going backwards in time. They agreed that, at a minimum, he should fill his own prescriptions and schedule his own doctor appointments, tasks that he had left to his mother. The patient showed some awareness by the end of the session that feeling child-like was part of a two-way interaction between his parents and himself, in which everyone was enacting an uncomfortable role.

Once again, family problem solving can be useful. For example, the 18-year-old who hid lithium tablets from his mother generated a plan in which she left the four tablets on a plate for him in the morning, and he agreed to take them at the correct times of day. The contingency was that she could not ask about the pills unless she found them around the house or recognized one or more of his prodromal symptoms (in his case, giggling, overeating, and staying up excessively late), or if his blood level results indicated subtherapeutic dosages. Eventually, he was able to take more responsibility for other aspects of his treatment, such as calling his physician for an appointment when his prescription needed to be refilled. All of these steps, however, required that she agree to reduce her "micromanaging" (her words).

### "Taking medicines means admitting I have an illness."

For some patients, agreeing to a regimen of mood stabilizers or second-generation antipsychotics feels like "being committed." It means admitting that their lives will be characterized by frequent trips to doctors, unpaid medical bills, hospitalizations, and the constant fear of being found out. They may have to acknowledge that their previous emotional reactions to social or family situations were inappropriate, despite feeling that they had been provoked by others. Taking medicines may mean admitting that their job or school problems were due largely to their own neurochemistry instead of nasty bosses and teachers, or that their inability to maintain romantic relationships was because of their impulsive, intrusive or inconsistent behavior rather than having chased "commitment phobics."

Admitting to a psychiatric illness means feeling different from everyone else, an especially big issue for teen and young adult patients. Psychiatric disorders still carry a significant social stigma. Patients may be haunted by hearing people speak in a derogatory way about the mentally ill (e.g., "That's all we need is for some psycho to show up here with a gun" or "Don't go all bipolar on me"). Furthermore, the stigma of the disorder can become equated with the stigma of taking medications. Among teens with bipolar disorder, lithium has a particularly bad reputation, which may explain why teens are more likely to accept drugs such as valproate.[21]

The first step in addressing these issues is to get into the mind-set of a person who is feeling stigmatized and having difficulty accepting the diagnosis. Feelings of shame, confusion, and resentment may be experienced intensely but are especially hard for the person to verbalize. If the patient has been diagnosed recently, then she may be trying to make sense of the doctor's and therapist's (possibly divergent) opinions, the meaning of blood tests, what the pills are and are not for, and why her family or friends are taking such a negative view of her behavior. In the example below, the psychotherapist validates the patient's viewpoint and clarifies the conditions under which she feels socially isolated by her illness. This 22-year-old woman had enrolled in community college after a depressed and psychotic episode.

> PATIENT: Taking any medicine makes me feel weird . . . like, different.
>
> CLINICIAN: Can you say more?
>
> PATIENT: I dunno, just like I'm marked, I'm taking crazy pills. I'm saying to the world that I'm mentally whacko and I need to be treated for it.
>
> CLINICIAN: That can't feel too good. Do you feel that way about just the pills, or these therapy sessions, too?
>
> PATIENT: Mostly the pills because they make me feel different, and I don't even know if they're working.
>
> CLINICIAN: How would you know if they're working? (*Redirects discussion toward the purposes of treatment.*)
>
> PATIENT: If I felt better. If I didn't feel anxious all the time, like I'm under a microscope . . . if I could sleep better, all the things we talked about.
>
> CLINICIAN: OK, I'm with you. I can see how you'd not want to take them if they made you feel different, or stigmatized, and you weren't even sure they were helping. (*Normalizes the patient's response.*)
>
> PATIENT: I won't say that I absolutely won't take them, I just don't want to. They make me feel bad about myself.

CLINICIAN: So, let's clarify what's making you feel this way. Was there something that happened that made you feel different because of your medications?

PATIENT: (*long pause, looks down*) I was eating lunch, and I remembered I hadn't taken my Adderall (dextroamphetamine mixed salts), and I was sitting with a group, and I kinda had to reach down into my backpack and find it, and then think of a way to swallow it without people seeing me. And I kind of choked on it, and somebody asked if I was OK. It was just really embarrassing, and I got upset. No one else was fishing around for pills in the middle of lunch. But then someone said that word I dread the most, "chill." Then I felt worse.

CLINICIAN: OK, let me see if I've got this right. It's not a particular pill, it's any pill where you end up feeling different from others, or where you might have to explain why you're taking them. Am I on the right track here?

The clinician has begun defining the problem: The patient felt like she was under a spotlight when taking medications at school. Later in the session, the clinician encouraged the patient to discuss her medication options with her physician. The patient was reluctant at first, believing that it was incorrect to challenge her doctor in this way. In fact, after hearing about her experiences, the treating physician made several changes to simplify the regimen, including substitution of extended release versions of her mood stabilizer and psychostimulant. Afterwards, the patient said she felt "empowered" by being able to solve this problem and liked feeling that she had collaborated in her own treatment planning.

### "Taking medications means giving up my hopes and aspirations."

Rarely do patients say this directly, but you may notice that when they discuss medications, it is accompanied by a sense of defeat. They may talk about having had to give up control over their lives, and revise their views of the future, so that it no longer includes having an education, a good marriage, children, or the quality of life they once took for granted. Caregiving relatives may contribute to these feelings of hopelessness. They may encourage the patient to apply for disability even though he can work, to take only one college class instead of the usual load of three or four, or not to trust himself to take care of his children.

The illness and its treatments can become mentally associated with giving up hopes and aspirations. The patient thinks about her life as bifurcated into the time before and after she became ill, or the time before or after she started taking medication. This process has been called *grieving over the lost healthy self*. [22] The prior self can be idealized as having been successful, beautiful, popular, and full of possibilities. The illness is then viewed as having destroyed all of these possibilities and replaced them with diminished potential and a lack of control over one's fate.

Some patients who discontinue their medicines are testing to see whether the prior self still exists. They may hope that their prior talents, energy, attractiveness, and potential will emerge once they are free of medicines. The risk of relapse is then denied altogether or seen as a low cost for regaining their more hopeful worldview. If you sense that these issues are in force, several interventions may be useful:

1. *Be empathic, but challenge cognitive distortions.* Patients usually feel validated by a clinician who acknowledges that, indeed, medicines can seem like the gatekeeper that prevents access to desired outcomes. But often implicit in grieving over the lost self are distorted beliefs about what it means to be ill and healthy. Some digging may be needed to bring those assumptions to light. For example, ask the patient to explain what is meant by words such as *control*. Does control over one's life mean never turning to anyone for help? Or can it mean availing oneself of opportunities to further one's life goals, which may include treatment? Enjoy with the patient her description of life before medications, but challenge the "black-and-white" thinking that may go along with her contrasts between the past and present. She may have had romantic relationships in the past that she remembers as fun, passionate, exotic, and exciting (and in all likelihood, mania-fueled). With additional details, she may admit that these relationships were short-lived, degrading, and damaging to her self-esteem. If she is partnered now, she may be able to see the value in a relationship that may not be as exciting and unpredictable as those in the past, but that may offer comfort, companionship, self-worth, and other benefits to her life and health.

2. *Help the patient adapt her goals to the realities of the illness.* Instead of giving up her desire to get a doctoral degree, she could adjust her academic timeline to avoid becoming overwhelmed by stress. These adjustments, which may require obtaining "reasonable accommodations" from teachers or educational counselors, may include taking a

lighter course load or obtaining approval to extend deadlines. True, she may not be able to stay up late at night like other degree-bound students, but with more time and mood stability and a regular daily and nightly routine, she may be able to finish her degree.

3. *Help the patient view medications as a route to achieving her life goals.* In motivational interviewing,[23] a treatment originally designed for individuals with addictive behaviors, the clinician helps the patient clarify her values and then evaluate the decision to abuse substances in light of these belief systems. The same approach applies to bipolar patients who are struggling with medicines. Ask the patient to consider whether there is any chance that the medicines will help her get where she wants. If she is still living with her parents, and has already had several mood episodes related to nonadherence, she may be able to see that consistency with treatment is a route to achieving greater autonomy rather than an obstacle.

## SUMMARY

Nonadherence may emerge at any time. In this chapter we have focused on the maintenance period, in which the patient has enough clinical stability and cognitive resources to think through the pros and cons of treatment. Intervening in the ways we have suggested here may or may not help the patient accept the long-term necessity of psychotropic medications for mood stability, but it may help the patient clarify her long-term goals and what the illness has meant for her life; understand the role of family members in her treatment decisions; and challenge pessimism regarding the illness and its implications for the future. On a more practical level, addressing nonadherence may open a discussion about the current regimen and whether the dosing patterns or medication choices are optimal. The patient may learn simple strategies for reminding herself to take pills at the right times. Finally, family members may learn how to be helpful without creating a backlash.

# ─── CHAPTER 9 ───

# Bipolar Disorder, Pregnancy, and the Postpartum Period

Pregnancy and the postpartum period pose special considerations for bipolar women. This unique period requires that clinicians weigh the risks of treatment for the mother against the risks for the baby. Moreover, untreated bipolar disorder carries its own risks for a developing fetus. Clinicians and patients have to consider multiple risk and protective factors in the woman's life before agreeing on appropriate treatment recommendations.

## BIPOLAR DISORDER IN WOMEN

There are a few important gender differences in the expression of bipolar disorder.[1] Although men and women are equally likely to have bipolar I disorder, bipolar women spend more time depressed than do bipolar men. Additionally, women are somewhat more likely to have bipolar II disorder, to show mixed states (as opposed to only euphoric manias) and, according to some studies, to show a rapid-cycling pattern of episodes (e.g., Schneck et al.[2]). Some medications prescribed for bipolar disorder show different side effects in women than in men. As examples: Valproate (Depakote) is associated with polycystic ovarian (PCO) disease in women. Although antipsychotics increase prolactin levels in both men and women, hyperprolactinemia in women can cause menstrual irregularities.[3]

None of these differences need alter the core approach to diagnosis and treatment that we have outlined in this book. The key consideration is that the typical age of onset of bipolar disorder—late teens to early 20s—coincide with the time in a woman's life in which she may become pregnant. Thus, the management of bipolar disorder during the childbearing years presents a unique set of dilemmas. In this chapter, we review medication considerations for the treating psychiatrist or obstetrician-gynecologist (OB-GYN), and psychosocial methods for the psychotherapist. The key pharmacological questions to be addressed include the following:

1. What is the course of bipolar disorder during pregnancy?
2. What are the risks for the bipolar mother in the postpartum period?
3. What are the risks to the fetus of the medications prescribed for the mother's bipolar disorder?
4. How should we think about the interaction of breastfeeding and psychotropic medications?

The key psychosocial questions include the following:

1. What is the psychosocial context of the pregnancy?
2. Are there adequate social supports for parenting should the mother develop a mood episode before or after delivery?
3. What is the status of the spousal relationship, if there is a spouse?
4. What has been the patient's history of having episodes that are related to major life changes?

Some patients decide to use psychotherapy as their sole treatment during and after pregnancy because of the potential teratogenic effects of mood-stabilizing medications. In that event, there must be clear and regular communication between the psychotherapist, treating psychiatrist (if there is one), and OB-GYN.

## THE COURSE OF BIPOLAR DISORDER
## DURING PREGNANCY

It is clinically wise to discuss pregnancy-related issues *before* a bipolar woman becomes pregnant. Of course, many women (and, probably, many more men) are less than rigorous about maintaining optimal birth control in order to avoid unwanted pregnancies. This may be especially the case for bipolar women who have higher rates of substance abuse than the population at large, potentially leading to impulsive sexual behavior. Additionally, when manic or hypomanic, sexual acting out—often without birth control—is very common. Therefore, a discussion about sexuality and birth control early in treatment is a very sound clinical practice. If appropriate and desired by the patient, this might evolve into a more detailed discussion about the specific medications that the patient is taking and the potential teratogenic risks of each of these individual agents, such that a plan is developed before the patient becomes pregnant. Furthermore, pregnancy-related issues are the most complex among all topics surrounding medication use in bipolar disorder, and each patient comes to the discussion with a different viewpoint. The involvement of a spouse/partner/significant other, if present, should be strongly encouraged.

In the past, pregnancy was considered a time of unusually good mental health for women. In this view, women were less vulnerable to mood difficulties while pregnant because of either or both of the following factors: (1) psychological protective factors, such as the positive feelings about being pregnant; or (2) biological factors, such as the positive mood effects of higher levels of hormones, especially estrogen. Extrapolating from these ideas, it was reasonable for bipolar women to consider discontinuing effective preventative mood agents before conception or upon pregnancy confirmation.

Unfortunately, more recent studies contradict these older myths. At this point, there is little consistent evidence to suggest that women with mood disorders are particularly psychologically healthy during pregnancy. Risk of a mood episode during pregnancy extends across all three trimesters.[4] Additionally, results from a large naturalistic study indicate that bipolar women show higher rates of mood episodes during pregnancy than do women with unipolar major depressive disorder.[5]

In the single best prospective study, the overall risk for bipolar women (some of whom were taking preventative medications, whereas others were not) to experience at least one mood episode during pregnancy was a startling 71%, with the highest risk for an episode in the first trimester.[6] Of note, depressive relapses during pregnancy were far more common than manic/hypomanic episodes, even in bipolar I disorder, consistent with the overall view that depression is the dominant pole of bipolar disorder.[6]

It is difficult to estimate the potential negative effects of mania during pregnancy on the fetus and the infant, since findings are confounded by other variables such as medication use (see below) and higher rates of cigarette smoking, which independently predict a poorer outcome in the neonate. Depression during pregnancy, whether part of bipolar disorder or not, is associated with higher rates of cigarette smoking, drinking alcohol, lower birthweight, and possibly higher rates of preterm delivery.[7]

Some, but not all, retrospective studies have found similar results:[8] Relapse rates among bipolar women during pregnancy are relatively high, although rates are usually lower than the 70+% in the study noted earlier. In contrast, a few case series and many individual clinical anecdotes testify to the smaller group of bipolar women who remain psychologically well with no medications during pregnancy. As expected, women with a more highly recurrent mood disorder, longer duration of illness, and a rapid-cycling pattern are at higher risk for pregnancy-related relapse.[5] Thus, the bipolar women who have the highest likelihood of doing well psychiatrically during pregnancy have milder symptoms and longer intervals between episodes.

Mood-stabilizer regimens seem to decrease episodes during pregnancy in bipolar women, just as they do in nonpregnant women. Although no randomized controlled studies have been done, all three of the prospective studies—which compared bipolar women who decided to discontinue their psychotropic medications either just before pregnancy, or when finding out about the pregnancy, to women who continued their medications—showed a clear protective effect of medications. In the best of the prospective studies, the rates of mood episodes in women with discontinued versus continued medications were 86 and 37%, respectively, a marked difference.[6] A more recent study found respective relapse rates of 40 versus 19%, lower relapse rates but a similar proportional difference.[9] Additionally, those who discontinued their medications more rapidly (i.e., within 2 weeks) relapsed far more quickly compared to those who tapered their medications slowly. Since unplanned pregnancies are, not surprisingly, associated with rapid medication discontinuation schedules, this points to the importance of an earlier discussion about pregnancy, preferably before pregnancy occurs, to allow the option of decreasing medications slowly.

## THE COURSE OF BIPOLAR DISORDER DURING THE POSTPARTUM PERIOD

Whereas there is some controversy as to the course of bipolar disorder during pregnancy, there is little doubt that the risk of mood episodes in the postpartum period is significantly higher than in any other time of a woman's life, much higher than during pregnancy, and higher than at any time in a man's life. Postpartum mood episodes are almost three times higher in the postpartum period compared to the relapse risk in an age-matched group of nonpregnant women with bipolar disorder.[10]

Soon after delivery, postpartum mood episodes must be distinguished from the milder and normal "baby blues," a syndrome characterized by affective lability and intense affect that occurs in 40–70% of women and is, by itself, nonpathological and self-limited.[11] Baby blues typically emerge within the first few days postpartum and resolve without treatment (except reassurance) by approximately the 10th day. Symptoms of genuine postpartum mood episodes may also begin within days to a few weeks postpartum, making the distinction between baby blues and postpartum mood episodes somewhat difficult in the first few days of symptoms. More severe and continuous (vs. intermittent) symptoms, psychotic symptoms, and the presence of any suicidal or homicidal thoughts (typically toward the infant) are all clear markers of a postpartum mood episode and should trigger more serious clinical evaluation and treatment.

The vast majority (90%) of *postpartum psychoses*, a term that refers to severe postpartum episodes with overt psychotic features that cut across diagnostic lines (major depression, bipolar disorder, schizoaffective disorder, etc.), typically emerge within the first 4 weeks postpartum.[12] In postpartum psychoses, delusions frequently involve the infant and may include homicidal fantasies (e.g., "It would be better if my child were dead given the coming catastrophes in the world"). Many, if not most, instances of infanticide in the postpartum period are associated with postpartum psychoses. Of note, when women with no prior mood history develop their first postpartum psychiatric episode during the postpartum period, and develop severe symptoms within 2 weeks (usually requiring hospitalization), they are likely to have a bipolar diagnosis later.[13] Thus, women with a first major psychiatric disorder in the immediate postpartum period should be carefully screened for bipolar mood symptoms.

Postpartum mood episodes in bipolar women may be manic/hypomanic, mixed, or depressive, similar to any other time. Similar to antepartum mood episodes, in the postpartum period, both bipolar I and bipolar II women are more likely to experience depression than mania or hypomania. In a naturalistic study that followed 2,252 women with mood disorders in two clinics specializing in pregnancy-related psychiatric disorders, 38% of bipolar I women and 34% of bipolar II women had major psychiatric episodes in the 6 months following delivery.[5] These rates were approximately twice as high as those seen in nonbipolar depressed women. In bipolar I women, half of the episodes were depression, almost one-fourth were manic/hypomanic, and 16% were mixed. In bipolar II women, the vast majority (85%) of postpartum episodes were depressive in nature.

The most important risk factor for a postpartum mood episode in women with either bipolar disorder or major depression is a past history of a postpartum mood episode. Other risk factors include having fewer children, younger age of illness onset, and, most importantly, a history of mood difficulties during pregnancy.[5] Interestingly, women with a history of only postpartum mood episodes (i.e., those who have never had a mood episode at any other time) seem to be at low risk for mood problems during or between pregnancies.[8] Women with mood problems during pregnancy and those with a past history of postpartum mood episodes constitute a rather high-risk group and should be carefully followed during the postpartum period.

## GENERAL CONSIDERATIONS FOR TREATING MOOD EPISODES DURING PREGNANCY

Given the relatively high rates of antepartum mood episodes in bipolar women and the even higher rates of postpartum episodes, issues of preventing and/or treating these episodes inevitably arise. All agree that, optimally, pregnant women should avoid any and all medications that might be associated with negative effects on the fetus. Therefore, psychotherapy should be considered for mild to moderate depressive episodes during both the antepartum and postpartum periods. Unfortunately, psychotherapy has virtually always been evaluated in the context of pharmacotherapy, and it is unclear whether it would have preventative effects in the absence of concurrent medications.

One approach that is applicable to pregnant and postpartum women with bipolar or unipolar depression is mindfulness-based cognitive therapy (MBCT).[14] This eight-session group treatment focuses primarily on teaching mindfulness meditation, and secondarily, on how to track and observe negative cognitions. It has been studied mainly in people with unipolar depression, where evidence suggests that it is more effective than usual care in preventing recurrences in patients who have had three or more prior episodes.[15] One study of 160 patients with major depressive disorder found that MBCT was just as effective in preventing recurrences as continuation therapy with antidepressants in "unstable remitters."[16] Thus, it may be applicable to pregnant or postpartum women with bipolar I or bipolar II disorder who have had recurrent periods of depression.

Group sessions of MBCT (or its close relative, *mindfulness-based stress reduction*) can often be obtained in community clinics for free. Because these are skills-oriented groups that do not delve into the patient's current interpersonal problems, it is less critical that other group members be pregnant or have mood disorders. The central premise is that individuals with histories of depression are vulnerable to recurrences of episodes of sadness, during which negative thinking patterns become reactivated and can trigger the onset of new depressive episodes. Mindfulness aims to interrupt the tendency to respond with strong negative emotions to pessimistic thoughts or bodily sensations that occur during sad mood. Interrupting these automatic processes requires individuals to notice and step out of their usual nonintentional response modes with intentional, nonjudgmental, and present-focused awareness.[14]

Consider how mindfulness applied in the treatment of a woman with bipolar I disorder.

---

Sarah, a 36-year-old woman with a husband and two children, was diagnosed with bipolar I disorder, with three severe major depressive episodes and one manic episode in the past 2 years. She had lost her job, and her relationship with her husband and children had become strained. At the time she started MBCT groups, she was (by choice) not taking any medications.

Being in a group with other patients with bipolar and unipolar disorder helped to "normalize" Sarah's experiences of depression, including her feelings of lethargy and fatigue, which she had previously attributed to laziness or weakness rather than to the nature of bipolar disorder. She also found mindfulness practice to be helpful in dealing with her racing thoughts. When practicing a sitting meditation, she was increasingly able to take a nonjudgmental "observing stance" toward her thoughts. When she did so, she reported the subjective sense that her thoughts were slowing down. She also used this strategy outside of her formal meditation practice when she noticed these racing thoughts returning.

Sarah reported that practicing directed awareness helped her to notice earlier when she was becoming upset and angry. Specifically, she found the practice of the 3-minute breathing space[14] (see Figure 11.1 in Chapter 11) to be useful. She began to use the 3-minute breathing space when she noticed physical sensations of anger (clenched jaw) or particular thoughts ("He always does this to me!"). Typically, such states would spiral to angry outbursts; however, using her mindfulness practice allowed Sarah to observe this cycle closely and to practice more effective alternative responses, such as articulating to her husband what had upset her. She reported that these changes were gradually having a positive impact on their relationship.

Sarah reported that, prior to the MBCT course, she had had difficulty recognizing the early warning signs of depression and mania. During the course, she began to recognize that experiencing everyone else as slow, observing an increased speed of her thinking, and feeling particularly good about herself were early signs of an oncoming manic episode. The reverse symptoms (e.g., experiencing others as too fast, a slowing down of her thinking) more typically heralded the beginning of a depressive episode.

At the end of the course, Sarah wrote a relapse prevention letter to herself, incorporating the early warning signs of mania and depression and the specific behavioral steps she could take when she noticed these occurring. Use of mindfulness skills played prominently in her plans. She listed "disclosing my mood changes to my husband and asking him for help"—for example, requesting his assistance with their children—as an important component of the relapse plan.[17] (pp. 379–380)

---

## PROS AND CONS OF PSYCHIATRIC MEDICATIONS DURING PREGNANCY

For many women with bipolar disorder, the decision whether to take medications or not during pregnancy is a very complicated one. There is no evidence that psychotherapy alone will prevent or treat manic episodes. Furthermore, many bipolar depressive episodes do not respond to psychotherapy. On the one hand, we should all be wary of any medication that may have potentially harmful (or more likely, unclear effects) on the fetus/infant. Any medication ingested by a pregnant woman will cross the placental barrier and expose the developing fetus to its effects. (The relative concentration in the fetal vs. maternal circulation differs across individual agents, but the fetus is always exposed to *some* amount of the medication.) On the other hand, untreated mood episodes during pregnancy and in the postpartum period can have significant adverse consequences on both mother and fetus, and later, the infant. Therefore, all decisions in this area should be made after careful consideration of the risks and benefits of each option, much discussion with the woman and her partner (if available), and equally clear documentation of the discussion.

In general, the more severe the bipolar disorder, the more reasonable it would be to continue preventative medications during pregnancy. Severity could be measured by either how frequently and/ or recently serious mood episodes occurred or by the intensity of the episodes themselves. Thus, a bipolar woman whose episodes occurred every 3 years without preventative treatment is more likely to do well during pregnancy without medications than a woman who cycles at least yearly. Similarly, a woman with bipolar II disorder who has relatively mild depressions and hypomanias can more easily consider being off mood stabilizers during pregnancy than a bipolar I woman who suffers psychotic manias and suicidal depressions.

---

Edith was 32 years old. Since her late teens, she had struggled with bipolar II disorder characterized by severe and frequent depressions and less severe hypomanic episodes. After trying many combinations of mood stabilizers and antidepressants, she did well on an initial combination of lamotrigine (Lamictal) and bupropion (Wellbutrin). A few years later, she discontinued the bupropion and for years was mostly euthymic on lamotrigine alone. When she and her partner decided to have a child, in consultation with her psychiatrist, Edith tapered and then discontinued her lamotrigine prior to conception. Off lamotrigine, she clearly became more "moody," with brief times of hypomania and some depression, but she was not incapacitated. During her first trimester of pregnancy, she continued to have mood swings that were uncomfortable but manageable. She resumed lamotrigine after the first trimester, became less moody, and continued the lamotrigine for the rest of the pregnancy. At birth, her baby was normal in all respects.

---

A key background fact that should always be discussed when considering medications during pregnancy is the 2–4% base rate (1 in 25 to 1 in 50) of major fetal malformations in healthy women who are not taking medications.[18] Inevitably, when problems arise, such as fetal malformations, there is an inherent tendency to look for a cause of the problem—or someone or something to blame. If medications have been taken during pregnancy, it is easy to attribute the malformation to the medication, even if that particular malformation is not associated with that particular medication. Awareness of the high base rate of fetal malformations does not preclude misattributions and blaming but may help balance the patient's and family's perceptions of risk.

Four different types of potential negative effects of medications on fetuses/infants, listed in Table 9.1, should be considered. The first type relates to potential effects on the overall course of the pregnancy, such as increased risk of miscarriage, higher rates of preterm birth, and/or lower birthweight. The second is that of classic fetal malformations or abnormalities of structure, almost always due to first-trimester effects. Avoiding these abnormalities gives rise to the option of discontinuing medications before conception and restarting them in the beginning of the second trimester, thereby avoiding early fetal malformations but not later pregnancy-related effects. Fetal abnormalities include congenital heart defects, neural tube defects (including spina bifida) that affect

**TABLE 9.1. Potential Short- and Long-Term Effects of Medication During Pregnancy**

Pregnancy-related parameters
- Risk of miscarriage
- Rates of preterm birth
- Birthweight

Teratogenic effects
- Fetal malformations, derived from first-trimester exposure

Neonatal toxicity
- Lung development, including primary pulmonary hypertension
- Toxicity at birth
- Withdrawal symptoms at birth

Developmental abnormalities (months or years later)
- Delays in developmental milestones
- Intelligence
- Motor coordination
- Attachment capability

the structure of the spinal cord, and hypospadias (abnormality in the development of the urethra in the penis).

The third type are the toxic effects on the fetus or newborn caused by exposure in the third trimester. These would include (1) abnormalities in the late stages of lung development, (2) hypothyroidism caused by exposure to a thyrotoxic medication (including lithium), and (3) irritability in the neonate as a side effect of a stimulating medication taken by the mother during pregnancy or withdrawn during the postpartum period.

The fourth group of potentially negative effects are developmental in nature and would not necessarily be apparent for months or years. These include abnormalities in IQ, psychomotor coordination, and attachment capabilities. Of course, in considering any of these outcomes, we must consider the inherent base rate of these abnormalities, and the potential effect of untreated psychiatric disorders as possible causes.

### Risks of Mood Stabilizers

Table 9.2 summarizes information on the effects of psychotropic medications on pregnancy and fetal development.

**TABLE 9.2. Medications for Bipolar Disorder in Pregnancy**

| Medication/ medication class | First trimester/ teratogenic concerns | Third trimester/immediate postpartum concerns |
|---|---|---|
| Lithium | Ebstein's anomaly (cardiac defects)— absolute risk low | Floppy-baby syndrome Neonatal hypothyroidism *Caution re*: lithium levels around delivery |
| **Anticonvulsants** | | |
| Valproate | Neural tube defects Facial abnormalities | Developmental delays Liver abnormalities |
| Lamotrigine | Cleft lip/palate | |
| Carbamazepine | Neural tube defects | Developmental delays Fingernail hypoplasia |
| Antipsychotics | | Tremors, increased muscle tone, restlessness, weight gain (with some agents) and its complications |
| Benzodiazapines | Cleft lip/palate (with diazepam) | Neonatal lethargy; decreased muscle tone; poor feeding; withdrawal symptoms such as tremor, irritability, diarrhea |
| **Antidepressants** | | |
| SSRIs | Heart defects (especially paroxetine) | Pre-term labor, lower birth weight Primary pulmonary hypertension (PPH) Neonatal adaptation syndrome |
| Other modern antidepressants | | Few studies |
| Tricyclics | Unknown | Maternal weight gain with some agents |
| MAO inhibitors | | Fetal growth abnormalities Hypertensive episodes |

## Lithium

Because it is the oldest of the mood stabilizers, there is a reasonable amount of information about lithium during pregnancy.[19] The major teratogenic effect of lithium is the higher rate of fetal cardiovascular abnormalities, especially *Ebstein's anomaly,* an abnormality characterized by structural changes in cardiac valves and ventricles in infants exposed to lithium during the first trimester. Ebstein's anomaly is 20–40 times more common in lithium-exposed infants than in the general population. At first glance, this sounds alarming. However the base rate of Ebstein's anomaly is 1 in 20,000; thus, a 20–40 times increase means that only 1 in 500 to 1 in 1,000 lithium-exposed infants will develop this abnormality. It is important that we help our patients distinguish between relative risk, 20–40 times higher in this case, and absolute risk, 1 in 500 to 1 in 1,000, which is low. Ebstein's anomaly can be diagnosed by ultrasound and fetal echocardiography at 16–18 weeks of pregnancy.

Lithium is also occasionally associated with "floppy-baby syndrome," characterized by poor muscle tone, lethargy and cyanosis, and neonatal hypothyroidism caused by exposure of the fetal thyroid gland to the known negative effects of lithium on thyroid function (see Chapter 6). These effects are generally assumed to be transient. Lithium has not been shown to affect developmental milestones negatively in the few small studies evaluating this question.

Lithium blood levels change, often substantially during the course of pregnancy and delivery. As pregnancy progresses, lithium excretion by the kidneys increases and lithium levels decrease, usually requiring an increase in the dose to maintain a steady lithium blood level. At delivery, this effect is dramatically and quickly reversed, and lithium doses must be decreased to avoid lithium toxicity. Dehydration significantly increases the likelihood of lithium toxicity and must be avoided. A reasonable approach would be to decrease the lithium dose by half at the beginning of labor. Above all, lithium levels must be monitored regularly during pregnancy and around the time of delivery to simultaneously avoid toxic and inadequate blood levels.

### Anticonvulsants

As a class, anticonvulsants are relatively teratogenic but with substantial differences across the individual agents. A *combination* of anticonvulsants, especially when one of the agents is valproate, increases the risk of malformations compared to the use of single-agent anticonvulsants.[20] Valproate plus lamotrigine is probably the most common combination of anticonvulsants for maintenance treatment of bipolar disorder.

#### VALPROATE

Of all the mood stabilizers, valproate is the agent most associated with clear negative effects on fetal development. In a dose-related manner, valproate significantly increases the risk of neural tube defects, with rates of 5–9% due to exposure specifically during the first month of pregnancy (when the spinal cord is being formed).[19] If at all possible, it should be avoided during pregnancy, especially during the first trimester. Furthermore, discontinuing valproate once pregnancy is confirmed is usually too late to avoid its effect on neural tube formation, making unplanned pregnancies particularly problematic. In general, folate supplementation in daily doses of 3–5 mg reduces the overall risk of neural tube defects, although it is still unclear whether it specifically reduces the risk of valproate-associated defects.

There is evidence of other, nonspecific anomalies associated with valproate exposure during pregnancy, including facial abnormalities, some of which resolve over time. Infrequently, valproate is associated with liver abnormalities in the neonate. Finally, there are suggestions that valproate may cause developmental delays.

## LAMOTRIGINE

Lamotrigine has a reasonable safe profile when taken during pregnancy. Virtually all studies in this area derive from women with epilepsy (which was the first FDA indication for lamotrigine) and not from those with bipolar disorder. Overall, major malformations are similar in infants exposed to lamotrigine during the first trimester compared to the general population. There is some evidence, however, that higher doses of lamotrigine may be associated with a slightly increased rate of malformations, notably cleft lip or cleft palate in infants exposed during the first trimester.[21] No behavioral problems or developmental delays have been seen so far in lamotrigine-exposed infants.

## CARBAMAZEPINE

Along with valproate, carbamazepine (Tegretol) has the most consistent evidence of teratogenic effects, and should be avoided in pregnancy if possible. Like valproate, it can cause neural tube defects, but at a lower rate.[22] It can also cause developmental delays and fingernail hypoplasia.

## Antipsychotics

There is a relatively large naturalistic database on the safety of antipsychotics in pregnancy. First-generation antipsychotics (FGAs) such as haloperidol (Haldol) and chlorpromazine (Thorazine) (described in more detail in Chapter 4) have been available for over half a century.

Overall, FGAs during pregnancy are not associated with fetal malformations (despite individual studies showing some risk). Some infants seem to show classic neurological side effects associated with FGAs, such as tremors, increased muscle tone, and restlessness. In the vast majority of cases, these side effects are transient and resolve within days after birth, assuming that there has been no further exposure to the medicine through breastfeeding. No developmental delays or diminished intelligence are found in infants exposed to FGAs *in utero*.[23]

Not surprisingly, there is less experience with SGAs in pregnant women because they have been available for less than half as long. No evidence to date suggests increased rates of fetal malformations, spontaneous abortions, or stillborns associated with SGAs taken during pregnancy, with the greatest amount of safety data available for risperidone (Risperdal), olanzapine (Zyprexa), quetiapine (Seroquel), and clozapine (Clozaril), the four oldest SGAs.[24] Of note, quetiapine crosses the placental barrier less well than the other antipsychotics, thereby exposing the fetus to lower levels of this medication than do the other agents.[25] So far, however, there is no evidence that this translates into greater safety. There are no good studies on developmental outcome or intelligence in infants exposed to SGAs *in utero*.

One other concern about antipsychotics taken during pregnancy is the likely higher risk of weight gain in the mother, particularly when taking olanzapine or quetiapine. Antipsychotics may increase the risk of weight-gain-related consequences including hypertension (high blood pressure) and gestational diabetes.

## Benzodiazepines

Benzodiazepines, such as clonazepam (Klonopin), lorazepam (Ativan), and alprazolam (Xanax) are often prescribed as sleep aids, tranquilizers, and adjunctively for manias/hypomanias. They may be prescribed for daily use or on an as-needed basis. The major concern about benzodiazepines during pregnancy is the inconsistent evidence of higher rates of cleft lips and palates in exposed fetuses, especially with diazepam (Valium).[26] Occasional (i.e., nondaily) use of benzodiazepines during the second and third trimester seems safe. However, infants born to mother who used benzodiazepines regularly during pregnancy may show transient lethargy, poor feeding, and diminished muscle tone soon after birth. Additionally, these infants may show transient symptoms consistent with benzodiazepine withdrawal, such as tremor, irritability, and diarrhea. Although there are few studies thus far, there is no evidence of developmental abnormalities in infants exposed to benzodiazepines *in utero*.

## Antidepressants

All information on the safety and risks of antidepressants during pregnancy are derived from studies of women with nonbipolar major depression. There may be additional risks in pregnant bipolar women that derive from taking antidepressants in conjunction with one or more mood stabilizers or atypical antipsychotics, but these differences have not been studied. Also, depression itself may be associated with some negative pregnancy-related outcomes such as lower birthweight or higher rates of preterm labor. Therefore, it is difficult at times to distinguish between the effects of depression in the course of bipolar disorder and the medication(s) used to treat it.

Overall, there is no evidence that antidepressants are consistently associated with increased fetal malformations or any specific malformation (e.g., in contrast to the association between valproate exposure and neural tube defects).[27] A few studies have shown a slightly higher risk of early miscarriage in depressed women taking antidepressants.[28] Other studies, but not all, have shown that depressed women taking antidepressants have higher rates of preterm birth (more prematurity) and lower birthweight in exposed infants compared to depressed women who are untreated (implying that the findings were due to the medications, not the depression).[29] However, the long-term health implications of these slightly premature births is unclear. Finally, there is no consistent evidence that *in utero* exposure to antidepressants causes any developmental delays, although there are few studies on this issue.[30]

We have more safety data on SSRIs than on any other antidepressant class due to their greater use during a time of more careful monitoring. Overall, SSRIs are not considered a medication class associated with fetal malformations.[31] A few studies show slightly increased rates of unusual abnormalities, such as omphalocele (an abnormality of the abdominal wall associated with extrusion of internal organs), but the absolute risk of this is very low. The more common concern is that of congenital heart defects, specifically, that of the septal wall. Some, but not all studies, have specifically implicated paroxetine (Paxil) as being associated with higher rates of cardiac defects.[32] Because of this, most experts recommend against the use of paroxetine as a new treatment for pregnancy-related depression.

Two third-trimester pregnancy-related concerns are (1) increased risk of primary pulmonary hypertension (PPH) and (2) neonatal adaptation syndrome. PPH, a syndrome at birth, manifests as difficulty in breathing in the newborn. There is inconsistent evidence that PPH is more likely in SSRI-exposed neonates.[33] Because it is still unclear whether there is a higher risk for PPH with SSRI-exposed neonates, there are no recommendations to alter third-trimester antidepressant treatment due to this concern. Neonatal adaptation syndrome, characterized by irritability/jitteriness, weak crying, temperature instability, and alterations in muscle tone, is seen in a minority of neonates exposed to SSRIs during the third trimester.[34] The cause of this syndrome is unclear and may reflect antidepressant withdrawal effects, antidepressant toxicity, or other unknown causes. These symptoms typically spontaneously resolve within 2 weeks.

## DUAL-ACTION ANTIDEPRESSANTS AND OTHER MODERN ANTIDEPRESSANTS

Much less information is available about the potential effects of other modern antidepressants on pregnancy. With the limited information we have, there are no known concerns regarding any of these medications, such as dual-action agents—venlafaxine (Effexor), duloxetine (Cymbalta), mirtazapine (Remeron), or bupropion (Wellbutrin). Given the smaller amount of safety information available for these medications during pregnancy, it is generally recommended that they be continued if an antidepressant is needed, but that they should not be the first antidepressant selected for pregnancy-related depression.

## OLDER ANTIDEPRESSANTS: TRICYCLICS AND MAO INHIBITORS

Tricyclic antidepressants are not known to be associated with negative effects on pregnant women and fetuses, but they typically are not used because of their overall side-effect profile.[26] If a tricyclic is prescribed, desipramine (Norpramin) and nortriptyline (Pamelor) are generally preferred due to lower rates of weight gain, sedation, and blood pressure changes. MAO inhibitors should generally be avoided during pregnancy, due to animal studies suggesting fetal growth abnormalities and concerns about the risk of hypertensive episodes associated with their use.[26] Given the infrequency of their use in the community in general, this issue rarely arises.

*Electroconvulsive Therapy*

As discussed in more detail in Chapter 6, ECT is generally considered a treatment for severe and/or treatment-refractory depression. It may also be effectively used to treat acute mania. Although it may seem jarring to consider its use during pregnancy, when used in pregnant women, it has few side effects and few adverse effects on the fetus or on the pregnancy.[35] There is no evidence of any long-term consequences in infants whose mothers had ECT while pregnant. Very infrequently, it can cause uterine contractions. Additionally, the medications used to facilitate ECT, such as the short-acting anesthetics, appear to be safe during pregnancy.

## GENERAL CONSIDERATIONS FOR TREATING POSTPARTUM MOOD EPISODES

As described earlier, bipolar women are uniquely vulnerable to postpartum mood episodes, both depressions and manias/hypomanias. Therefore, all bipolar women should be monitored closely in the postpartum period, especially during the first few weeks to 1 month after delivery, when the risk for mood episodes is highest. Considerations about the setting—outpatient, inpatient, or partial hospital for treatment of postpartum mood episodes—are the same as described in Chapters 4 and 5. The key difference in a postpartum and a nonpostpartum mood episode, of course, is reflected in the need for a plan to care for the infant, since very depressed and manic postpartum women may not be able to care properly and safely for their newborns.

Additionally, for those women taking medication postpartum, the issue of breastfeeding versus formula feeding arises. During pregnancy, it is not possible to separate medication exposure in the mother from that of the fetus, since all medications cross the placental barrier (albeit in different amounts). In the postpartum period, these risks can be separated, since, in the absence of breastfeeding, the mother can take medications without inherently exposing her infant to them. Thus, the risk of exposing the infant to the medication via breastfeeding must be balanced against the benefits of breastfeeding to the child and mother. Additionally, right after birth, infants' livers, kidneys, and blood–brain barriers are immature and not functioning nearly as effectively as they will even 6 months later. This translates into potentially higher blood levels of ingested medications and more of the medications crossing into the brain. As an example of the inefficient metabolism of newborns, the *half-life* of caffeine (which is indeed a psychotropic drug), defined as the amount of time it takes for half of the substance to be metabolized, is 90 hours in a neonate vs. 2.6 hours in a 6-month-old baby![36]

One general strategy for women who are breastfeeding is to take their psychiatric medications after feeding their infant or before the infant takes a long nap. Some women also pump their breast milk before they have taken their morning or evening dose. These strategies reduce the amount of medication to which the infant is exposed.

Another general issue about preventing and treating postpartum mood episodes is the sensitivity of individuals with bipolar disorder to sleep deprivation as a trigger or exacerbating factor for manic/hypomanic episodes. A mother of an infant who wants to breastfeed around the clock and/or take care of the bottle feeding in the middle of the night will inevitably be sleep deprived. Therefore, help from a significant other, a relative or a baby nurse, will allow the new mother to get enough sleep to avoid the mood consequences of sleep deprivation.

Finally, in considering the risks and benefits of medications in the postpartum period for bipolar women, we should distinguish between two situations:

1. A woman who has been taking a mood stabilizer regimen throughout pregnancy. In this situation, it is assumed that the same medication will be continued after birth, since the bipolar disorder was serious enough to warrant exposing the fetus during pregnancy. Here, the only question is whether to breastfeed.
2. A woman who has discontinued her medications pre-pregnancy or early in the first trimester. The options in this situation are whether to start the medication right after giving birth or only if mood symptoms arise. If medications are prescribed preventatively, they should be started as soon after birth as medically possible and usually with the same regimen as before pregnancy (except possibly lithium; see below).

Although there are few systematic studies in this area, preventative mood stabilizers lower the risk of postpartum mood episodes and should be strongly recommended if the woman is not breastfeeding.[37] For bipolar women who want to breastfeed and have not taken medications during pregnancy, the risk–benefit ratio for breastfeeding should be discussed with them and their partners during pregnancy, so that a plan is in place prior to delivery. Optimally, if no medications are prescribed during pregnancy or soon after delivery, they will be restarted once breastfeeding is discontinued.

### Psychiatric Medications and Breastfeeding

Just as all medications cross the placental barrier, all medications similarly cross into breast milk, albeit at different amounts. Table 9.3 summarizes information in this area.

### Lithium

Lithium is the best established medication for preventing postpartum mood episodes. Unfortunately, it crosses easily into breast milk, with levels at approximately 50% of maternal levels, and newborn lithium

**TABLE 9.3. Breastfeeding and Medications for Bipolar Disorder**

| Medication/medication class | Transmission into breast milk/infant blood levels | Potential side effects |
|---|---|---|
| Lithium | +++ | Lethargy, decreased muscle tone, hypothermia (low temperature), cyanosis |
| Anticonvulsants Valproate/ carbamazepine | ++ | Few |
| Lamotrigine | +++ | Few; *caution re*: potential rash risk |
| Antipsychotics First-generation agents | + | Few; occasional sedation |
| Second-generation agents | + | Few; occasional sedation |
| Benzodiazepines | + | Few; occasional sedation |
| Antidepressants | + | Few; occasional lethargy or agitation |

levels averaging 25% of the mother's levels. Furthermore, dehydration, to which infants are vulnerable, increases lithium levels further. Therefore, usual recommendations are for mothers either not to breastfeed when taking lithium or to do so with caution.[38] Symptoms/side effects consistent with lithium ingestion in newborns are lethargy, decreased muscle tone, low temperature, and increased creatinine (a measure of kidney function). If a woman taking lithium does breastfeed, lithium levels in the mother and infant should be monitored regularly.

## Anticonvulsants

Ironically, since they are the most teratogenic of all mood stabilizers, both valproate and carbamazepine are generally considered to be compatible with breastfeeding based on extensive experience in women with epilepsy.[38] Although both medications achieve measurable concentrations in breast milk, breastfeeding infants seem to have relatively low levels, and adverse events are rather infrequent.

Lamotrigine crosses into breast milk easily, with levels in the infant approximately 60% of those of the mother. Nonetheless, adverse events in newborns of mothers taking lamotrigine are few.[38] Because of concerns about severe rash in youngsters taking lamotrigine (see Chapter 6 for details), these infants should be monitored for skin eruptions.

## Antipsychotics

There are relatively few studies that have examined the safety of either FGAs or SGAs in breastfeeding women.[39] These meager data are complicated by the need to distinguish between infants exposed to the medication *in utero* and additionally during breastfeeding, and infants exposed during breastfeeding alone. However, individual case reports suggest that an occasional infant will show either higher than expected medication blood levels or some unusual side effect.

## Benzodiazepines

Benzodiazepines may be used to treat agitation—usually adjunctively to other agents—in postpartum mania. There are surprisingly infrequent reports of sedation in a breastfeeding neonate when the mother is taking benzodiazepines.[40] The other clinical concern is that if the breastfeeding mother takes benzodiazepines regularly, the infant is vulnerable to benzodiazepine withdrawal effects either when the medication is discontinued or when breastfeeding is stopped. Benzodiazepines with no active metabolites (e.g., lorazepam or clonazepam) are generally preferred for breastfeeding mothers. However, because of its relatively longer half-life, clonazepam may accumulate in breastfeeding infants.

## Antidepressants

Overall, antidepressants have a relatively benign side-effect profile in breastfeeding.[41] Again, all antidepressants are excreted into breast milk in measurable levels. Yet the blood levels of these antidepressants in breastfed infants are very low to nondetectable (which means the amount is low enough to be below the threshold for measurement; this is not the same as a level of zero). Consistent with this, the great majority of breastfed infants show no negative effects from maternal antidepressants. Occasional individual case reports describe an infant with both high blood levels of antidepressants and/or symptoms consistent with antidepressant side effects, such as either sedation or colic and crying. These, however, are exceptions to the general finding of low blood levels and no side effects.

## CLINICAL RECOMMENDATIONS

Given all the information reviewed earlier, we can derive some general guidelines. Of course, the nuances and details of individual patients' histories and personal convictions, such as "I do not want to expose my baby to any medications at all" versus "I will do anything to ensure that I do not have a manic or major depressive episode during pregnancy or after I deliver," will ensure that a different specific clinical plan will be chosen with each patient.

### Bipolar Women on Mood Stabilizers, Prepregnancy

In this situation, the question of whether to continue medication around the time of conception and/or the first trimester is the first topic to discuss. As noted earlier, with women with a more severe disorder—more frequent, more severe, or more difficult-to-treat episodes—the usual recommendation would be to continue on maintenance treatment unless the ongoing treatments are valproate or carbamazepine. In the latter circumstance, a gradual switch (i.e., cross-titration) to a different mood stabilizer well before attempting to conceive should be the first choice. The only reason to continue on either of these two mood stabilizers during conception and the first trimester would be the unusual circumstance of the patient having failed to respond to maintenance treatment with virtually all of the other mood stabilizers.

Bipolar women with a milder disorder may consider discontinuing their medications before conception. In this circumstance, a slow tapering over 2–4 weeks with monitoring is recommended. Any method to increase the likelihood of conception, so the woman can remain off medications as briefly as possible, should be discussed with the woman and her obstetrician. Some women want to remain off medications for as long as possible, often during the entire pregnancy. In others, staying off medication during the first trimester only to avoid teratogenic effects may suffice, and medications may be restarted in the beginning of the second trimester.

An unanticipated pregnancy while the bipolar woman is taking medication(s) presents a trickier set of options. Frequently, the awareness of pregnancy occurs after the majority of the first trimester has passed and the time of risk associated with first-trimester teratogenic effects has already occurred. Because sudden discontinuation of mood stabilizers predicts an earlier relapse, precipitously stopping mood stabilizers during weeks 10–12 of pregnancy may cause more problems than it solves. In this circumstance, a discussion about the previously described risks and benefits should take place as soon as the pregnancy is discovered.

### Breakthrough Episodes

Breakthrough mania during pregnancy should be treated with an antipsychotic as a first choice, either risperidone, olanzapine, quetiapine or the FGA, haloperidol. Each has specific advantages and disadvantages in side effects, such as sedation, weight gain, tardive dyskinesia, and extrapyramidal symptoms (see Chapter 4). Lithium should be considered a second-line treatment for a pregnant manic woman, whereas valproate should be avoided. ECT should be considered for very treatment-resistant mania.

Breakthrough depression during pregnancy may be treated in a number of ways. If at all possible, psychotherapy should be considered, since it may be helpful and is not known to have any negative effects on mother and/or fetus! Among the mood stabilizers, lamotrigine has the best efficacy for depression and, other than a potential risk for cleft palate/lip with first-trimester exposure (and even this risk is unclear), appears to be relatively benign in pregnancy. As noted earlier, other than paroxetine, SSRIs are relatively safe during the first trimester and have no obvious risk during the second trimester. Bupropion may be considered, especially if the woman has a past history of response to this agent. Finally, although currently only anecdotal data exist, transcranial magnetic stimulation (TMS) may be considered as a treatment for depression during pregnancy, since no medication is given during TMS, there are no known systemic effects, and the treatment occurs only around the skull/brain.[42]

Because of the controversies surrounding potentially negative effects of SSRIs during the third trimester, some experts recommend withdrawing antidepressants during that time. However, avoiding the potential negative effects of antidepressants during this time should be weighed against the potential advantage of taking the antidepressant preventatively just before the postpartum period given its high risk of depression.

## Preventing Postpartum Mood Episodes

When we first started to talk about having another child, my tendency toward postpartum depression was a big factor. Being depressed had been hard not only on me; it had been really hard on my husband too, seeing me go through it, worrying about me, having to do a lot of the child care, and dealing with the ways in which I treat him when I'm depressed. I knew I was at risk for getting depressed again if I had another baby—I wasn't sure if I should even try to get pregnant. I wanted to be a mother again, but I was afraid of what it would do to the people around me. I cried a lot. I'm glad we went ahead, but it was a hard decision.
       —A 39-year-old mother with bipolar I disorder[43] (p. 266)

Of course, the primary treatment goal in the postpartum period is the prevention of mood episodes. Thus, either the continuation of antepartum medications or the restarting of a previously effective regimen soon after birth is optimal. For the treatment of breakthrough episodes—either mania or depression—the usual options described in Chapters 4 and 5, respectively, should be considered. If the woman is breastfeeding, the ongoing use of lithium presents the greatest concern. Antipsychotics and valproate can be considered relatively safe options to treat mania in a breastfeeding woman.

Although bottle feeding can be recommended, the decision to breastfeed or not is often a very emotional one. The woman's decision may be linked to her feelings about the stigma of mental illness and guilt about the possibility of passing an illness on to her children. Overall, clinical strategies for preventing and treating mood episodes during and after pregnancy should be flexible and, if needed, creative. We present two cases, one treated pharmacologically and the other with psychotherapy.

## Preventing a Postpartum Mood Episode with Lithium and Quetiapine during the Antepartum Period

Marissa, now 30 years old, has had bipolar I disorder since age 19. After an early stormy course with three manic episodes and poor medication adherence, she has been mostly well for the last 5 years on lithium 1,200 mg daily, with a serum lithium level of 0.7. Because she was planning to become pregnant soon after recently getting married, she and her husband discussed the issues of bipolar disorder and medications with her psychiatrist. Marissa insisted on discontinuing her lithium in anticipation of conception. After a 4-week taper and discontinuation of lithium, Marissa became pregnant in her second month off lithium. During the first trimester of pregnancy, she was somewhat moody but was otherwise felt reasonably well. During her fifth month, however, she had a full manic episode. She agreed to take quetiapine given its relatively low rate of crossing the placental barrier into the fetal circulation. She responded well to daily doses of quetiapine 350 mg. After further discussion following the resolution of the manic episode, Marissa agreed to resume lithium, since she was beyond the first trimester, and was reassured that risk of Ebstein's anomaly was associated only with first-trimester exposure. With careful monitoring of her lithium level, Marissa did well for the rest of her pregnancy. She elected not to breastfeed and stayed on lithium after her baby was born (healthy). She did not have a mood episode during the postpartum period.

## Treating Postpartum Depression with MBCT

Eunice, age 29, had bipolar II disorder, and had gone off of her mood stabilizer and antidepressant to become pregnant. She had been episode-free during her pregnancy. She noticed the return of her depressive symptoms about 4 weeks after the baby was born. At first, she was able to manage these symptoms with weekly individual and couple sessions with her partner, Tom, following the IPSRT approach. The social rhythm regularity component of IPSRT posed significant challenges: How could one sleep regularly with a baby who would be up at irregular intervals? In a couple therapy session, Eunice and Tom devised a strategy that involved trading off nights, so that Eunice could get regular sleep on the nights she was not on duty. She would pump her breast milk during the day, and Tom would do the night feedings. During the day, Eunice made sure she had enough relaxed time when she was not with the baby, such as talking to a close friend who also had a baby.

Things took a turn for the worse when Eunice's mother became severely ill with pneumonia. Eunice, who felt caught between the needs of her infant and those of her mother, began to lose sleep. She could feel her depression returning but did not want to resume her medications. Her clinician focused their work on her assumptions about mothering (and "daughtering") and how she felt like a failure when either was not going well. She tended to "catastroph-ize" when she had a negative interaction with Tom, jumping to the conclusion that everything was falling apart. Eunice had taken mindfulness classes prior to her delivery, and she resumed a half-hour sitting meditation each morning. The goal was to observe her thoughts nonjudgmentally, as passing events in her mind, rather than trying to change them or worrying about their severity.

Eventually, Eunice learned to experience her thoughts as "like playing cards. . . . it's like I turn one over and some negative thing appears on each card, but I can also look at the card or turn it back over. . . . I'm able to react mindfully before I am emotionally hijacked." As her mother's illness began to stabilize, Eunice's postpartum depression began to subside.

## SUMMARY

As we have illustrated in this chapter, managing pregnancy and the postpartum period is a careful balancing act. The medications selected, the timing and dosing of those agents, and the introduction of psy-chotherapy can all contribute to a positive outcome for the mother and the baby. In future iterations of treatment guidelines, physicians may be able to help pregnant patients select treatments based on a numeri-cal weighing of costs and benefits. At present, the data to guide these decisions are not available. Psychotherapy is a viable alternative, but it should not be presented to the patient as an alternative to pharmaco-therapy; we have even fewer data indicating that bipolar disorder can be successfully managed with therapy alone. Nonetheless, appreciation of the psychosocial context of the pregnancy will help the clinician and patient to develop an integrated (and likely, more successful) treatment plan.

# CHAPTER 10

# Bipolar Disorder and Suicide

Suicide is the negative outcome of greatest concern for all psychiatric disorders. When a patient exhibits significant suicidal thinking or has made a suicide attempt in the recent past, heightened vigilance, increased anxiety and worry, and the psychological burden of caretaking increase dramatically for family members and mental health professionals alike. The risk of suicide is greater for people with mood disorders than for people with any other psychiatric disorder. Thus, suicide is especially relevant for those involved in the care of bipolar patients. In this chapter, we use the term *suicidality*, which refers to the group of clinical expressions related to suicide, and includes suicidal ideation (thinking about suicide), suicidal intent (having the will to commit suicide), self-harm (with nonsuicidal intent), suicide attempts, and completed suicide.

Not surprisingly in a disorder that is dominated by depressive symptoms, suicidal ideation is very common in bipolar disorder, with studies reporting that prevalence rates range from 14 to 59%.[1] This chapter provides an overview of what we know about suicide and its relationship to bipolar disorder, followed by a more detailed discussion of the evaluation and management of suicidality, including both psychological and pharmacological approaches.

## RATES, BIOLOGICAL PREDISPOSITIONS, AND RISK FACTORS FOR SUICIDE

Globally, it is estimated that at least 1 million people commit suicide yearly.[2] Suicide rates differ substantially across countries.[3] Some of this difference in estimates is due to variability in reporting, such as disparities in autopsy rates. Beyond methodological issues, cultural and possibly biological factors explain some of the differences in suicide rates. In the United States, over 30,000 individuals commit suicide yearly.[4] In Western countries, women make more suicide attempts but men commit suicide more frequently, by a ratio of approximately 4:1. Older individuals, especially older men, are at higher risk for suicide than younger individuals.[3] Adolescents are also a high-risk group for suicidal behavior, both boys and girls. Within the United States, suicide rates are highest in Native Americans, particularly males. White individuals in the United States have higher rates of suicide than black individuals. In the Northern hemisphere, suicide rates peak in the late spring to early summer (May through June).

Suicide runs in families, with almost half the risk statistically explainable by genetic factors. As an example, the monozygotic (identical) twin of an individual who has committed suicide is more likely to commit suicide than the dizygotic (nonidentical or fraternal) co-twin of someone who commits suicide.[5] Adoption studies have shown that the risk for suicide among the biological relatives of adoptees who committed suicide is six times greater than the rate in biological relatives of nonsuicidal adoptees.[6]

Since there is no suicide gene, it is reasonable to ask what factors might be inherited that could explain the familial nature of suicide. Two factors seem to be particularly relevant. The first, of course, is the genetic risk for the disorders that are associated with suicide. Because the psychiatric disorders most associated with suicide risk—mood disorders, schizophrenia, and drug–alcohol abuse—all run in families due substantially (but certainly not entirely) to genetic factors, families with these disorders are more likely to have individuals with completed or attempted suicide. The overwhelming majority (more than 90%) of individuals in Western countries who kill themselves are suffering from one or more psychiatric disorders.[7] Thus, "rational" or existentially based suicides are relatively rare. Cultural factors are also relevant. In China, suicides unrelated to psychiatric disorders are more common, indicating the role of culture in suicide vulnerability.[8]

Second, *impulsive/aggressive* behaviors and personality traits are potentially heritable and cut across diagnostic categories. Both lifetime aggressiveness and impulsivity independently predict suicidal behavior and run in families, with substantial genetic input into these traits.[9] Thus, whereas some families are loaded with individuals with mood disorders but exhibit little to no suicidality, other families may have the same number of individuals with mood disorders but, because of additional impulsive/aggressive traits, have a much higher number of suicidal individuals.

A number of clinical risk factors (Table 10.1) are associated with suicidal ideation and attempts. The single most powerful factor is a history of suicide attempts, with at least 40% of those who commit suicide having made past attempts.[7] Among clinical symptoms, severe agitation, insomnia, and hopelessness are most associated with suicide risk. Of course, these predictors provide opportunities for clinical intervention (which we discuss later) to diminish these symptoms and, we hope, decrease suicide risk in vulnerable persons.

An important historical predictor—and one that is often neglected by clinicians—is a recent discharge from a psychiatric hospital.[10] Sometimes, considerable efforts have gone into arranging a patient's hospitalization, and it is often assumed that the patient has converted to low suicide risk upon discharge. Unfortunately, the posthospital period is a time of considerable suicide risk and requires closer monitoring by the family members and outpatient clinicians.

Not surprisingly, psychological factors play a huge role in suicide.[11,12] Proximal risk factors can include recent separation or loss experiences (e.g., marital breakups, death of a spouse, loss of a job), social alienation, and lack of social supports (e.g., feeling rejected by one's family; moving to a residential home in older age and losing one's sense of community). More distal risk factors can include prior trauma, including early sexual or physical abuse; or more recent trauma, such

---

**TABLE 10.1. Clinical Predictors of Suicide**

Historical and symptom predictors
- History of past attempts
- Hopelessness cognitions (e.g., "Nothing will ever get better")
- Persistent insomnia
- Agitation/profound anxiety
- Recent discharge from psychiatric hospital

Psychological and psychosocial predictors
Early traumatic life events
Recent stressful life events, especially loss
Significant family conflict with one or more parents or spouse
Social isolation or alienation

as war, torture, or events in which patients experience "survivor guilt." Thus, older patients who have experienced recent stressors, have a background of trauma, and are socially isolated are at particularly high risk.

Of course, risks factors should not be viewed in isolation: Some factors are most powerful as predictors when another risk factor is present (interactive risks). A recent study demonstrated that among adoptees whose biological parent showed suicidal behavior, the risk was highest if the adoptive mother had been psychiatrically hospitalized.[13] As another example of interactive risks, alcohol abuse may increase the risk for suicide more profoundly in an individual who is already depressed than in a person with no history of depression. Similarly, a recent loss experience, which may create the conditions of increased hopelessness and suicidal thinking, will be more impactful if there is little or no social support in the person's life.[12,14]

## BIPOLAR DISORDER AND SUICIDE

Among the psychiatric disorders, depression is associated with the highest suicide risk, with more than half of all people who die by suicide suffering from a current depressive disorder. The exact percentage of individuals with mood disorders who commit suicide over a lifetime is unclear. Earlier estimates of 15–20% are assuredly too high for a number of reasons:

1. Suicide rates may be given as either proportionate mortality (the percentage of suicides among those who have died) or case fatality (the percentage of patients followed over a certain time period who commit suicide).[15] Many of the early studies that calculated high rates of suicide among depressed individuals used proportionate mortality rates. Because young people only infrequently die from medical causes, proportionate mortality overestimates the actual percentage of bipolar individuals who commit suicide.

2. Compounding this difficulty, a number of early studies examined suicide rates in those who had been hospitalized, thereby studying only patients with the most severe mood disorders.[16] Adding this factor to the issue of proportionate mortality, and the relatively short periods of follow-up in studies of young bipolar individuals makes suicide rates appear very high.

Recent studies that use longer follow-up periods and a more broadly defined group of mood disorder patients find that suicide rates range from 2% in all mood patients to 9% among those previously hospitalized for suicidal behavior.[16] It is also possible (and hoped for!) that the lower suicide rates among those with mood disorders in more recent studies indicate the availability of treatments that have decreased suicide risk. In a 44-year follow-up of bipolar and unipolar individuals in Switzerland, lithium, neuroleptics, and antidepressants significantly reduced the long-term risk of suicide.[17] (See below for a discussion on medications as modifiers of suicide risk.)

Suicide rates of people with bipolar and unipolar depressive disorders have generally been found to be equal, although the Swiss study found higher rates of suicide completion in depressed than in bipolar persons, especially those for whom mania predominates.[17] Bipolar I and bipolar II patients have approximately the same rate of suicide attempts.[18] Mood cycling and, most likely, rapid cycling are independent predictors of suicide attempts and completed suicide within a bipolar population. Similar to the findings for all mood disorders, suicide attempts and completed suicides are relatively more common early in the course of bipolar disorder, which does not always correspond to a young age.[19]

Not surprisingly, suicide is most likely (80%) in bipolar disorder during the depressed phase, with approximately 10% of suicides occurring during mixed periods in which depressed mood, irritability, and increased/manic energy combine to create a relatively high suicide risk.[20] Suicides during euphoric manias are rare. When deaths occur during euphoric manias, they are typically a consequence of a person's dangerous behavior and bad judgment, without the specific intent to end one's life.

---

Raymond experienced his second manic episode when he was in his late 20s. His first manic episode occurred at age 22 and required hospitalization. Following recovery from that episode, Raymond discontinued his mood stabilizer and, other than two mild depressions, had no other mood episode until this second episode, which was characterized by the typical symptoms of increased energy, decreased sleep, grandiosity, increased money spending, and driving recklessly. Despite his family's appropriate concern and worry about him, Raymond refused hospitalization and was inconsistent in taking antimanic medication. As part of his grandiosity, Raymond thought he could make a great deal of money quickly by buying illegal drugs, then selling them in his upper-middle-class neighborhood. He bought these illegal drugs in one of the more dangerous neighborhoods in the city. In the fourth week of his manic episode, he was found shot to death in an alley in the area where he was attempting to buy drugs. Although his death was not ruled a suicide, it was clearly a consequence of manic-driven, dangerous, and impulsive behavior.

---

Despite our knowledge of individual predictors of suicide in general and in bipolar populations, it must be acknowledged that predicting suicide for any individual is exceedingly difficult.[21] The individual predictors for suicidal behaviors are neither common enough (sensitivity) nor exclusive enough (specificity) to help very much with any given patient. Even the red flag of a past history of suicide attempts—the most reliable predictor of future attempts—tells us little about the timing of a future suicide attempt or about how to intervene to prevent that attempt.

## EVALUATION OF ACUTE SUICIDALITY

We find that it is best to assess suicidality in patients with bipolar disorder even if there is no immediate evidence of it. It is surprising how many patients who present with elevated mood and grandiosity also admit to thinking about ending their lives. In most cases, it is best to explore suicide openly with the patient and, whenever possible, with his family members.

### Open Inquiry

The first challenge in suicide assessment is to be open and direct. This means showing the patient that you are not afraid of his self-destructive impulses, morbid fantasies, or feelings of hopelessness. Figure 10.1 gives examples of ways to ask about suicidality, most of which will be of no surprise to the seasoned clinician. Note that we do not recommend talking around suicidality, as in "those bad feelings" or "when you get really down on yourself." Try to determine whether the patient uses specific language to express his suicidal impulses, such as "thinking about checking out" or "cashing my check."

### Assessing Lethality and Risk Factors

As with any patient under one's care, it is important to assess the lethality of the patient's suicidal impulses, notably, the presence of a specific plan, the means, and a stated intent to carry out the plans.

- "Do you have very morbid thoughts about dying or, more specifically about ending your life?"

- "Do you ever feel that the world or your family would be better off without you?"

- "When you get really depressed, do you ever think about killing yourself or hurting yourself?"

- "Some people, especially when they get depressed, think about suicide, even though they might not think about this in other moods. How has it been for you—are you thinking about killing yourself now?"

- "How would you do it? Prompts: do you own a gun? Overdose? Hanging, jumping?"

- "Have you ever tried to kill yourself before? How about intentionally harming yourself, even if you didn't really want to die? Ever cut/burn yourself because you were feeling so bad?"

- "Have you made any specific plans? Can you tell me about them?" (If a family member is present, offer the patient the chance to talk with you without the relative present.)

- "Why would you want to do this? What motivates these thoughts?"

- To family members: "Are you worried that she'll hurt or kill herself? Why now?"

**FIGURE 10.1.** Questions to clarify a patient's suicide risk.

From *Clinician's Guide to Bipolar Disorder* by David J. Miklowitz and Michael J. Gitlin. Copyright 2014 by The Guilford Press. Permission to photocopy this figure is granted to purchasers of this book for personal use only (see copyright page for details). Purchasers can download a larger version of this figure from *www.guilford.com/miklowitz5-forms*.

A comprehensive assessment of risk factors will inform the degree of immediacy the situation requires.

## Degree, Persistence, and Frequency

Assess whether the morbid ideation is constant or seems to come and go with cycling mood, and whether it occurs multiple times per day as opposed to one to two times per week. Distinguish between thoughts of dying (e.g., "I often think of what it would be like to be gone") and concrete thoughts of ending one's life. Of course, more persistent or severe suicidal ideation is more closely associated with actual attempts. Patients who have written suicide notes, given away their possessions, or made attempts to hide their suicidal intent from others are at particularly high risk.

## Prior Attempts

One or more prior attempts is the best predictor of future attempts. Determining whether a prior incident was an actual suicide attempt, however, may require detailed probing.

## Hopelessness Cognitions

Hopelessness thinking centers on themes of misery that are never expected to lift (e.g., "I don't see anything getting better," "I will eventually kill myself; it's gonna happen someday"). The self-rated Beck Scale for Suicide Ideation[22] or the Suicide Ideation Questionnaire[23] may be useful supplements to a clinical interview.

## Mood State

Assess whether the patient is currently depressed, and particularly whether this state has worsened. Suicidal thoughts that previously have not reached the threshold for action can cross that threshold when depression worsens.

## Relationship of Suicidal Ideation to Comorbid Syndromes

If the patient is regularly drinking or using drugs (which includes abuse of prescription medicines), the risk for suicide is substantially increased. Patients who have severe anxiety disorders, such as panic disorder or posttraumatic stress disorder (PTSD), are also at heightened risk. Assess whether the triggers for anxiety (e.g., financial woes) also increase suicidal ideation.

### Presence of Social Supports

Assess the degree to which, in a given week, the patient interacts with others, including therapists or support groups. Does the patient have any contact with a spouse (current or former), children, or parents? Is there a social support network (e.g., a church or temple group; AA meetings)? Are the patient's friends primarily online acquaintances? Are these social supports available in the next few days? Note that social connectedness may reduce the translation of suicidal thoughts into acts. A patient who has the thought, "I would never want to hurt my kids" is at lower risk than one who has no such reason to stay alive (see "Reasons to Stay Alive," below).

In gathering this information, assess whether the patient truly wishes to die or whether the thoughts seem closely connected with making a statement to others. The degree to which there is true suicidal intent may be reflected in the seriousness of past attempts. Ask patients with well-formulated plans whether they have imagery regarding their own funeral or its aftermath, such as whether a former lover or a neglectful child feels guilty.

The main consideration in assessing patients with bipolar disorder compared to other populations is the volatility of moods. Patients who leave your office in one state may have a worsening of mood later that same day. They may have self-adjusted their medications or stopped them altogether. As stated in Chapter 8, patients who rapidly discontinue medications are at especially high risk for suicide. Moreover, patients with bipolar disorder often have access to medications with a high potential for lethality.

### Assessing Motivations for Suicide

The lethality assessment should include an exploration of the reasons one is motivated to commit suicide. Although the causes of suicidal acts are virtually limitless, motivations can be roughly classified as follows: (1) a true wish to die; (2) a desire to escape loneliness, distress, or other negative mood states; (3) a desire for attention; (4) a desire to make life easier for others; or (5) a way to express hostility or induce guilt in others.

It is not difficult to understand how the level of pain of a severe bipolar depressive episode, often with crippling anxiety, panic, or lethargy, would motivate a desire to escape. In fact, framing the patient's suicidal wishes as a desire to escape rather than to die is itself a useful intervention. For example, clinicians can validate the patient's feelings with statements such as "So you don't want to die as much as get away from some pretty awful feelings and experiences. When you feel hopeless about anything changing, I can understand why you'd consider doing that. But let's look at whether more can be done to alleviate the pain you're in."

We have often noted the close connection between suicidality and family dynamics in mood disorders. Sometimes a patient may believe that others in her family would be better off if she were dead ("altruistic suicide"). This is especially likely if the patient has a resentful spouse or adult child who has become a caregiver. A patient who has both bipolar disorder and borderline personality disorder may have suicidal impulses that are fueled by real or imagined separations from close attachments (typically, romantic relationships, but also extending to family members, friends, or even therapists). A patient whose family relationships have become hostile, aggressive, or otherwise highly conflictual—especially in the aftermath of an illness episode—may contemplate suicide as a means of escape or exacting revenge.

### Chain Analysis

When an assessment protocol allows one to go beyond the basic questions about immediate risk, it is nearly always helpful to conduct an antecedent–behavior–consequence (ABC) "chain analysis."[24] This assessment attempts to identify the sequence of events—both external and internal—that lead to suicidal thoughts, attempts, or self-harm. The basic assessment questions take the form, "What events, followed by what feelings or thoughts, led you to hurt yourself?" In many cases, the triggering event may have seemed minor, but in the context of unstable mood (often complicated by substance abuse), the event may become magnified in importance.

Teresa, an 18-year-old with bipolar I disorder, became hypersocial and hypersexual during her manic episodes. A typical trigger for self-harming behavior was when her parents told her that she couldn't go out at night, which often led Teresa to sneak out of the house and, in one case, jump off a balcony. On one particular night, Teresa's father restrained her when she tried to leave. She ran upstairs and cut her wrists with a broken bottle. Upon hospital admission, she denied wanting to die but admitted to wanting to hurt her parents.

If there are family members, ask whether they observed any of the "buildup" phase and attempted to intervene at any point in the chain. Some family members have become inured to the patient's suicidal thoughts or even acts, believing that she is highly manipulative and better off ignored. It is important to determine whether ignoring the behavior decreases or increases its intensity; in our experience, it is more often the latter.

Suicidal events are usually related to interpersonal events, but a chain analysis may also reveal that the triggers are internal:

---

Nestor, a 37-year-old whose 10-year relationship ended abruptly, would frequently search for his ex-girlfriend online and read her Facebook entries. When it became obvious that she was in a new relationship, he lapsed into a severely depressed period during which he attempted suicide. His ex-girlfriend visited him in the hospital, but her visit, which further confirmed her lack of interest in continuing their relationship, made him feel worse. His therapist helped him identify the thoughts "I will never be with anyone who makes me happy" and "I cannot hold down a good relationship" as key cognitions that increased his anxiety and depression. His suicidal wishes, in turn, were triggered by a desire to escape from these tortuous thoughts.

---

Finally, it is just as important to examine the consequences of suicidal events as the antecedents. Suicide attempts may generate more attention and open expressions of caring from others (including clinicians), relief from job demands, and a temporary alleviation of negative emotional states. A worksheet such as Figure 10.2 may help summarize the evaluation of the patient's risk factors and the chain analysis as an aid to prevention planning.

## CLINICAL MANAGEMENT OF SUICIDAL STATES

### Hospitalization

Hospitalization should be considered for any bipolar patient whose safety is at risk. Although suicides do occur in inpatient settings, they are relatively infrequent because of greater monitoring by staff and the dramatic restriction of the means for self-destructive behavior. In inpatient settings, guns, knives, and ropes are, of course, unavailable. Patients are closely watched after taking medications, thereby making it more difficult to sequester enough pills for overdoses. Within locked units (increasingly common in today's psychiatric hospitals), jumping from high places is rare. And, finally, refinements in the prevention of

1. List the patient's *early warning signs* of a recent suicidal episode (e.g., sleep disturbance, anxiety, panic, lethargy, mood cycling, anhedonia, insomnia, psychotic thinking, hopelessness cognitions).

_____

_____

2. List *risk factors* in the patient's illness history and any recent psychosocial factors or life events that may be contributing to the current state: history of suicide attempts, availability of lethal means of self-harm, specific suicide plans that involve precautions against discovery, history of impulsive or aggressive behaviors, substance/ alcohol abuse, social isolation, recent loss or change events.

_____

_____

3. List *current protective factors* that may mitigate the likelihood of a suicide attempt (e.g., patient expresses hopefulness; acknowledges responsibility to spouse, children, parents, or pets; describes strong and protective social or familial network; fears social disapproval for suicide attempts; fears the suicide act itself; has religious or spiritual beliefs; expresses a commitment to follow a crisis intervention plan).

_____

_____

4. *Chain analysis.* Using the most recent suicidal act or period of ideation as an example, list the chain of events, thoughts, and feelings that led up to, and that followed this act or period.

Antecedent events:

_____

_____

Behaviors (i.e., What did the patient do when the antecedents occurred? When and under what circumstances did the suicidal act/impulse occur?):

_____

_____

Consequences (i.e., What happened after the patient made the attempt or had suicidal impulses? How did others react?):

_____

_____

**FIGURE 10.2.** Suicide prevention plan: Assessment phase. From M. M. Linehan et al.[25] *Cognitive and Behavioral Practice*, 2012;19:218–232. Copyright 2012 by Elsevier. Adapted by permission.

From *Clinician's Guide to Bipolar Disorder* by David J. Miklowitz and Michael J. Gitlin. Copyright 2014 by The Guilford Press. Permission to photocopy this figure is granted to purchasers of this book for personal use only (see copyright page for details). Purchasers can download a larger version of this figure from *www.guilford.com/miklowitz5-forms*.

self-hanging, such as curtain rods that break if enough weight is put on them, minimize the risk further. Consistent with these safety considerations, most inpatient suicides occur outside the hospital when patients are on a pass or are absent without leave.[26]

Because suicidal ideation is far more common among bipolar patients than serious suicide attempts, it is neither reasonable nor possible to hospitalize every patient who acknowledges suicidal ideation. Considering our enormous difficulty in predicting suicide, the important clinical question becomes: When should we decide that the suicide risk for a bipolar patient is serious enough to warrant hospitalization? The previously described predictors/correlates of suicide help but provide only general guidelines. Certainly, clinical wisdom suggests that the manifestations of hopelessness—what the patient says and behaviors associated with giving up, such as rewriting a will or other preparations for death—are important signs. Statements consistent with the notion that "the world [or my family] would be better off without me" should similarly trigger serious consideration of hospitalization, even when patients deny overt intention of self-harm. Use any and all signs, including historical variables such as past suicide attempts, to ascertain suicide risk as best as possible.

---

Frank, 56 years old, had bipolar II disorder since his early 20s, with a number of relatively mild hypomanias and three depressive episodes of moderate severity. He hated taking medications and never accepted any maintenance treatment. On several occasions, he presented for treatment during an acute episode and, within a month of becoming euthymic, self-tapered his medications. Throughout his adult life and during all of his mood episodes, Frank had been able to function at work; he owned a successful business.

Over a 3-month period prior to his hospitalization, Frank became more severely depressed than at any previous time, with the usual classic vegetative features, but for the first time was unable to work. Despite taking mood stabilizers, an antidepressant, and seeing a therapist regularly, he became noticeably worse. Initially, Frank denied any current suicidal ideation as well as any history of self-destructive ideas during any prior episodes. By the third month of the depression, however, he began to see his life as a failure, to believe that he was of no use to his wife and children, and that his business was doomed to failure (because of his inability to work, Frank's business had financial difficulties but was not in dire jeopardy). He had vague, distant fantasies of shooting himself but did not own a gun and did not know how to buy one. Other than taking a short walk and seeing his doctors, he stayed in the house all day and did little else.

Frank never made an overt suicidal threat, but expressed an intense feeling of hopelessness and a sense that the world would be better without him.

With enormous urging from his wife, his therapist, and his psychopharma-cologist, Frank agreed to be hospitalized. By his second day in the hospital, he acknowledged that his suicidal thoughts were far more intense than he had described while living at home, but he had been too embarrassed to talk about them. According to Frank, his anhedonia and depressive fatigue were all that kept him from killing himself.

---

Of course, not all bipolar suicidal patients who should be in hospital agree to go voluntarily. Although nuances differ across states, the core requirement for involuntary hospitalization is that the potential for self-harm is imminent—typically within days, allowing for three days of inpatient evaluation and treatment. If possible, it is always better to have a patient agree to a voluntary hospitalization. However, the capacity to hospitalize patients against their will is sometimes imperative to protect them from impulsive, self-destructive behavior.

The inpatient treatment of the phase of bipolar disorder that gives rise to suicidality—usually depression or a mixed state—is identical to its outpatient treatment. No medication should be considered as protective against suicide risk in the immediate situation. However, given the strong link between profound agitation/anxiety and suicide risk, it is best to treat agitated suicidal inpatients aggressively, typically with antipsychotics or tranquilizers such as benzodiazepines.

After hospitalization, patients with a recent history of significant suicidal ideation or a past attempt should be monitored very closely, given that the highest suicide risk related to hospitalization is in the first 2–4 weeks after discharge.[10] Simple interventions that express concern and caring, such as clinician-initiated phone calls, letters, or even postcards, have been found to protect against suicide attempts in patients who have just been discharged from the hospital.[14]

### Medications

We have no "antisuicide" medications. As discussed earlier, the factors associated with suicidal risk are complex, involving genetics, biology, psychology, and culture. Nonetheless, it is legitimate to consider whether some medications decrease the likelihood of suicide. Paradoxically, the opposite is also true: some medications may *increase* suicidality in *some* patients. The medications for which we have some positive information, as well as some concern in this regard, are, not surprisingly, mood medications—mood stabilizers, antidepressants, and antipsychotics.

The biological mechanisms by which medications might decrease suicidal risk in bipolar disorder are hypothetical at best. Conceptually, one can consider either of two pathways. First, effectively treating the negative psychological state that gives rise to suicidal thoughts should decrease suicide risk. Thus, any medication that treats (or prevents) depression should decrease suicidal risk. Within this category would be mood stabilizers that decrease the likelihood or intensity of depression, or antidepressants that prevent or treat depression. Second, medications that diminish the underlying symptoms of impulsivity and/or aggressiveness may diminish the risk of suicide attempts regardless of their efficacy in treating bipolar disorder.

Direct and conclusive evidence on the efficacy of any medication in decreasing suicide risk is lacking. Additionally, even if some antisuicide efficacy can be demonstrated for a specific medication, it is still unclear whether the positive effects are due to the medication's mood stabilizing properties, its capacity to diminish impulsive aggressive behavior, or both simultaneously. The three medications that have been examined with regard to altering suicidal risk are lithium, clozapine (Clozaril), and antidepressants.

## Lithium and Other Mood Stabilizers

By far, lithium has been the medication evaluated in the greatest number of trials for its antisuicide effects. Over 40 studies have compared rates of suicide and/or suicide attempts or self-harm in those taking lithium versus a control group not taking lithium.[27,28] Some studies evaluated patients with bipolar disorder, others with major depression, others with both mood disorders. In some of the studies, comparison groups took other medications, such as antidepressants or anticonvulsant mood stabilizers, whereas in other studies, patients took no medications. Yet another group of studies compared the rate of suicide attempts or suicides in groups of bipolar individuals during periods of time when they took lithium, to other times (either before or after the lithium-treated periods) when they did not take lithium.

Adding up the results of all these studies makes clear that patients with mood disorders who take lithium continuously are less likely to commit suicide and make fewer suicide attempts than those who do not take lithium or who discontinue it, with a reduction of suicide events of approximately 80%. A meta-analysis found that in 31 studies involving 85,229 "person-years of risk-exposure," patients taking lithium were five times less likely to attempt or complete suicide compared to those not treated with lithium.[27] A more recent meta-analysis of 48 randomized controlled trials concluded that lithium reduced suicide risk in mood disorder patients by almost eightfold, and was generally better than other comparators; however, lithium did not have clear effects on deliberate self-harm.[28,29]

These studies do not help distinguish between lithium's effects on mood stability, depression, impulsiveness, or aggressiveness. Additionally, the vast majority of these studies were not intended to evaluate lithium's antisuicide effects. It would therefore be instructive to see whether lithium decreased suicide risk in nonbipolar patients. Here, too, lithium seems to reduce suicide risk. As an example, one randomized trial examined a group of patients primarily with depressive (not bipolar) disorders who had been hospitalized for suicide-related behaviors and were treated with lithium in conjunction with their other medications. These patients showed a greater decrease in suicides than a group treated with other medications but without adjunctive lithium.[30] A separate series of studies makes clear that, even in the absence of mood disorders, lithium reduces aggressive behaviors in groups such as children with conduct disorders and aggressive adult prisoners.[31]

Another key question is whether lithium reduces suicidal behavior more effectively than do other mood stabilizers. Here, too, the answer is unclear. In patients without bipolar disorder who have impulse control disorders (e.g., those with borderline personality disorder or intermittent explosive disorder), anticonvulsants have a stronger track record than lithium in decreasing impulsive/aggressive behaviors. (To be fair, this reflects the sheer lack of studies of lithium in treating borderline personality disorder patients compared to the number of studies of anticonvulsants in this population. There are no head-to-head studies comparing lithium to anticonvulsants in patients with borderline personality disorder.) Thus, anticonvulsants might be expected to decrease suicide risk in bipolar individuals through the mechanism of reducing impulsiveness.

One nonrandomized trial using a pharmacy database of 20,638 health plan members suggested that lithium had a considerably lower suicide risk than valproate (Depakote).[32] However, a more recent study that randomly assigned bipolar patients with a history of suicide attempts to take either lithium or valproate found no difference in suicidal behavior over the next 2 years.[33] Paradoxically, there are also some concerns—and much controversy—as to whether anticonvulsants (e.g., valproate, lamotrigine [Lamictal], and carbamazepine [Tegretol]) may *increase* suicidality in patients with epilepsy.[34]

For now, it is reasonable to conclude that the strongest evidence supports lithium's antisuicide effects, but it is still unclear whether this effect is unique among the mood stabilizers. It is equally unclear whether lithium's ability to diminish suicidality is due to its mood-stabilizing effects, its antidepressant efficacy, its anti-aggressive/impulsive behavior effects, or a combination of these factors. Given our current information, it is reasonable to add lithium to the regimen of a bipolar patient who is considered to be at high risk for suicide, even if other mood stabilizers are the primary medications.

### Antipsychotics

Some evidence suggests that patients with schizophrenia who are treated with antipsychotics have a lower risk of suicide than those not taking antipsychotics. No such data exist for bipolar patients. The best evidence for an antisuicide effect among antipsychotics is for clozapine which, as described in Chapter 6, is prescribed almost exclusively for treatment-resistant schizophrenia or bipolar disorder. Most of the studies demonstrating clozapine's antisuicide effects—even those that have compared it to olanzapine—have been in schizophrenia populations.[35] In the one relevant study, the rate of hospitalization due to a suicide attempt decreased by over 60% in bipolar patients treated with clozapine.[36] Given the dangers and difficulties of clozapine treatment (see Chapters 4 and 6), it would be highly unusual for a bipolar patient to be treated with clozapine solely on the basis of its antisuicide effects.

### Antidepressants

Given that antidepressants are the most common pharmacological treatment for depressed individuals at high risk of suicide, a first intuitive conclusion would be that, of course, antidepressants prevent suicide by treating the most common disorder that gives rise to suicidality. This statement *may* be true, but it has never been demonstrated in any convincing manner by any study. The occasional uncontrolled study seemingly demonstrates that depressed individuals treated with long-term antidepressants are less likely to commit suicide than those who do not stay on antidepressants.[37] Unfortunately, in uncontrolled naturalistic studies, patients treated with antidepressants differ from patients who are not treated in many other relevant ways (e.g., their prior depressive episodes may have been less responsive to other forms of treatment). Also, antidepressants are often given along with psychotherapy or at least brief supportive contacts. For now, it is impossible to state from research that antidepressants prevent suicide.

The relationship between antidepressants and suicidality has become even more complicated recently, highlighted by the FDA's official "black-box" warning that these medications may paradoxically *increase* suicidality in individuals up to age 25. Although all of the studies in this area have evaluated nonbipolar depressed individuals, this issue is still highly relevant for the use of antidepressants in the treatment of bipolar depression (Chapter 6) or suicidality.

For decades, clinical wisdom has suggested carefully monitoring suicidal depressed patients as they begin to improve, with the underlying concern that suicide risk increases as patients regain their energy, yielding the potentially dangerous situation of a still depressed mood but with the energy to follow through on a suicide plan. This scenario, often referred to as the "rollback phenomenon" (since it is thought that depressed symptoms improve—or roll back—in the reverse order of their emergence, with energy improving before mood), has not been systematically studied, and its validity is unknown. Additionally, in the early 1990s, soon after the release of the SSRI antidepressants, a number of small case series described the emergence of new onset obsessional/suicidal/violent thoughts in the beginning of SSRI treatment in adults.[38] Then, approximately 10 years ago, after a study indicated a lack of efficacy of paroxetine (Paxil) in depressed children and a small increase in new-onset suicidal thoughts, a review of all antidepressant studies in children and adolescents and the emergence of suicidality during treatment was mandated by the FDA. The question, "Do antidepressants increase suicidality?" was then examined using a variety of methods in studies of depressed patients of all ages.

To summarize a large group of controlled studies: Antidepressants are associated with twice the rate of new-onset suicidality in depressed children, adolescents, and young adults up to age 25, compared to those treated with placebo (4 vs. 2%).[39] In these controlled studies, *no* completed suicides occurred, only increases in suicidal ideation, self-destructive behaviors, and suicide attempts. Therefore, when antidepressants are prescribed for younger patients, it is appropriate in the first weeks of treatment to monitor closely for this relatively unusual side effect. Strikingly, this finding of increased suicidality (but not suicide) disappears in studies of depressed individuals over age 25. In fact, the older the patients studied, the more one sees a *decrease* in suicidal thinking and behavior in those treated with antidepressants versus placebo, with geriatric patients showing the greatest decrease in suicidality when treated with antidepressants.[40]

The mechanism(s) by which antidepressants occasionally increase suicidal thinking in younger depressed individuals (but not in those

**TABLE 10.2. Mechanisms of Action of Treatment-Emergent Suicidality with Antidepressants**

- Stimulation effects (akathisia), compounded by young people's lack of awareness that negative feelings may be side effects
- Improvement in energy and psychomotor retardation prior to mood improvement (rollback phenomenon)
- Decrease in serotonergic neurotransmission due to immediate rather than delayed effects of SSRIs
- Shift into mixed manic or mixed depressive state

over age 25) is still unclear. A number of hypotheses, listed in Table 10.2, have been suggested, none of which has been systematically evaluated.[41] Stimulation side effects, common with SSRIs and other modern antidepressants, may increase depressive, irritable, or anxious feelings that may in turn increase suicidal thinking. This may be especially true in younger individuals, who may not recognize that new uncomfortable feelings are side effects of a medication and may respond to these feelings with self-destructive thoughts or behavior. As patients age and become better able to label their internal states as side effects, they may become better able to discuss changes to their regimen with the prescribing physician.

Biologically, in the central nervous system, the most immediate reaction to an SSRI (which, overall, *increases* serotonin function) is to *decrease* serotonin function (in order to maintain homeostasis, or sameness). If this compensatory mechanism of decreasing serotonin function is too vigorous, it is possible that, transiently, some patients have a net decrease in serotonergic tone that is associated with decreased impulse control and potentially self-destructive behavior.

For a discussion on suicidality, antidepressants, and bipolar disorder, the potential switch into mixed states is the most important hypothesis to consider. Since the age of onset of bipolar disorder is typically the late teens to early 20s, a greater percentage of younger depressed individuals (age 25 or less) have unexpressed bipolar disorder than do older depressed patients, most of whom have passed through the age of risk. Consistent with this hypothesis, switch rates with antidepressants in depressed, nonbipolar patients are higher in younger patients than in older patients.[42] If only a small percentage of the younger individuals in the depression studies switched into an unrecognized mixed state with irritability, impulsivity and new-onset suicidal thinking or self-destructive behavior, that would be consistent with the small difference in new-onset suicidality (only 2%) in the pediatric depression studies.[39] To be clear: No study has yet evaluated this hypothesis and it remains speculative. Nonetheless, it suggests the need for especially careful monitoring in young patients treated with antidepressants who are at high risk for bipolar disorder, such as those with a family history of bipolar disorder in a sibling or parent.

Another method of evaluating the potential risks of antidepressants in younger individuals would be to examine whether young people who committed suicide were treated with antidepressants. This would not give us information on the risk to a specific individual, but it would provide clues as to the extent of the risk for the general population. In the Western world, coroner's offices, which are responsible for evaluating causes of death, routinely obtain toxicology screens in which medication blood levels, including antidepressants, are measured at the time of death. In the four coroners' series from the United States and Europe examining youth (teenagers and younger) suicides, just over 2% of those who committed suicide had any measurable antidepressant in their body at the time of their death. Thus, 98% of these youngsters were not taking antidepressants at that time.[43–46] Presumably, many, if not most of these youngsters were suffering from depression.

As noted earlier, these studies are not immediately relevant to treating bipolar depression, but they provide evidence that inadequate treatment of mood disorders is a far greater problem than the small increase in suicidality (but not actual suicide) seen in the studies of young depressed individuals taking antidepressants. In fact, the very youngsters who are at highest risk for suicide appear to be the least likely to receive antidepressants.

Overall, then, in contrast to lithium, antidepressants have not been shown to be associated with decreases in suicidal thinking and behaviors, and they may increase suicidal thinking and behaviors in a few younger depressed individuals. For bipolar suicidal patients, this indicates the need for caution in the use of antidepressants, especially in youngsters. As described in Chapter 6, mood stabilizers decrease the risk of antidepressant-induced switches into mixed states and should minimize the theoretical risks of antidepressants increasing suicidality in younger patients.

### Electroconvulsive Therapy

ECT is often considered and appropriately recommended for the bipolar patient who is severely depressed and suicidal. Because of the relative rapidity of its antidepressant effects (see Chapter 6), ECT is associated with a rapid reduction in suicidal ideation when used in patients with acute suicidal depression. In contrast to antidepressants, there has been no concern that ECT increases suicidal thoughts. No controlled studies have examined ECT's long-term efficacy in reducing suicide attempts or completed suicides.

As previously noted, involuntary ECT is exceedingly rare due to legal protections to avoid its use coercively; thus, its use is limited to patients who are capable of providing informed consent and who give that consent. As an example, a psychotically depressed suicidal patient who considers ECT a punishment for past sins and wants the treatment for that specific reason does not understand the nature and purpose of the treatment, and would therefore be deemed incapable of giving consent. However, a depressed patient who is psychotic—for example, believes that he is bankrupt when he is not or thinks he has cancer, but understands that ECT is a treatment for depression and not a punishment—*is* capable of providing informed consent.

### Psychosocial Approaches

There is a considerable literature on the psychosocial treatment of suicidality. In our view, the best-articulated are the dialectical behavior therapy (DBT), CBT, and mindfulness-based cognitive therapy (MBCT) approaches. Many of the recommended interventions for borderline personality disorder can be adapted for managing a current suicidal episode or preventing a future one in persons with bipolar disorder. Here, we summarize some of the main considerations when the clinician is treating a patient with bipolar disorder and is either trying to prevent the patient from killing himself (suicide management), or to prevent the future occurrence of a suicidal episode (suicide prevention).

### Take Your Own Pulse

One of the first strategies is to be aware of the desire to avoid discussing a patient's suicidal wishes. Understandably, clinicians are worried about being held responsible—legally or otherwise—for a patient's death. Often accompanying this worry are concerns that discussing suicide or its precipitants will make the patient more suicidal, or bring to consciousness thoughts or impulses that would have otherwise stayed underground. It is well established, however, that most people who commit suicide did not talk to a clinician in the days before the act (see earlier discussion). Having a strong working alliance with a patient who is suicidal, and communicating an openness to discussing her feelings of despair and hopelessness, even when they have been discussed multiple times before, is one of the best things you can do to prevent suicide.

The clinician's own avoidance strategies may foster "quick fix" solutions to the patient's preoccupations. The most common of these is the "no suicide contract" or "safety plan." While we generally agree with the intent of a safety plan, it must go well beyond the simple "I want you to agree to call me if you feel suicidal again." Empirical studies show that no-suicide contracts have little if any value in preventing actual suicide.[47,48] They probably do more to reassure the clinician than to keep the patient safe.

Although patients may feel some comfort in knowing that the clinician is available, many will not call, or do not believe that the clinician really wants them to call. Also, many clinicians do not know what to say when the patient actually does call, or they express frustration that the patient's suicidal feelings—seemingly in remission at the last visit—have reappeared.

Instead, start by observing your own internal process when the patient discusses suicide. Be aware of your desire to change the subject, or to get a quick reassurance that she will not kill herself, or that she will continue to take her medications. It is important for the patient not to feel that she must take care of the clinician by making promises she may not be able to honor. Instead, focus on validating the patient's feelings and showing a deep level of empathy with her pain.

## Validation

*Validation*, discussed at length by Marsha Linehan[24] and others, is the process of communicating to the patient that his responses to current life circumstances are understandable and logical. Linehan describes validation as having three steps: First is *active observing*, which occurs when the clinician gathers information about the current life circumstances (and if relevant, the triggers of current suicidal behavior), and summarizes the sequence of the patient's thoughts, emotions, and behaviors (the chain analysis, discussed earlier). Second is *reflection*, which means paraphrasing in a nonjudgmental way the thoughts, beliefs, or emotions the patient has expressed without necessarily expressing agreement with those thoughts or beliefs. Third is *direct validation*, which means underlining the wisdom or logic in the patient's choices, and making clear that these choices make sense within the context of the patient's life situation, even though you may see many other options that do not involve self-harm. The process of validation may occur over one or many sessions. It sets the stage for examining what the patient can do differently when the same environmental triggers, feelings, and thoughts present themselves.

---

Janelle, a 27-year-old woman with bipolar II disorder, attempted suicide with an overdose of sertraline (Zoloft). Her attempt was in response to a boyfriend who rejected her at a vulnerable moment, just when she was acknowledging her bipolar disorder for the first time. His reaction had been stilted and unpleasant; his only statement after she had described her symptoms and history of hospitalizations was "That explains a lot." An argument ensued, and he left shortly thereafter. She then swallowed the pills.

Her clinician asked her to recount the sequence of events leading up to the suicide attempt, including what she felt and thought at each stage. Janelle acknowledged that she chose to disclose her illness after an argument, in which she had become very upset and accused her boyfriend of not caring about her. She and her boyfriend had been moderately intoxicated at the time. The details of the sequence were sketchy, so the clinician emphasized those points where she felt strong emotions, accompanied by pessimistic thoughts such as "This is what will happen to me every time I tell anyone about my illness—they'll run away."

Janelle tearfully recounted having felt empty and abandoned when she found the pill bottle nearby. Rather than immediately pursuing the question of what else she might have done at that moment, her therapist quietly said, "I can understand why you'd have felt that way, and why that experience made you think about ending it all. You were feeling horrible, and you didn't feel like there was anything else you could do." This statement elicited a noticeable change in Janelle's posture, and she stopped crying. Janelle "tested" the clinician by saying, "Yeah, but I didn't call you like I was supposed to." The clinician nodded and added, "It can be very hard to reach out when you're that upset and feel like you don't matter to anyone else." The clinician did not say or imply that the suicide attempt was a wise decision—only that it was understandable in the context. The subsequent discussion focused on what alternatives Janelle felt she had if the same sequence occurred in the future: choosing a different time to discuss her illness with her boyfriend, avoiding alcohol when doing so, keeping only a limited number of pills at her house, and calling a close friend when she felt suicidal.

---

## Problem Solving

If you are seeing the patient individually, it is nearly always helpful to develop a list of strategies she could use when depressed, anxious, or aggressive feelings dominate. "Improving the moment" strategies refer to a number of tools that can be introduced before, during, or immediately after the suicidal sequence.[24] Examples of improving the moment strategies are listed in Figure 10.3, a handout for generating alternatives when one feels suicidal.

Many of these behaviors will be helpful when the patient first becomes depressed, as a means of staving off further mood deterioration. It is best to develop this list of response options when the patient is not at the height of a suicidal crisis; she may be unable to generate a list of viable options at those times. Explore with the patient the behaviors that might be distracting or introduce different feeling states (e.g., paying attention to one's breathing), and those that involve interpersonal connectedness and cognitive mechanisms (e.g., challenging negative thinking patterns).

Keep in mind that many patients hone these strategies over time. It is rare for a patient to select a group of strategies and immediately be able to use them during the next crisis. It is important to reinforce even minor attempts at using healthy alternative responses ("shaping"), even if the patient believes that she failed miserably. So, for example, if she says, "I wanted to call you but I couldn't find your phone number," praise her for having considered that alternative. If she says, "I tried deep breathing but I was way too distracted by my anxiety and all the street noise," validate the difficulty that many people experience in meditating under such circumstances, and explore whether there were other places she could have gone that were quieter and less stressful.

### Reasons to Stay Alive

Linehan and others have conceptualized suicide as being about not having enough reasons to live rather than wanting to die.[49] For patients with bipolar disorder, the negative feelings, loss, and failed expectations brought about by episodes of illness—often magnified when destructive decisions were made—create a sense of hopelessness about the future. When this sense of hopelessness pervades the individual's consciousness, he may have difficulty accessing reasons to stay alive. Nonetheless, a person can be protected from suicide when he can access reasons to live. Thus, an additional *improving the moment* strategy is to construct with the patient a list of reasons not to commit suicide when he feels like it.

The Reasons for Living Inventory (Figure 10.4) contains items generated by people who were not suicidal but had previously considered suicide.[49] They were asked to write down the reasons they did not act on these thoughts at the time, the reasons they do not want to commit suicide now, and why they believe other people did not commit suicide. Like other improving the moment tools, it is best to construct this list when the individual is not acutely suicidal; during the acute

Describe the feeling state that often accompanies feeling suicidal (depression? anxiety? irritability or anger?). _____

Place a checkmark next to those strategies you can use when you have depression, anxiety, or suicidal thoughts or impulses.

___ Meditation exercises that involve attention to the body and breathing

___ Progressive muscle relaxation (may involve self-instructional tapes)

___ Prayer (or attending church/temple)

___ Exercise (specify type: _____ )

___ Challenging negative thinking, writing down adaptive thoughts

___ Review my reasons for wanting to stay alive

___ Contact my therapist (phone numbers: _____ )

___ Contact my psychiatrist (phone numbers: _____ )

___ Call or text a friend (potential names and contact information: _____

_____ )

___ Call a family member (names and contact information: _____

_____ )

___ Spend time with pets

___ Spend time with children

___ Computer/Internet (video games, Facebook, etc.)

___ Take shower, bath, sauna

___ Other strategies

_____

_____

_____

_____

_____

_____

**FIGURE 10.3.** Strategies for improving the moment.

From *Clinician's Guide to Bipolar Disorder* by David J. Miklowitz and Michael J. Gitlin. Copyright 2014 by The Guilford Press. Permission to photocopy this figure is granted to purchasers of this book for personal use only (see copyright page for details). Purchasers can download a larger version of this figure from *www.guilford.com/miklowitz5-forms*.

Check the statements below that indicate why you would *not* commit suicide if the thought were to occur to you or if someone were to suggest it to you.

___ I have a responsibility and commitment to my family.

___ I believe I can learn to adjust to, or cope with, my problems.

___ I believe I have control over my life and destiny.

___ I believe only God has the right to end a life.

___ I am afraid of death.

___ I want to watch my children as they grow.

___ I have future plans I am looking forward to carrying out.

___ No matter how bad I feel, I know that it will not last.

___ It would not be fair to leave the children for others to take care of.

___ My religious beliefs forbid it.

___ It would hurt my family too much and I would not want them to suffer.

___ I am concerned about what others would think of me.

___ I consider it morally wrong.

___ I am afraid of the actual act of killing myself (the pain, blood, violence).

___ I still have many things left to do.

___ I would not want my family to feel guilty afterward.


List other reasons for living:

_____

_____

_____

_____

_____

_____

**FIGURE 10.4.** Reasons for Living Inventory. From M. M. Linehan et al.[50] *Journal of Consulting and Clinical Psychology.* 1983;51:276–286. Copyright 1983 by the American Psychological Association. Adapted by permission.

From *Clinician's Guide to Bipolar Disorder* by David J. Miklowitz and Michael J. Gitlin. Copyright 2014 by The Guilford Press. Permission to photocopy this figure is granted to purchasers of this book for personal use only (see copyright page for details). Purchasers can download a larger version of this figure from *www.guilford.com/miklowitz5-forms*.

crisis, the individual may be unable to generate good reasons. However, reminding patients of the reasons for living that they previously endorsed can be protective at key moments.

### Suicide Prevention Plans That Incorporate Family Members

Although suicide attempts may appear to be quite impulsive, they are often planned by the patient weeks or months in advance. The people who are most likely to observe the behavior changes associated with suicidality are immediate family members. Family members may describe a sequence in which the patient first expresses low-level suicidal thoughts (e.g., "I would be better off dead") but no suicidal intent, followed by more specific plans (e.g., behaviors that involve preparing for the suicidal act, such as buying weapons, stockpiling pills, writing letters, giving away possessions), and then periods of withdrawal. Others may emphasize the seemingly impulsive nature of the attempt, but on questioning may report that the behavioral signs of depression or anxiety were evident weeks before.

### Educating the Family

If the patient has been suicidal recently, and the attempt can be clearly connected to a mood episode, bring in one or more caregivers (spouse, parents, siblings) for a few sessions to educate them about bipolar disorder and their potential role in helping to prevent the patient's suicide. During these sessions, it is important to frame suicidality as one of the symptoms of bipolar disorder. Explain that when a person with bipolar disorder becomes more depressed, feelings of despair and hopelessness often follow; this cluster of feelings is often part of the biological changes associated with a mood episode. Some family members benefit from learning that levels of serotonin in the brain are lower when people become suicidal.[51]

Key to the discussion is to make clear that the patient does not necessarily have control over these impulses. An instance of self-harm does not necessarily mean that the patient is being manipulative or trying to control or hurt members of his family.

### The Family and the Chain Analysis

As discussed earlier, try to determine whether there are particular early warning signs and triggers that caregivers recognize from past suicidal events. Understanding the sequence of events will be most relevant to the family if the patient has attempted suicide recently and is now in partial or full remission. Caregivers often have difficulty discussing suicide openly, so the clinician can say: "This is difficult, but in the end it may save her life for you (relatives) to know what she's going through and how to help her cope with it."

Caregivers often recognize early warning signs such as irritability, increases in anxiety or worry, agitation, social withdrawal, outright aggressiveness (e.g., slamming doors, shoving people), or morbid ruminations (e.g., talking incessantly about the meaninglessness of life). Ask whether they have observed specific triggers that precede the actual attempt: severe arguments between a young adult and her parents regarding freedoms outside the home; interactions between a patient and his spouse in which the patient expressed feeling like a burden to the family.

It is equally relevant to examine what happens after the patient has attempted suicide. In families with adolescents or young adults, parents may become overly solicitous of the ill offspring and neglect the patient's siblings. Adolescents may report that their siblings are treating them worse since the event, and that these interactions contribute to their feeling of being a burden. In family sessions, you can encourage the siblings to express their frustration directly to their parents and highlight their competing desires for the parents' attention, which is often the real source of their anger. A sibling who says, "I feel like you don't care or don't even want to know what I'm doing" may hurt a parent's feelings, but it suggests a course of action. It will be far less damaging to the patient than saying, "You only care about Larry and his stupid bipolar disorder." In turn, parents can be coached to explain, "Yes, we're worried about Larry and want to make sure he gets through this phase safely, but that doesn't mean we don't care about you. Let's talk about how we can spend more time together."

## Communication Enhancement Training

As discussed in Chapter 7, opening up clogged lines of communication can enhance the protective effects of family relationships. In family or marital sessions, coach the patient and caregivers on how to talk about suicidality. The following steps can be helpful in developing a family-oriented safety plan:

1. Encourage the patient to verbally express his suicidal despair, loneliness, hopelessness, and feelings of guilt and shame to family members.

2. Encourage family members to respond calmly and validate the patient's feelings (see above) without becoming angry, punitive, or anxious.

3. Encourage the patient and family members to problem-solve about how to ensure the patient's continued safety. The results of this problem-solving are written into an overall suicide prevention contract (see below) that the patient, caregivers, and clinician signs.

Consider the following therapy vignette involving Elizabeth, age 26, and her mother (Marjorie) and father (Earl). Elizabeth had just made her third suicide attempt as she was recovering from a bipolar depressive episode.

> CLINICIAN: Marjorie, can you say more about what's hard about this for you?
>
> MOTHER: (*tearful*) I just don't know what to do.
>
> CLINICIAN: What feelings do you have when you don't know what to do?
>
> MOTHER: (*Pauses.*) I don't know . . . helpless, I guess. Dumb. I want Lizzy to tell me what to do.
>
> CLINICIAN: Can you tell Liz that now, more directly?
>
> MOTHER: Lizzy, when you get that way, I feel helpless. I want to help you but I don't know how. You're going to have to tell me how.
>
> ELIZABETH: Mom, I wish I knew myself. I don't know how to make myself feel better. But just sitting like this and talking without getting all upset helps a lot.

Elizabeth and her parents were encouraged to list triggers for suicidal thoughts or actions, early warning signs, and preventative plans involving the patient, the family, and the clinicians. Earl had difficulty with this more focused discussion, often lapsing into long diatribes about how "we only have one life to live." Liz tended to shut down when he spoke. She was eventually able to say to her father that she would value "having you there to hold my hand" during crisis times, instead of feeling like he had to say something.

The family-oriented suicide prevention plan developed for Liz is shown in Figure 10.5.

**Date:** _____

**Liz's early warning signs of a suicidal episode (include here depressive, mixed, or other symptoms that precede suicidal thinking or actions):**

She gets anxious, paces a lot, seems tearful, shuts down. (Mom)
I get tired but wired, can't sleep, my thoughts eat me alive. (Liz)
She gets confrontational, snaps easily. She seems tired a lot. (Dad)

**Circle the things Liz can do when she starts feeling suicidal or even just depressed.**

1. Call her psychiatrist and therapist and set up an appointment.
2. Set up a daily schedule with rewarding activities, and plan them for hard times of the day (going to coffee shop, watching a movie, taking dogs to park).
3. Use the following "improving the moment" strategies:

    Meditation or relaxation

    Light exercise (walking, StairMaster)

    Review my "Reasons for Living" list

    Take a bath or shower

    Get together with Amy and do something distracting (art museum, shopping)

    Ask friends or family members to talk with me

    Agree not to hurt myself if they haven't gotten back to me or if they haven't been as helpful or responsive as I expected

**Things that family members can do:**

1. Take all dangerous weapons out of the house; lock up gun cabinet. (Dad)
2. Talk to Liz, ask her how I can help, listen and empathize. (Mom)
3. Call her therapist or psychiatrist; go to a session with her if useful. (Mom)
4. Avoid being critical or judgmental, avoid lecturing. (Dad)
5. Notify friend Amy (213-555-1212).
6. Take Liz to emergency room if she doesn't think she can stay safe. (Dad or Mom)
7. Be available by cell phone when I'm at work. (Dad)

**Things Liz's therapist can do:**

1. Agree to see her on an emergency basis, help her understand why suicidal thoughts are coming up now.
2. Help her communicate with Dr. Miller about potential need for change in medications.
3. Help arrange hospital stay if necessary.

**Signatures:** _____

_____

**Relevant phone numbers:** _____

_____

**FIGURE 10.5.** Suicide prevention plan for Liz.

## SUMMARY

The risk of suicide has been and will remain a central concern in the treatment of bipolar disorder. Even with optimal psychotherapy, pharmacotherapy, the engagement of families, and sufficient financial resources to afford this care, mood swings can always heighten the risk of morbid thinking, self-destructive thoughts, and suicide attempts. As in the treatment of any and all other serious disorders, be they medical or psychiatric, patients sometimes die of their disease. However, with optimal care of patients with bipolar disorder, we can decrease this risk through the multimodal approaches described in this chapter.

# CHAPTER 11

## Strategic Interventions in Challenging Situations

*Comorbidity and the Use of Split Treatment*

I n this last chapter, we cover two sets of topics that are clinically relevant and interrelated but do not fit easily in the earlier chapters. The first part of the chapter covers illness comorbidity, the situation in which a bipolar patient also has another psychiatric disorder. Clinical work would certainly be easier if disorders presented in isolation: The clinician would make a single diagnosis and a single treatment plan would be constructed. The reality, of course, is that most illnesses—both medical and psychiatric—present in bunches, clouding both the clinical picture and relevant treatment approaches. The psychiatric disorders we discuss here that are frequently comorbid with bipolar disorder are ADHD, substance abuse, personality disorders, and anxiety disorders. We also review the situation of a bipolar patient with significant medical problems. The key question is: How does the presence of non-mood comorbid disorders alter the overall treatment approach described in previous chapters?

In the second part of the chapter, we focus on issues surrounding "split" treatment and, specifically, the relationship between the psychopharmacologist and the therapist, assuming that the two roles are not filled by one individual. What are the strengths, and what are the problems and pitfalls in this interaction? Which issues are most important for each of the professionals? How much and what type of communication does each want from the other? Because we each represent one of these groups of professionals, we try individually to answer these questions, then respond to the other's concerns, so that the relationship can be fully explored from both sides.

## BIPOLAR DISORDER AND COMORBID DISORDERS

Whether we are considering psychiatric or medical disorders, comorbidity in bipolar disorder is the rule rather than the exception. In a recent World Health Organization study, over 80% of bipolar I and bipolar II patients had at least one other psychiatric disorder, the most common of which were anxiety disorders.[1] Of course, in considering comorbidity, the question arises as to the causal relationship between two co-occurring disorders. Does one disorder make the individual more vulnerable to the other disorder? Can either disorder make the other one more likely to occur? Can both disorders be expressions of the same core vulnerability? And finally, is this just diagnostic overlap, in which the symptoms of one disorder are being counted as symptoms of the other, making it appear as if there are two disorders when only one exists? As an example of the latter, ADHD shares a number of features with bipolar disorder: impulsivity, physical hyperactivity, distractibility, and pressured speech. Finally, if another psychiatric disorder exists along with bipolar disorder, it may change the expression of the mood disorder and will almost certainly alter treatment strategies.

### Attention-Deficit/Hyperactivity Disorder

Both in child and adult studies, bipolar disorder and ADHD seem to coexist more frequently than would be expected by chance.[2] It does not seem to matter whether the individuals evaluated are drawn from a bipolar population or an ADHD population. In either circumstance, the other disorder is often diagnosed. As noted earlier, the overlap in symptoms between bipolar disorder and ADHD has made many observers suspicious that we are simply diagnosing one unitary set of symptoms and calling it two disorders. Compounding the problem is the increasing evidence that many adult bipolar patients show clear cognitive deficits (i.e., attention, memory, and executive function) when euthymic that cannot be fully explained by medication side effects. Thus, the types of cognitive impairment often seen in bipolar disorder are similar to those commonly seen in ADHD.

Coexistence of the two disorders is more common in children than in adults, with an estimated 62% of bipolar youth also having ADHD.[3] For adults, comorbid ADHD, seen in 9–10% of bipolar individuals, may be particularly common in those with an early onset (i.e., before age 13) of bipolar disorder.[4] Those with comorbid bipolar disorder and ADHD are also at higher risk for more severe depression and other psychiatric disorders such as substance abuse or anxiety. Additionally, family studies consistently find a higher prevalence of ADHD in the families of bipolar individuals than in control populations, and a higher prevalence of bipolar disorder in the families of individuals with ADHD.[2]

Despite evidence of high comorbidity between bipolar disorder and ADHD, no treatment approach for individuals with these disorders has been systematically explored.[5] The general recommendations for medication treatment, based mainly on clinical case series, is to treat the bipolar disorder with mood stabilizers first and *then* add appropriate ADHD treatment, such as stimulants or bupropion (Wellbutrin). Although there are concerns about the potential of these medications to destabilize mood, at least one randomized trial has shown that children with mania can be safely treated with adjunctive stimulants after being treated to remission with valproate (Depakote).[6]

The clinician should consider various forms of *cognitive rehabilitation* to help build attentional skills. A therapist may help the patient learn to use a daily calendar, to break large tasks down to smaller ones, and to address the negative thoughts and frustration that may accompany cognitive limitations. Concrete problem solving about time management, ways to avoid distraction and improve recall, and enhance longer-term planning (e.g., writing out the steps of tasks to be completed) may be useful supplements to a patient's psychostimulant regimen.

---

Regina, now age 36, was a wild and challenging child and adolescent. She was ill-behaved in school and her grades were poor. Her behavior was similar at home, where she was impulsive and oppositional. She was moody and had short periods of depression, but these were typically ascribed to her overall intense and chaotic life, and the frequent punishments from parents and teachers because of her unruly behavior. She had a brief trial of stimulants at age 11, but her parents were ambivalent at best about giving Regina medications. Her response to the stimulant was unclear. As an adolescent, she used a variety of street drugs and alcohol, but always in a social setting and without any evidence of addiction.

As a young adult, she continued to be disorganized and chaotic but held some jobs, got married, and had one child. In her 20s, Regina began to have clear depressive episodes lasting for months, with all the classic symptoms. Preceding these episodes, however, were periods typically lasting a few weeks in which she became irritable and her energy level increased. She would also spend money impulsively, become hypersexual, and speak rapidly. With a diagnosis of comorbid bipolar II disorder and ADHD, it was recommended that Regina take a mood stabilizer and then, once she was relatively stable, add a stimulant. She and her husband were also offered education, coping skills training, and parent training. Regina was started on lamotrigine

(Lamictal), with the dose gradually increased to 200 mg. Two months later, mixed amphetamine salts (Adderall) were added in doses up to 40 mg. Regina's mood cycling stabilized markedly but not completely.

During family sessions, Regina and her husband discussed the necessary steps for following through on her career plans, such as writing a resume and selecting a summer program for their children. With the combination of the problem solving and the psychostimulant, she became much more effective, both at work and as a parent. There has been no evidence of increased mood cycling since Regina started taking the stimulant.

---

### Substance Abuse

From a clinical perspective, substance abuse and dependence are the comorbidities of greatest concern. This concern reflects both the frequency of these disorders and their destructive potential in interaction with mood disorders. Bipolar patients are at higher risk for comorbid substance abuse than patients with any other psychiatric disorder, with rates ranging up to 60%.[7] Patients with bipolar I disorder show higher rates of substance abuse than do patients with bipolar II disorder, who, in turn, are at higher risk than those with major depression. The rates of substance abuse are higher in bipolar men than in bipolar women, but relative to the nonbipolar population, bipolar women show a greater proportional risk (seven times that of the population) than do bipolar men (almost three times the population risk).[8]

Bipolar patients with comorbid substance abuse have more severe mood symptoms; more complex presentations, such as rapid-cycling courses and mixed states; and more substance withdrawal difficulties than those without this comorbidity.[9] They also tend to be less treatment adherent and to have poorer responses to many different medications. Most importantly, they are at higher risk for suicide than people with either disorder alone.

The relationship between mood disorders and substance abuse disorders is complex. Some patients show early substance problems and later develop a mood disorder, while for others, the order is reversed. For those with a first expression of bipolar disorder, it is tempting to see the substance use as a form of self-medication to combat mood symptoms. As the substance abuse and bipolar disorder persist over time, this view becomes more firmly held in mind by the patient (and sometimes the family members). This myth persists, we suspect, because it provides a neatly packaged explanation: The patient is hurting inside, and once the hurt is treated, the substance abuse will disappear.

If the self-medication hypothesis were the case, one would expect greater use of stimulants when depressed and greater use of tranquilizing substances, such as alcohol, when manic. However, this is not consistently true. One study found that bipolar patients used more alcohol when depressed and more marijuana when manic.[10] Patients tend to use more cocaine and other stimulants when manic than when depressed.[11] Manic patients do most things to excess, including any and all drug and alcohol use. Furthermore, in up to half of dual-diagnosis patients, the course of bipolar disorder and either alcohol or cannabis abuse is divergent.[10]

Although generally not considered a substance of abuse, it is clear that nicotine-containing products, most commonly inhaled cigarettes, are addictive and associated with predictable craving and withdrawal symptoms. Bipolar patients smoke far more than the population at large, but not as frequently as do those with schizophrenia. In a recent large study, 44% of bipolar individuals smoked, compared to 64% of those with schizophrenia and less than 20% of those without a psychiatric disorder.[12] Although there is no evidence that nicotine contributes substantially to the course of bipolar disorder, it assuredly increases the risk for a variety of medical disorders and therefore contributes to the overall poorer outcome of bipolar individuals. Perhaps most disturbingly, one study found that current smoking was associated with a greater likelihood of having previously attempted suicide, even after adjusting for a number of covariates, such as lifetime history of substance abuse.[13]

## Pharmacological Treatment

The goal of treatment in dually diagnosed patients focuses on both greater mood stability and sustained abstinence. Despite the frequency of drug–alcohol abuse complicating bipolar disorder, only a handful of studies have examined treatment approaches for those with comorbidity, thereby making all recommendations tentative at best.[7] Most medication studies have focused on the specific comorbidity of alcohol abuse/dependence and bipolar disorder. Valproate may be effective in reducing alcohol abuse when prescribed by itself or when added to lithium. In a few studies, quetiapine (Seroquel) has also shown some modest efficacy with these patients. Classic medication treatments for alcohol abuse, such as naltrexone (Revia), acamprosate (Campral) or even disulfiram (Antabuse), may be safely used in bipolar patients when added to a mood stabilizer regimen. Their efficacy is still unclear due to a lack of studies.[7]

Other than nicotine substitution therapies (e.g., gum or patch), the two medications most commonly used to aid in cigarette smoking cessation are bupropion (marketed as Zyban) and varenicline (marketed as Chantix).[14] Although there has been no systematic study of the use of bupropion to aid in smoking cessation in bipolar individuals, the risk of switching into mania/hypomania should always be considered. Therefore, if bupropion is prescribed for smoking cessation in bipolar I disorder, it is safest if the patient is already on a mood stabilizer. Varenicline may also be effective in decreasing cigarette smoking. However, it may be associated with a number of psychiatric side effects, including treatment-emergent mania, and should therefore be prescribed with caution.

## Psychosocial Approaches

A cognitive-behavioral group approach called *integrated group therapy* (IGT) has been developed for patients with alcohol or drug abuse and bipolar disorder.[15] The approach treats bipolarity and substance abuse as if they are one disorder. The groups emphasize abstinence and instruct patients in identifying and fighting triggers for substance use, recognizing early warning signs of recurrence of either disorder, practicing "refusal skills," and restructuring self-defeating thoughts. IGT has been validated in two short-term, randomized trials of bipolar adults with dual diagnoses. In both trials, patients in IGT showed a reduction in alcohol and drug abuse over 3- to 8-month intervals compared to patients in single-focus drug education groups. Paradoxically, in one of the trials, patients in IGT had higher subsyndromal mood symptom scores at follow-up than patients in the drug education groups. The meaning of this finding is not clear. Possibly, reductions in substance use worsened mood symptoms in these patients, or the integrated treatment may have increased the frequency with which patients identified and reported their mood symptoms.

There is a version of family-focused treatment (FFT) for adolescent bipolar patients with a substance use disorder (FFT-SUD).[16] The goals of the FFT-SUD approach include (1) promoting substance-free homes in which substance use by parents is addressed as a risk factor; (2) framing substance abuse as a health-compromising behavior and challenging the notion that it reflects self-medication; (3) identifying high-risk situations in which the patient may be exposed to substances; and (4) developing strategies for avoiding these triggers and/or managing cravings. There are no randomized trials of this approach, although open-trial data are encouraging.[16]

Groups such as AA and Narcotics Anonymous (NA) should always be considered for dual-diagnosis patients. Although no data exist on their effectiveness in bipolar disorder, there is considerable evidence in the general population that these groups save lives. One long-term follow-up study found that bipolar patients with alcoholism—particularly those who attended AA and maintained contact with a family doctor—tended to have better outcomes than depressed patients with alcoholism.[17] However, it is important to refer patients to AA or NA groups that recognize the validity of dual-diagnosis conditions (e.g., "Double Trouble in Recovery" groups). One cannot assume that the groups always support the patient's need for psychiatric medications.

Other group or individual approaches may be helpful if the goal of complete abstinence seems impossible. An example is the Self-Management and Recovery Training (SMART) group program and its associated Web-based intervention, Overcoming Addictions.[18] A program of individual motivational interviewing to address the patient's ambivalence about discontinuing substances may also be helpful.[19]

### Personality Disorders

Every clinician working with individuals with bipolar disorder recognizes the complications of comorbid personality pathology in these patients. Comorbidity between bipolar disorder and personality disorders is relatively common, with rates ranging rather broadly between 12 and 84%, with an average of just under 50%.[20–21] No single personality disorder seems to be the most common in bipolar patients. In this section we focus mostly on the interaction of bipolar disorder and borderline personality disorder (BPD), since this comorbidity is the most challenging. The key complications in the treatment of comorbid BPD patients include (1) diagnostic confusion, such as deciding when the presenting clinical picture represents bipolar disorder, borderline personality disorder (or features), or a combination of the two; and (2) management of the multiple sources of symptoms in these patients. Clinicians often have to parse behaviors that (1) appear to be reflections of personality pathology that might respond best to psychotherapy, (2) reflect the more biological components of personality pathology (such as impulsivity or affective lability) and that might be optimally treated with a change in medications, or (3) are primarily a reflection of mood disorder symptoms that have not stabilized with medications and/or psychotherapy.

As we discussed in Chapter 2, the first issue in evaluating and treating comorbid bipolar disorder and BPD is making a proper diagnosis, or diagnoses, given the overlap in symptom pictures. Impulsivity (e.g., excessive spending, sexual behavior, drug use), affective lability, and suicidality are common features of both disorders. Confounding the diagnostic question is the likelihood that some personality features present differently depending on the patient's mood state. As an example, in the midst of a mania/hypomania, provocative features associated with narcissistic or borderline personalities may be accentuated in a patient, whereas when depressed, the same patient may show few of these characteristics. Therefore, when possible, personality traits should be evaluated when the patient is euthymic, or by using information about the patient's personality characteristics when *not* in a mood episode. One way of assessing trait stability is to ask, for each of the major interpersonal behaviors consistent with personality disorder, "Has this behavior (impulsive sex, rage reactions, wanting to be the center of attention) been true of you for most of the past 5 years, even when you weren't clearly depressed or manic?"

Overall, and as expected, patients with comorbid bipolar disorder and BPD show an overall poorer outcome compared to those with pure bipolar disorder. Those with both disorders tend to have a greater number of suicide attempts, poorer treatment adherence, poorer function, and less response to medications.[20]

## Psychosocial Approaches

We first described DBT in Chapter 10 in relation to suicide. Arranging DBT for a patient—at least as conceptualized in the original model—involves weekly individual skills training sessions and weekly group sessions. If the patient has BPD, a supervisory team is often needed to manage the reactions the clinician(s) may have to these patients and to integrate the treatment plans. Thus, DBT requires considerable resources. The skills taught in DBT include interpersonal effectiveness, distress tolerance, emotion regulation, and mindful awareness. One research group has successfully adapted DBT for bipolar disorder in adolescence,[22] but no studies have examined the effects of DBT on bipolar patients with comorbid BPD.

IPSRT has been evaluated in a small study of adult bipolar patients with BPD.[23] Those with both disorders took almost three times as long to stabilize with IPSRT, and required greater use of atypical antipsychotics than did bipolar patients without BPD. They were also more likely to drop out of treatment.

A new approach to psychotherapy for BPD, mentalization-based therapy (MBT), may be applicable to patients with bipolar disorder.

MBT is based on research indicating that individuals with significant emotional dysregulation have deficits in the ability to *mentalize*—the process by which we make sense of ourselves and others, either explicitly or implicitly, in terms of thoughts and feelings.[24,25] In this framework, significant stress leads to increases in emotional arousal, which interfere with the patient's ability to make sense of interpersonal events and cause temporary losses in mentalization (i.e., loss of perspective in interpreting one's own or others' motivations). This process, combined with ongoing or recurrent depression, results in an increase in self-defeating thoughts, leading to more significant depression, social withdrawal, and an urgent desire to escape through self-harm.[26]

MBT typically proceeds with regular individual therapy sessions that focus on the patient's social experiences and resulting mental states. Through exploration and clarification, patients learn to manage anticipated interpersonal challenges, particularly those involving separation or loss. Although the approach may sound a lot like IPSRT, it is based in psychodynamic formulations. The clinician emphasizes failures of mentalizing as the key trigger for mood swings, rather than sleep–wake or social rhythm irregularity. Although no studies of bipolar patients have been done, MBT has a good track record in alleviating self-harming behavior in adults[25] and adolescents[26] with BPD.

## Pharmacological Treatment

Luckily, many of the medications that are most effective in treating BPD overlap substantially with those prescribed for bipolar disorder. Unluckily, there are no studies examining the efficacy of any medication approach for those with bipolar disorder plus BPD (or any other personality disorder). Ironically, there are almost no good studies on lithium for BPD. Anticonvulsants and SGAs are the best validated medications for BPD.[27,28]

Anticonvulsants show substantial efficacy in decreasing impulsive aggressive behavior (in the absence of mania) and reactive anger. This seems to be a medication class effect: All anticonvulsants (valproate, lamotrigine, topiramate [Topamax], oxcarbazepine [Trileptal], etc.) seem to be effective in reducing aggressive outbursts, in contrast to the differential efficacy of specific anticonvulsants in alleviating mood symptoms in bipolar disorder (Chapters 5 and 6). Therefore, in picking a specific anticonvulsant for bipolar patients with BPD, it would make sense first to use an agent with efficacy in both disorders, such as valproate or lamotrigine. As always, side-effect profiles need to be considered given the poor medication adherence of comorbid patients.[29]

SGAs may also be effective in patients with comorbid bipolar disorder and BPD, especially in decreasing anger. Studies on SSRIs in borderline patients show weak positive effects in decreasing anger and anxiety. I (M. J. G.) have had positive experiences with SSRIs in these patients, especially in diminishing affective reactivity (the ability to tolerate negative events without becoming overwhelmingly depressed, upset, or suicidal). Because the SSRIs are relatively benign in their side-effect profile, many experienced clinicians (including M. J. G.) often prescribe them as first-line treatments if affective reactivity and lability are dominant features of the personality disorder. Of course, since SSRIs are antidepressants, the usual caveats about potential antidepressant-induced mood switching apply.

---

Maggie had struggled with bipolar I disorder since her early 20s, with two hospitalized manias, other milder hypomanias, and many depressions. Some depressions were triggered by life events, usually a romantic breakup or, when she was younger, a bad fight with her parents. Lithium had markedly decreased the frequency of her manic and hypomanic episodes, but Maggie continued to have very stormy and chaotic relationships, with mood lability alternating with periods of depression and self-destructive behavior. Because of the continued depressive symptoms and their intimate relationship with her borderline personality features, lamotrigine was prescribed in doses gradually increasing to 200 mg daily (in addition to the lithium).

Within 2 months, Maggie felt more "settled"; her relationships were still somewhat chaotic but she was less impulsive and less overwhelmed after fights with her boyfriend. She had a marked decrease in her self-destructive urges and behaviors. At that point, she felt more ready to take on the tasks of DBT, such as attending group sessions, practicing meditation, and filling out a daily diary card. Thus, lamotrigine was effective in stabilizing her mood and chaotic behavior to the extent that she could benefit from psychotherapy.

---

## Anxiety Disorders

It is not intuitive that bipolar individuals are at higher risk for full-syndrome anxiety disorders (as opposed to anxiety symptoms frequently seen in both manic and depressive states). Yet up to 60% of bipolar individuals meet criteria for one or more anxiety disorders over their lifetimes.[30] Bipolar II individuals seem to be at higher risk than bipolar I patients for anxiety disorders.[31] Panic disorder and obsessive–compulsive disorder (OCD) are the most common anxiety disorders seen in bipolar individuals, but generalized anxiety disorder, social anxiety disorder, and PTSD are also common.[30,32] Some, but not all studies have found that patients with comorbid bipolar disorder plus anxiety disorders do less well clinically than those without anxiety disorders, and are at risk for other comorbidities such as substance abuse.[33]

Anxiety disorders can be effectively treated with medications, psychotherapy, or a combination of the two. For panic disorder, benzodiazepines and SSRIs are both effective. Benzodiazepines do not destabilize bipolar disorder, but they are not optimal treatment for those with comorbid substance abuse. OCD is typically treated with exposure and response prevention and/or high dose SSRIs or clomipramine (Anafranil; a tricyclic antidepressant with strong effects on serotonin). As described, SSRIs may occasionally destabilize bipolar disorder, but tricyclics are much more likely to do so. Additionally, the side-effect burden of clomipramine is far greater than that of any SSRI. Therefore, adding an SSRI to a mood stabilizer should be the first medication strategy chosen for bipolar individuals with comorbid OCD. When patients have an inadequate response to high-dose SSRIs for OCD, treatment can be augmented with low-dose antipsychotics, which should pose no additional risks for bipolar individuals.

---

Megan had severe bipolar I disorder, with multiple hospitalizations for psychotic manias but no depressive episodes. After breakthrough episodes on lithium, valproate, a combination of the two, and antipsychotics, she eventually stabilized on clozapine (Clozaril). Unfortunately, she developed new-onset OCD (which is an occasional side effect of clozapine). Terrified of having another manic episode, she was treated with intensive behavior therapy in a partial hospital program, but with no improvement. After 3 years of comorbid OCD and no mood episodes, she reluctantly agreed to a trial of high-dose (60 mg) citalopram (Celexa) added to her clozapine. After 3 months, she had a clear reduction in her rituals. Although she continued to have OCD symptoms, they were much milder. Over the next 10 years, she had only one mild manic episode, and Megan continues to improve on the combination of clozapine plus citalopram.

---

## Cognitive-Behavioral Therapy

CBT approaches have become the treatments of choice for patients with anxiety disorders, although, of course, findings with anxiety patients cannot necessarily be generalized to bipolar patients with comorbid anxiety disorders. Although various brands of CBT exist, most include an educational component (i.e., understanding how anxiety is fueled by one's avoidance behavior), exposure (i.e., gradually introducing the patient to the feared stimulus, which may be external [e.g., novel situations in people with social phobia] or internal [i.e., imagery in PTSD; bodily sensations in panic disorder], and a cognitive restructuring component [e.g., challenging one's beliefs that a rapid heart rate will lead to a heart attack]).[34] The treatments usually involve *in vivo* exposure exercises. For example, a patient with panic disorder might be asked to spin in a chair to re-create the physical sensations that often precede panic. A patient with PTSD might be asked to return gradually to the setting where a traumatic event occurred. These approaches have been empirically validated in multiple trials of patients with anxiety disorders,[34] but their effectiveness in bipolar disorder has not been examined.

Many clinicians report that CBT specialists are not available in their communities, have long waiting lists, or are unaffordable. As indicated in prior chapters, introducing mindfulness exercises into sessions can offer the patient temporary respite from anxiety until proper CBT (or more extensive mindfulness training) can be obtained. For example, the clinician can take the patient through a 3-minute breathing exercise at the beginning of each session (Figure 11.1).

The exercise may feel awkward or staged at first; meditation is like a muscle that has to be developed over time. If the patient has responded well and says that his anxiety has been temporarily lowered, the clinician can consider referring the patient to one of the mindfulness groups that are becoming increasingly available (and often free) in communities. The patient can also obtain instructional DVDs that guide mindfulness exercises, along with a self-guided text that puts these exercises in context (e.g., Williams et al.[37]).

Regardless of the form that the behavioral treatment takes, the patient should be encouraged to track his daily anxiety on a mood chart (perhaps with a separate line or box) and the events, mood states, and sleep patterns that contribute to it (see Chapter 7). Mood charts kept over months often reveal unexpected patterns: For example, the patient feels more anxious when hypomanic than depressed; his anxiety level is correlated with sleeping too much; or he is more likely to drink or smoke marijuana when anxious than when depressed.

### Medical Disorders

Medical disorders are routinely present in more than half of bipolar patients and occur at higher rates than would be expected in an age-matched healthy population. Many other serious psychiatric disorders, such as schizophrenia and major depression, are also characterized by unusually high rates of comorbid medical disorders. In a recent study,

When the patient reports feeling mildly anxious or down, ask him to sit comfortably in the chair, with his back upright and hands on his thighs, not touching the back of the chair. He can also lie on his back if he prefers. Then, slowly give the following instructions:

- Close your eyes or stare at an object in the room. Spend 60 seconds being aware of the noises in your room—the sound of the air conditioner or heating, sounds from the street, music, people's voices. Ask yourself, "What am I experiencing in my thoughts, my emotions, and my body?" Acknowledge to yourself each sensation, thought, or feeling, whether pleasant or unpleasant.

- Now, for the next 60 seconds, focus on your breathing. Keep focusing on your in-breath and out-breath, like you were riding a wave. It's inevitable that your mind will wander. If your attention shifts to thinking of other things, notice what took you away but gently escort yourself back to your breathing.

- Now, for the next 60 seconds, shift your attention to your entire body—your belly, feet, legs, thighs, buttocks, stomach, chest, neck, and facial expression. Notice your posture and the sensation in different parts of your body as you breathe in and out. If your mind wanders, gently escort your awareness back to your body and breathing.

- Slowly open your eyes and come back in contact with the room.

**FIGURE 11.1.** A 3-minute mindfulness breathing exercise. From D. J. Miklowitz and E. L. George.[36] *The Bipolar Teen: What You Can Do to Help Your Child and Your Family.* New York: Guilford Press; 2008. Copyright 2008 by The Guilford Press. Reprinted by permission. (Adapted with permission from Z. V. Segal et al.[35])

58% of bipolar patients also had a medical disorder, with neurological disease, cardiac disease, thyroid disease, or diabetes being the most common. Bipolar patients with an earlier onset, more lifetime episodes, and those who smoke cigarettes and/or have a history of substance abuse are at greater risk for one or more chronic medical disorders.[38]

Bipolar individuals with medical disorders have relatively more lifetime depressive episodes and a greater severity of depressive symptoms.[39] In older adults, it is less clear that medical comorbidities are more common in bipolar individuals than in those without a mood disorder. However, in one study, 49% of older adults with bipolar disorder were obese (with its attendant medical risks) compared to 30% for the national average.[40]

This pattern of findings raises the question of how best to understand the comorbidity between bipolar and medical disorders. Does a mood disorder somehow make an individual more vulnerable to certain medical disorders? Activation of hormonal changes during manic and/or depressive episodes might, over long time periods, increase the risk of some medical disorders. Additionally, there is considerable research on the role of inflammatory processes as part of the underlying biology of psychiatric disorders, with recent evidence in bipolar disorder.[41] These processes might also predispose some to medical disorders, such as cardiac disease or diabetes. Given the early onset of bipolar disorder compared to significant cardiac and metabolic disorders, it seems more likely that bipolar disorder predisposes people to medical disorders rather than the reverse, but the causal direction has never been studied.

Another critical factor is the role of medications (specifically, antipsychotics that cause weight gain) in causing medical disorders such as obesity, cardiovascular disease, diabetes, and hypertension; or, for lithium, thyroid and/or renal problems. Unhealthy lifestyles associated with mood disorders, such as less exercise, poor diet, and smoking and drug–alcohol abuse, may increase the risk of a number of medical disorders. Patients with mood disorders often have poorer access to health care due to insurance issues, resulting in later diagnoses of medical disorders and less medical follow-up.

When medical disorders and bipolar disorder coexist, they may interact with each other in a number of ways, as shown in Table 11.1. The most important of these (and the easiest to lose sight of) is the sheer additive results of side effects of all medications, both medical and psychiatric. These concerns are especially important in older adults because not only are they more likely to be taking multiple medications for multiple disorders but also they are less resilient. A young person whose balance is affected by medication(s) may fall but will typically grab onto something and perhaps be bruised; the older person may fall hard and break a hip. Additionally, one medication may be only slightly sedating, with no clinical significance, but four of these medications might make someone very sleepy, and at risk for car accidents, falling or other adverse outcomes. The potential interactions between psychiatric medications and treatments for medical disorders are more straightforward and are listed in Table 11.1.

---

Bob had his first manic episode at the unusual age of 48. In retrospect, he had probably suffered from mild but unrecognized hypomanias and a few

**TABLE 11.1. Interactions between Medical Disorders and Treatment of Bipolar Disorder**

Nonpsychiatric medications that can exacerbate preexisting mood disorders
- Steroids, causing depression or mania
- Tamoxifen (Nolvadex), tretinoin (Retin-A) for breast cancer, causing depression

Medical disorders that alter treatment choices for bipolar disorder
- Obesity, limiting the prescription of psychiatric medications that cause weight gain
- Renal (kidney) problems, potentially making lithium contraindicated

Liver cirrhosis, making valproate and/or carbamazepine relatively contraindicated

Seizure disorder, making bupropion contraindicated

Side effects of psychotropic medications that worsen medical disorders
- Weight gain that may worsen diabetes, heart disease, metabolic syndrome, or back pain
- Worsening renal function from lithium

Additive side effects of medical and psychiatric medications (particularly in older adults)
- Sedation
- Orthostatic hypotension (dizziness upon standing up) with antipsychotics and antidepressants
- Poor balance
- Cognitive side effects

Pharmacokinetic interactions (one medication affects blood levels of another)
- Some SSRIs or duloxetine (Cymbalta) decreasing tamoxifen levels
- Carbamazepine and oxcarbazepine decreasing levels of oral contraceptives

life-event-triggered depressions that were untreated and short-lived. His manic episode was relatively severe and required an involuntary hospitalization, during which he was emergently treated with olanzapine (Zyprexa) with positive effect. During the hospitalization, it became clear that Bob also had hepatitis C, with only a small increase in his liver enzymes. Because of the hepatitis C, it was strongly recommended that Bob start lithium because it is not metabolized by the liver (it is excreted unchanged through the kidneys) and cannot worsen hepatitis C. Although Bob was initially reluctant to take lithium, having heard horror stories about it, he ultimately agreed for these health reasons. After a mild postmanic depression, he has been euthymic for over 3 years. His hepatitis C continues to be quiescent.

## SPLIT TREATMENT

### Relationships between Psychopharmacologists and Psychotherapists

The high frequency of comorbid disorders in bipolar disorder underlines the importance of collaboration between multiple mental health and medical professionals in treating a patient. *Split treatment* refers to the situation in which a patient's pharmacotherapy is conducted by a psychiatrist and therapy is conducted by another psychiatrist, psychologist, social worker, or other professional.

Twenty to 30 years ago, when we began our clinical careers, splitting treatment into psychiatric and psychological components with two separate professionals was fraught with problems. The theoretical models underlying the two treatments were very different and, in the minds of some professionals, incompatible. There were theoretical concerns that one treatment might undermine the efficacy of the other: Would medication decrease the motivation for therapy and seduce the patient into wanting only a "quick fix"? Would psychotherapy stir up unnecessary affect and undermine mood stabilization therapy? With some, there was an undeniable professional rivalry, with concerns that the other practitioner might undermine the professional's treatment approach and that one's clinical practice (and livelihood) would be negatively affected by split treatment.

Decades later, these potential pitfalls, although still problematic on occasion, are much less of a concern. First, with rare exception, the sheer experience of most mental health clinicians with split therapy has desensitized us and made us more comfortable with the model. We have all seen the model work successfully many times. Second, the increasing emphasis on comorbid disorders has forced all of us to think more broadly and flexibly about psychopathology in general, and to acknowledge that most of our patients have problems that require a variety of therapeutic approaches. Third, research studies have demonstrated that one form of treatment almost never undermines another, simultaneous form of treatment. (The only exception, which is not particularly relevant to bipolar disorder, is that benzodiazepine tranquilizers may diminish the efficacy of desensitization/exposure therapy for phobias.) Fourth, there is solid evidence that the efficacy of pharmacotherapy and psychotherapy is additive. As the most relevant example for bipolar disorder, the psychotherapies described in Chapter 7 consistently provide benefit beyond that seen with medication alone (for a recent review, see Geddes & Miklowitz[42]).

**TABLE 11.2. Advantages of Split Treatment**

- Allows each treatment modality to stay focused.
- Different interviewing techniques may lead to broader acquisition of clinical data.
- Transference issues may be diffused by the presence of two mental health professionals.
- The nuances of everyday situations and changes in the course of the illness over time can be observed by both professionals, leading to earlier identification and treatment of recurrences.

Splitting the treatment into components provided by two different professionals may be helpful for a number of other reasons[43] (see Table 11.2). First, with a split treatment, each therapy can stay focused. Somatically preoccupied patients may dwell on physical symptoms and side effects, distracting the psychotherapy. With a split model, the somatic concerns can be addressed by the psychopharmacologist, allowing the therapist to stay on track with psychological issues. Second, different interviewing styles and clinical requirements may be more easily managed with a split treatment. Medication management sessions, which often must be conducted in less than half an hour, tend to be structured and directive, with concrete questions on symptoms and side effects as essential components. Psychotherapy—even behavioral approaches—is less structured. Third, all mental health professionals have had the experience of incredibly difficult patients (e.g., those with bipolar disorder plus BPD and/or substance abuse) with whom the therapeutic relationship can be very difficult to manage. The presence of two treating professionals can be mutually supportive and dilute some of the difficulties in the therapeutic interaction. A single, conjoint session involving the patient, prescribing physician, and therapist can often break a therapeutic impasse.

Finally, in treating bipolar individuals with psychotherapy plus medication, there is a need for both the intensive, microcosmic examination (What did the patient do or think this week?) and the broader macrocosmic view (What is the pattern of mood symptoms over weeks and/or months?) Having two professionals with different vantage points allows both views to be examined.

### The Prescriber's Perspective

Having worked with the split-treatment model for over 30 years, I (M. J. G.) am more than comfortable with it. When it works well, it is a pleasure to collaborate with a colleague, to see keen attention paid to both psychological and pharmacological aspects of therapy, and to see a patient improve due to combined efforts. From my viewpoint, a number of key elements underlie the success of split treatment.

First, it is mandatory that the two professionals believe in the helpfulness of the other treatment (and the other practitioner), and that they convey these beliefs to the patient. Without this mutual respect and encouragement, "splitting" will occur (i.e., one provider is good and the other is bad) and undermine the collaborative efforts rather quickly. Of course, there is always a first time working with a new colleague, and split treatment is rarely seamless at the beginning. Over time, as with any team, professionals develop a more comfortable collaborative style. However, communication must be optimal in frequency: neither too infrequent nor too much.

## Optimal Communication

Communication between the two treating clinicians should occur at important treatment junctures:

1. When there is a change in clinical condition, such as when the patient becomes manic or depressed, and there is a clear need to change the treatment strategy based on the mood shift.
2. If the patient becomes suicidal. Considerations about whether the patient can be safely treated in an outpatient setting should be addressed. If the patient has a substantial amount of medication at home and there is concern about overdose potential, a legitimate therapeutic plan would be for the therapist, who is likely to see the patient more frequently, to keep the medication in her office and distribute 1 week of medication at a time to minimize the medical risk of overdose. Of course, the patient must agree to this plan.
3. When there is a major change in diagnosis, usually necessitating an equally major change in pharmacological—and often psychological—treatment. An example might be the emergence of a hypomanic episode in a patient previously treated for unipolar depression, shifting the diagnosis to bipolar disorder.

James's diagnosis was recurrent major depressive disorder. Both his therapist and his psychopharmacologist agreed on this. After his most recent and severe depression, he improved dramatically with a course of ECT, after which he was placed on mirtazapine (Remeron) and venlafaxine (Effexor) to prevent a depressive relapse. Two weeks after the discontinuation of ECT, his therapist noted that James was not just better, but "moving in fast-forward." His sleep had decreased to 6 hours per night, only slightly less than his usual 7 hours, but he was flirting with women (uncharacteristic of this married man) and was more confident than he had ever been before. He was considering a change in his business and was unusually bold in his thinking. The therapist and psychopharmacologist conferred and agreed that James was having a first hypomanic episode. The therapist decided to work with James on his sleep–wake rhythms, and the psychopharmacologist added a low dose (2.5 mg) of aripiprazole (Abilify) to his antidepressant. When the two clinicians talked again a week later to check in on James's status, they concluded that he was no longer hypomanic. This change in treatment plan may have prevented the occurrence of a more serious manic episode.

---

Communication needs to be optimal, not excessive. Part of the problem in having reasonable and mutually consistent expectations regarding communication between two professionals is the inherent imbalance in the number of patients each one follows. A psychiatrist who practices psychopharmacology exclusively and sees patients for 15- to 20-minute sessions may follow hundreds of patients. In contrast, a therapist may see only a few dozen patients per week. Because of this, each therapy patient comprises a larger part of the therapist's practice. Consequently, the therapist often wants to talk about the patient more often and for a longer time than does the psychopharmacologist.

Many psychopharmacologists dread the phone call of the therapist who wants/needs to tell at great length about all of the details of the psychological traumas the patient has suffered, minor changes in the transference relationship, slight behavioral changes in sessions that may or may not indicate improvement, or endless nuances of the patient's marital difficulties. These are certainly relevant issues for the therapy, but the psychopharmacologist is usually thinking: "What is the current problem? What do I need to do differently to help?" Details about the past traumas or relationship problems do not typically alter the questions that the psychopharmacologist needs to address. He may also be thinking about 10 pharmacy calls and 12 calls from patients about side effects that he must return. Therefore, from the psychopharmacologist's viewpoint, communication needs to be brief and efficient.

Another pet peeve of psychopharmacologists is when the therapist recommends a specific medication to the patient and urges the psychiatrist to follow through on this recommendation. As an example, a patient called the prescribing physician relaying the message (accurately) that her therapist thought that sertraline (Zoloft) was the right antidepressant to be added, not the bupropion that the physician had just recommended. The therapist was right to recognize the patient's depression and to communicate to the physician that a medication change should be considered. The direct recommendation to a patient of a specific treatment or, even more, of a specific medication within a treatment class, is not reasonable from the psychopharmacologist's viewpoint and predictably creates resentment. Encouraging the therapist to limit recommendations to classes of medications—and to communicate these specific recommendations to the physician before recommending them to the patient—will reduce this kind of conflict.

## The Therapist's Perspective

Split-treatment arrangements can work very well and are essential when working with relapse-prone or suicidal bipolar patients. Many therapists do not work with bipolar patients at all because their practice does not have an emergency infrastructure (e.g., a psychopharmacologist who can administer emergency medications and has hospital admitting privileges; 24-hour paging or answering services) for high-risk patients. This has always disappointed me (D. J. M.); many psychologists and social workers who are talented clinicians have not considered the value of a split-treatment arrangement with an MD colleague, or are intimidated by this arrangement.

The intimidation may be borne of experience. Many therapists cite occasions when they felt inadequate when interacting with psychiatrists, as if their treatment were viewed as less powerful or less important than the pharmacotherapy. Many of us hear "Who's the real doctor?" ringing in our ears from previous exchanges. Some therapists report that they have to work exceptionally hard to get a physician to call them back, and when they finally reach him, he is brusque and impatient. Therapists also report that they conscientiously share clinical information with the physician, especially at crisis times, but then do not hear from the physician when the patient has been hospitalized, a major change in medication has been undertaken, or there has been a suicide attempt. This communication problem can be compounded when patients or family members believe that only the physician needs to know about crises, since the necessary intervention will likely be pharmacological.

Paralleling the annoyance of physicians when a therapist recommends a certain medication, the biggest pet peeve of therapists is a physician who recommends to the patient forms of therapy other than the one the therapist has been providing, interrupting a productive therapeutic alliance. Sometimes this occurs when there is a lack of information exchange between the therapist and pharmacologist about the goals and expected duration of therapy. For example, Alec, a 55-year-old man with bipolar disorder, BPD, and substance abuse was doing well in individual IPSRT. His therapist had been conscientiously communicating with the psychiatrist, although his phone calls often went unanswered. Then, during a crisis, Alec's physician told him that he really should be getting DBT because "there is no evidence that bipolar disorder can be treated with interpersonal therapy." Although Alec stayed in IPSRT, this event caused him to doubt the treatment plan and engendered a degree of mistrust with his therapist. When the therapist discussed the matter with the physician, the physician said, "I didn't know you were still seeing him."

In my experience, therapists do best when they pair up with a specific physician or physician practice. By doing so, they can collaborate on multiple cases and establish regular conversations about the progress of cases. Some therapeutic dyads meet for case discussions over lunch, or at least schedule a weekly or biweekly time to review all cases. However, as discussed earlier (by M. J. G.), the therapist must keep in mind the time limitations of the physician. If the physician is seeing dozens of cases in a single day, then knowing the details of the psychotherapy with any one case will be viewed as too much information and an unnecessary distraction.

The therapist should examine her expectations about what the physician needs to know to reconsider the medication regimen. Organizing the clinical information into current symptoms (e.g., recent prodromal symptom behaviors, a return of substance abuse), stressors (e.g., marital breakup, loss of job), evidence of medication nonadherence, and side effects (e.g., weight gain) will help the discussions go more efficiently. Indeed, therapists are usually quite time-burdened themselves, and brief, efficient discussions may be more realistic than extensive case analyses.

Prescribing physicians are more likely to refer other patients to psychotherapists who are able to organize communication in a way that not only appreciates the goals of the pharmacotherapy but also recognizes the physician's time limitations. Likewise, the therapist is more likely to refer patients to a psychopharmacologist who appreciates the role of psychotherapy in stabilizing the patient, and the unique vantage point that therapeutic contacts provide. On the whole, we believe the split-treatment arrangement to be a powerful approach in the management of bipolar disorder, albeit one that needs careful planning, regular information exchange, and appropriate boundary setting.

## LOOKING TO THE FUTURE

In this book, we have attempted to take readers through the stages of bipolar treatment—from diagnosis to acute treatment to long-term maintenance. We have tried to convey the complexity of the condition; the different needs of patients who are perinatal, medically ill, or have comorbid psychiatric disorders; the important role of families in maintaining consistency with treatment and even in preventing recurrences; and the importance of integrated pharmacological and psychosocial treatment, especially in instances when suicidality is a factor.

We recognize that the treatment of patients with bipolar disorder may increasingly occur in general practice or family medicine clinics. Our recommendations will require adaptation in general practice, such as when a doctor can only see the patient once every few months. If medical care goes in the direction of the "medical homes" model (i.e., all health providers in a single location), some of the difficulties with split treatment or lack of access will be minimized, but we suspect that most of our recommendations will still apply.

We are beginning to see technological advances in the ability of professionals to monitor patients' mood states and incorporate the results of this monitoring into treatment planning.[44] These are positive developments, as is the appearance of online medical record keeping and prescription management. Nonetheless, the personalized care we have recommended, in which patients are provided with careful, systematic diagnosis and thoughtful, integrated pharmacological and psychosocial treatment, will never be fully automated.

# ─────── APPENDIX A ───────

## Resources for Clinicians and Patients

This section contains information—including national organizations, websites, and books—that may be of help to clinicians looking for referrals for their patients, as well as to patients who are either looking for treatment or are already in treatment and want to learn more about their disorder.

### SUICIDE HOTLINES

Suicide Prevention Hotline (national)
800-273-TALK

Suicide Hotlines by State
*www.suicidehotlines.com*

### PSYCHIATRIST AND THERAPIST REFERRALS

American Psychiatric Association (psychiatrist referrals)
Washington, DC
*www.psych.org*
*apa@psych.org*
888-357-7924 and press 0

American Psychological Association (therapist locator tool)
Washington, DC
*www.apa.org*
*http://locator.apa.org*
800-964-2000

Association for Behavioral and Cognitive Therapies (behavioral therapist locator tool)
New York, NY
*www.abct.org*
212-647-1890

National Association of Social Workers (social worker referrals)
Washington, DC
*www.naswdc.org*
*www.helppro.com/nasw/basicsearch.aspx*
202-408-8600

National Network of Depression Centers
Ann Arbor, MI
*www.nndc.org/health-resources/appointments-referrals*
*nndc@nndc.org*
734-332-3914 or 734-332-3989

Substance Abuse and Mental Health Services Administration (state-by-state treatment locator)
Rockville, MD
*http://findtreatment.samhsa.gov/mhtreatmentlocator/faces/quicksearch.jspx*
877-SAMHSA-7

Balanced Mind Foundation (for locating child psychiatrists and psychologists/social workers)
Chicago, IL
*www.thebalancedmind.org*
847-492-8510

## BIPOLAR DISORDER SPECIALTY CLINICS

UCLA Child and Adolescent Mood Disorders Clinic (CHAMP)
UCLA School of Medicine, Los Angeles, CA
*www.semel.ucla.edu/champ*
310-825-2836

Robert D. Sutherland Clinic for the Treatment of Bipolar Disorder
University of Colorado, Boulder, CO
*http://rdsfoundation.org*
303-492-5680

Child and Adolescent Bipolar Services Clinic
University of Pittsburgh Medical Center, Pittsburgh, PA
*www.pediatricbipolar.pitt.edu*
877-526-2629

University of Cincinnati Mood Disorders Center
Cincinnati Children's Hospital Medical Center
Cincinnati, OH
513-558-7700 (adults); 513-558-2989 (children and teens)

Family Center for Bipolar
Beth Israel Medical Center
New York, NY
*www.bpfamily.org*
212-420-2302

Stanford Adult and Pediatric Bipolar Disorders Clinics
Stanford University School of Medicine
Stanford, CA
*http://bipolar.stanford.edu*
650-498-9111, 650-725-6760, or 650-736-2688

## NATIONAL AND INTERNATIONAL ORGANIZATIONS

**American Foundation for Suicide Prevention**
*www.afsp.org*
212-363-3500

The leading national not-for-profit organization exclusively dedicated to understanding and preventing suicide through research, education and advocacy.

**Balanced Mind Foundation**
*www.bpkids.org*
847-492-8519

A parent-led organization that provides information and support to family members, health care professionals, and the public concerning bipolar disorders in young people. Formerly known as the Child and Adolescent Bipolar Foundation, the organization advocates for health services and research on the nature, causes, and treatment of early-onset bipolar disorder. Visitors can locate mental health providers who see bipolar children and adolescents in different areas of the United States. The Learning Center contains examples of mood charts, articles on how to prepare for initial doctor visits, and information on research studies.

**Danny Alberts Foundation**
*www.albertsfoundation.org*

Funds research on alternative treatments for bipolar disorder. Their current studies emphasize mindfulness meditation as an adjunct to pharmacotherapy. The Resources section of the website is highly informative.

## Depression and Bipolar Support Alliance
*www.dbsalliance.org*
800-826-3632

Devoted to educating consumers and their family members about mood disorders, decreasing the public stigma of these illnesses, fostering self-help, advocating for research funding, and improving access to care. DBSA has chapters in many cities that offer free, peer-led support groups.

## Equilibrium: The Bipolar Foundation
*www.bipolar-foundation.org*

An international/nongovernmental organization based in the United Kingdom that seeks to increase understanding and reduce the societal stigma of bipolar disorder through funding research, providing educational webinars, and other endeavors.

## International Bipolar Foundation
*www.internationalbipolarfoundation.org*
858-764-2496

Seeks to better understand, prevent, and treat bipolar disorder through research; to promote care and support services for individuals and caregivers; and to erase stigma through public education. It publishes an e-newsletter called "My Support" with information about talks, clinical referrals, webinars, and recent advances in research. A "Get Help" section provides resources around the world.

## International Society for Bipolar Disorders
*www.isbd.org*
412-802-6940

Aims to promote awareness of bipolar conditions in society at large, educate mental health professionals, foster research on bipolar disorder, and promote international collaborations. Its journal, *Bipolar Disorders—An International Journal of Psychiatry and Neurosciences*, has become a primary outlet for new research on the diagnosis, etiology, and treatment of bipolar conditions. ISBD publishes a newsletter and has several online chat rooms, including an "ask the experts" exchange.

## Juvenile Bipolar Research Foundation
*www.bpchildresearch.org*
866-333-JBRF

The first charitable organization dedicated solely to the support of research on the etiology, treatment, and prevention of juvenile-onset bipolar disorder. JBRF has organized a consortium of collaborating research groups and individual investigators from a number of medical schools and treatment centers around the country. Information is provided concerning educational forums for parents and teachers, how to subscribe to professional e-mail listservs for physicians and therapists, how to enroll in research studies, and new research findings pertinent to childhood-onset bipolar disorder.

## MDF the Bipolar Organization
*www.mdf.org.uk*
+44 207793 2600 (U.K.)

A user-led charitable organization in the United Kingdom that offers self-help groups, publications, and other practical information for living with bipolar disorder. There is a useful link for employment services and an "e-Community" with online message boards.

## National Alliance on Mental Illness
*www.nami.org*
800-950-NAMI

A grassroots mutual support and advocacy organization for people with severe mental illnesses (including bipolar disorder, recurrent depression, and schizophrenia) and their family members or friends. NAMI offers parent support groups all over the United States and a structured educational program taught by parents of people with severe psychiatric disorders called "Family to Family."

## National Alliance for Research on Schizophrenia and Depression/ Brain and Behavior Research Foundation
*www.narsad.org*
800-829-8289

The largest donor-supported, nongovernment organization dedicated to raising and distributing funds for research into the nature, causes, treatments, and prevention of severe mental illnesses, including bipolar disorder, schizophrenia, depression, and severe anxiety disorders. Its website includes up-to-date information about the diagnosis and treatment of major psychiatric disorders, with an emphasis on biological/genetic mechanisms and new drug development.

## National Institute of Mental Health
*www.nimh.nih.gov/publicat/index.cfm*
866-615-6464

The mental health organization for the U.S. National Institutes of Health. The website provides up-to-date publications on the symptoms, course, causes, and treatment of bipolar disorder. Separate sections of the website are devoted to child and adolescent bipolar illness, suicide, medical treatments and their side effects, co-occurring illnesses, psychosocial treatments, sources of help for individuals and families, and clinical research studies. For referring to a clinical trial, see *www.clinicaltrials.gov*.

**National Network of Depression Centers**
*www.nndc.org*
734-332-3914

A collection of comprehensive care centers for depression and bipolar disorder, coordinated by the University of Michigan. Its member universities are committed to implementing state-of-the-art treatment protocols and research. Currently, the network includes specialty clinics at Brigham & Women's Hospital, Duke University, Emory University, Johns Hopkins School of Medicine, Massachusetts General Hospital, Medical University of South Carolina, Mayo Clinic, McLean Hospital, Stanford University, University of Cincinnati and Lindner Center, University of Colorado–Denver Health Sciences Center, University of Illinois at Chicago, University of Iowa, University of Louisville (Kentucky), University of Massachusetts, University of Michigan, University of Pennsylvania, University of Texas Southwestern, and Weill Cornell Medical College. Information about contacting these centers for appointments can be obtained at *www.nndc.org/health-resources/appointments-referrals.*

## INTERNET RESOURCES

The following websites offer a variety of information and often interactive features, such as chatrooms and forums, but have no physical presence in the community and no phone contact.

**Bipolar Significant Others**
*www.bpso.org*

Offers an e-mail exchange group in which members—relatives or friends of persons with bipolar disorder—share information about the illness, provide support to one another, and problem-solve about treatment options and issues related to the impact of the illness on families. The website contains much helpful information on treatment, book reviews, and Web links to additional resources.

**BP (Bipolar) Magazine**
*www.bphope.com*

Available in online and print form and contains articles on issues relevant to patients and caregivers, such as how to cope with bipolar disorder as a couple.

**Bipolar World**
*www.bipolarworld.net*

Provides information on bipolar diagnosis, treatments, and suicide, an "ask the doctor" link, personal stories, information on disabilities and stigma, community and family support, relevant books, a bipolar message board, and chat rooms.

## The Bipolar Child
*http://bipolarchild.com*

Developed by Demitri and Janis Papolos. Offers up-to-date research findings pertaining to bipolar children, a newsletter on new treatment approaches, samples of individualized educational programs for children, information on upcoming conferences, and tips on how to start a support group.

## Bipolar Disorder Sanctuary
*www.mhsanctuary.com/bipolar*

Includes educational articles on bipolar disorder, an "ask the therapist" discussion forum, first-person accounts, chat rooms for patients and family members, a clinician's forum, links to new research studies, and an online bookstore.

## Depression Central
*www.psycom.net/depression.central.bipolar.html*

Offers links to the Mayo Clinic's bipolar home page; answers frequently asked questions about bipolar disorder; discusses treatment guidelines; gives up-to-date information on topics such as novel treatment approaches, use of lithium during pregnancy, sleep deprivation, differential diagnosis, adjunctive therapy, suicide, and seasonal mood disorders; and provides a self-screening tool.

## Harbor of Refuge Organization, Inc.
*www.harbor-of-refuge.org*

Provides peer-to-peer support for individuals diagnosed with bipolar disorder who are undergoing treatment. There is a discussion forum/chat room and information on self-care and illness management strategies.

## Internet Mental Health
*www.mentalhealth.com/dis/p20-md02.html*

A strength of this site is the direct links between specific topics and published research abstracts pertaining to the topics. It is a particularly good site for new research on medications. Downloadable self-rated mood questionnaires and mood charts are available.

## Jed Foundation
*www.ulifeline.org*

Dedicated to promoting emotional health and preventing suicide among college students. Self-evaluation tools are available, as are the numbers of various suicide prevention hotlines.

## Mayo Clinic's Page on Bipolar Disorder
*www.mayoclinic.com/health/bipolar-disorder/ds00356*

Information about the disorder and links to videotaped patient testimonials.

## McMan's Depression and Bipolar Web
*www.mcmanweb.com*

A comprehensive website with substantial links to current research, essays on first-person experiences, and an opinion page. The webmaster, John McManamy, is an award-winning mental health journalist and author.

## Medline Plus Health Information
*www.nlm.nih.gov/medlineplus/bipolardisorder.html*

Offers links to National Institute of Mental Health publications and clinical trials. A link is provided to the Medline search engine for the most recent research articles on bipolar disorder.

## Pendulum Resources
*www.pendulum.org*

Offers information about DSM-5 diagnostic criteria, current medical treatments, books favored by mental health consumers and family members, articles on how to cope with depression or bipolar disorder, writings and poetry, and updates on research studies.

## Ryan Licht Sang Foundation
*www.ryanlichtsangbipolarfoundation*

Dedicated to fostering awareness, understanding, and research for early-onset bipolar disorder. The primary goal of the Foundation is to find an empirical biomarker test for bipolar disorder ("Quest for the Test") so that early detection and early intervention become more feasible.

## BOOKS ON BIPOLAR DISORDER

### *Informational Guides*

Amador X, Johanson AL. *I Am Not Sick I Don't Need Help!* Peconic, NY: Vida Press; 2000.

Basco MR. *The Bipolar Workbook: Tools for Controlling Your Mood Swings.* New York: Guilford Press; 2005.

Bauer M, Ludman E, Greenwald DE, et al. *Overcoming Bipolar Disorder: A Comprehensive Workbook for Managing Your Symptoms and Achieving Your Life Goals.* New York: New Harbinger; 2009.

Birmaher B. *New Hope for Children and Teens with Bipolar Disorder.* New York: Three Rivers Press; 2004.

Brondolo E, Amador X. *Break the Bipolar Cycle: A Day-By-Day Guide to Living with Bipolar Disorder.* New York: McGraw-Hill; 2007.

Carlson T. *The Life of a Bipolar Child: What Every Parent and Professional Needs to Know.* Duluth, MN: Benline Press; 2000.

Fast JA, Preston JD. *Loving Someone with Bipolar Disorder: Understanding and Helping Your Partner.* Oakland, CA: New Harbinger; 2004.

Fawcett J, Golden B, Rosenfeld N. *New Hope for People with Bipolar Disorder.* Roseville, CA: Prima Health; 2000.

Findling RL, Kowatch RA, Post RM. *Pediatric Bipolar Disorder.* Boston: Boston Medical Publishers; 2000.

Frank E. *Treating Bipolar Disorder: A Clinician's Guide to Interpersonal and Social Rhythm Therapy.* New York: Guilford Press; 2005.

Fristad MA, Goldberg Arnold JS. *Raising a Moody Child: How to Cope with Depression and Bipolar Disorder.* New York: Guilford Press; 2004.

Geller B, DelBello MP, eds. *Treatment of Bipolar Disorder in Children and Adolescents.* New York: Guilford Press; 2008.

Goodwin FK, Jamison KR. *Manic–Depressive Illness.* 2nd ed. New York: Oxford University Press; 2007.

Greenberger D, Padesky CA. *Mind over Mood.* New York: Guilford Press; 1995.

Jamison KR. *Touched with Fire: Manic–Depressive Illness and the Artistic Temperament.* New York: Maxwell Macmillan International; 1993.

Jamison KR. *Night Falls Fast: Understanding Suicide.* New York: Vintage Books; 2000.

Jamison KR. *Exuberance: The Passion for Life.* New York: Knopf; 2004.

Lowe C, Cohen BM. *Living with Someone Who's Living with Bipolar Disorder: A Practical Guide for Family, Friends, and Coworkers.* San Francisco: Jossey-Bass; 2010.

Lynn GT. *Survival Strategies for Parenting Children with Bipolar Disorder.* London: Jessica Kingsley; 2000.

Miklowitz DJ. *Bipolar Disorder: A Family-Focused Treatment Approach.* 2nd ed. New York: Guilford Press; 2010.

Miklowitz DJ. *The Bipolar Disorder Survival Guide: What You and Your Family Need to Know.* 2nd ed. New York: Guilford Press; 2011.

Miklowitz DJ, George EL. *The Bipolar Teen: What You Can Do to Help Your Child and Your Family.* New York: Guilford Press; 2008.

Newman C, Leahy RL, Beck AT, et al. *Bipolar Disorder: A Cognitive Therapy Approach.* Washington, DC: American Psychological Association Press; 2001.

Papolos DF, Papolos J. *The Bipolar Child: The Definitive and Reassuring Guide to Childhood's Most Misunderstood Disorder.* 3rd ed. New York: Broadway Books; 2006.

Phelps J. *Why Am I Still Depressed?: Recognizing and Managing the Ups and Downs of Bipolar II and Soft Bipolar Disorder.* New York: McGraw-Hill; 2006.

Smith HT. *Welcome to the Jungle: Everything You Ever Wanted to Know about Bipolar Disorder but Were Too Freaked Out to Ask.* Newburyport, MA: Conari Press; 2010.

Stahl SM. *Depression and Bipolar Disorder: Stahl's Essential Psychopharmacology.* 3rd ed. Cambridge, UK: Cambridge University Press; 2008.

Torrey EF, Knable MB. *Surviving Manic Depression: A Manual on Bipolar Disorder for Patients, Families, and Providers.* New York: Basic Books; 2005.

Waltz M. *Bipolar Disorders: A Guide to Helping Children and Adolescents.* Sebastopol, CA: O'Reilly & Associates; 2000.

Whybrow PC. *A Mood Apart: The Thinker's Guide to Emotion and Its Disorders.* New York: HarperCollins; 1998.

### First-Person Accounts

Behrman A. *Electroboy: A Memoir of Mania.* New York: Random House; 2002.

Cheney T. *Manic.* New York: HarperCollins; 2009.

Greenberg M. *Hurry Down Sunshine: A Father's Story of Love and Madness.* New York: Vintage Press; 2008.

Hines K, Reidenberg DJ. *Cracked, Not Broken: Surviving and Thriving after a Suicide Attempt.* Lanham, MD: Rowman & Littlefield; 2013.

Hinshaw SP. *The Years of Silence Are Past: My Father's Life with Bipolar Disorder.* Cambridge, UK: Cambridge University Press; 2002.

Hornbacher M. *Madness: A Bipolar Life.* Mariner Books; 2009.

Jamison KR. *An Unquiet Mind.* New York: Knopf; 1995.

Pauley J. *Skywriting: A Life Out of the Blue.* New York: Ballantine Books; 2005.

Simon L. *Detour: My Bipolar Road Trip in 4-D.* New York: Washington Square Press; 2002.

Solomon A. *The Noonday Demon: An Atlas of Depression.* New York: Touchstone; 2001.

Steele D. *His Bright Light: The Story of Nick Traina.* Des Plaines, IL: Dell; 2000.

Styron W. *Darkness Visible: A Memoir of Madness.* New York: Vintage Books; 1992.

Weiland MF, Warren L. *Fall to Pieces: A Memoir of Drugs, Rock 'n' Roll, and Mental Illness.* New York: Morrow; 2009.

# — APPENDIX B —

## Medication Names and Classes

| Medication name | Trade/generic | Medication class |
|---|---|---|
| Abilify (*see* aripiprazole) | Trade | |
| Adapin (*see* doxepin) | Trade | |
| Adderall (*see* mixed amphetamine salts) | Trade | |
| Adipex-P (*see* phentermine) | Trade | |
| Akineton (*see* biperiden) | Trade | |
| alprazolam | Generic | BZP antianx/hyp |
| amantadine | Generic | Antipark, anti-SE |
| Ambien (*see* zolpidem) | Trade | |
| amitriptyline and perphenazine (combination) | Generic | AD |
| amitriptyline | Generic | Cyclic AD |
| amoxapine | Generic | Cyclic AD |
| Anafranil (*see* clomipramine) | Trade | |

*Explanation of abbreviations:* AD, antidepressant; ADHD, attention-deficit/hyperactivity disorder; antianx, antianxiety; antihist, antihistamine; antipark, antiparkinsonian; antipsych, antipsychotic; anti-SE, anti–side effect; barb, barbiturate; BZP, benzodiazepine; hyp, hypnotic; MAO, monoamine oxidase; OCD, obsessive–compulsive disorder; SSRI, selective serotonin reuptake inhibitor; stim, stimulant; TS, Tourette syndrome.

| Medication name | Trade/generic | Medication class |
|---|---|---|
| Antabuse (*see* disulfiram) | Trade | |
| aripiprazole | Generic | Acute mania, maintenance treatment |
| armodafinil | Generic | Stim |
| Artane (*see* trihexyphenidyl) | Trade | |
| asenapine | Generic | Acute mania |
| Asendin (*see* amoxapine) | Trade | |
| Atarax (*see* hydroxyzine) | Trade | |
| atenolol | Generic | Antianx, anti-SE |
| Ativan (*see* lorazepam) | Trade | |
| Aventyl (*see nortriptyline*) | Trade | |
| Benadryl (*see* diphenhydramine) | Trade | |
| benztropine | Generic | Antipark |
| biperiden | Generic | Antipark |
| Brintellix (*see* vortioxetine) | Trade | |
| buprenorphine | Generic | Opiate abuse |
| bupropion | Generic | Cyclic AD |
| Buspar (*see* buspirone) | Trade | |
| buspirone | Generic | Antianx |
| Calan (*see* verapamil) | Trade | |
| carbamazepine | Generic | Mood stabilizer |
| Catapres (*see* clonidine) | Trade | |
| Celexa (*see* citalopram) | Trade | |
| chloral hydrate | Generic | Hyp |
| chlordiazepoxide | Generic | BZP antianx/hyp |
| chlorpromazine | Generic | Antipsych |
| Cibalith-S (*see* lithium) | Trade | |

| Medication name | Trade/generic | Medication class |
|---|---|---|
| citalopram | Generic | AD |
| clomipramine | Generic | Cyclic AD, OCD |
| clonazepam | Generic | BZP antianx/hyp |
| clonidine | Generic | Antianx,TS, ADHD |
| clorazepate | Generic | BZP antianx |
| Clorazil (*see* clozapine) | Trade | |
| clozapine | Generic | Antipsych |
| Cogentin (*see* benztropine) | Trade | |
| Concerta (*see* methylphenidate—extended release) | Trade | |
| Consta (*see* risperdone) | Trade | |
| Cylert (*see* pemoline) | Trade | |
| Cymbalta (*see* duloxetine) | Trade | |
| Dalmane (*see* flurazepam) | Trade | |
| *d*-amphetamine | Generic | Stim |
| Depakene (*see* valproate) | Trade | |
| *Depakote (see divalproex, valproate)* | Trade | |
| desipramine | Generic | Cyclic AD |
| desmethylvenlafaxine | Generic | AD |
| Desoxyn (*see* methamphetamine) | Trade | |
| Desyrel (*see* trazodone) | Trade | |
| Dexedrine (*see* *d*-amphetamine) | Trade | |
| diazepam | Generic | BZP antianx/hyp |
| diethylpropion | Generic | Stim |
| diphenhydramine | Generic | Antihist, antianx/hyp, antipark |
| disulfiram | Generic | Alcohol abuse |

| Medication name | Trade/generic | Medication class |
|---|---|---|
| divalproex | Generic | Mood stabilizer |
| Doral (*see* quazepam) | Trade | |
| Doriden (*see* glutethimide) | Trade | |
| doxepin | Generic | Cyclic AD |
| duloxetine | Generic | AD |
| Effexor (*see* venlafaxine) | Trade | |
| Elavil (*see* amitriptyline) | Trade | |
| Eldepryl (*see* selegiline) | Trade | |
| Emsam (*see* selegiline) | Trade | |
| Endep (*see* amitriptyline) | Trade | |
| Equetro (*see* carbamazepine) | Trade | |
| Eskalith (*see* lithium) | Trade | |
| Eskalith-CR (*see* lithium) | Trade | |
| estazolam | Generic | BZP hyp |
| Fetzima (*see* levomilnacipran) | Trade | |
| fluoxetine | Generic | SSRI AD |
| fluphenazine | Generic | Antipsych |
| flurazepam | Generic | BZP hyp |
| fluvoxamine | Generic | SSRI AD, OCD |
| gabapentin | Generic | Anticonvulsant, antianx |
| Geodon (*see* ziprasidone) | Trade | |
| Glucophage (*see* metformin) | Trade | |
| glutethimide | Generic | Nonbarb hyp |
| guanfacine | Generic | ADHD |
| halazepam | Generic | BZP antianx |
| Halcion (*see* triazolam) | Trade | |

| Medication name | Trade/generic | Medication class |
|---|---|---|
| Haldol (*see* haloperidol) | Trade | |
| haloperidol | Generic | Antipsych |
| hydroxyzine | Generic | Antihist, antianx/hyp |
| imipramine | Generic | Cyclic AD |
| Inderal (*see* propranolol) | Trade | |
| Invega (*see* paliperidone) | Trade | |
| Isoptin (*see* verapamil) | Trade | |
| Klonopin (*see* clonazepam) | Trade | |
| Lamictal (*see* lamotrigine) | Trade | |
| lamotrigine | Generic | Maintenance treatment, bipolar depression |
| Latuda (*see* lurasidone) | Trade | |
| Lexapro (*see* S-citalopram) | Trade | |
| levomilnacipran | Generic | AD |
| Librium (*see* chlordiazepoxide) | Trade | |
| lisdexamfetamine | Generic | Stim |
| lithium | Generic | Mood stabilizer |
| Lithobid (*see* lithium) | Trade | |
| Lithonate (*see* lithium) | Trade | |
| Lithotabs (*see* lithium) | Trade | |
| lorazepam | Generic | BZP antianx/hyp |
| loxapine | Generic | Antipsych |
| Loxitane (*see* loxapine) | Trade | |
| L-tryptophan | Generic | Hyp |
| Ludiomil (*see* maprotiline) | Trade | |
| lurasidone | Generic | Bipolar depression |
| Luvox (*see* fluvoxamine) | Trade | |

| Medication name | Trade/generic | Medication class |
| --- | --- | --- |
| maprotiline | Generic | Cyclic AD |
| Mellaril (*see* thioridazine) | Trade | |
| meprobamate | Generic | Nonbarb antianx/hyp |
| mesoridazine | Generic | Antipsych |
| metformin | Generic | Weight loss agent |
| methamphetamine | Generic | Stim |
| methylphenidate | Generic | Stim |
| methylphenidate–extended release | Generic | Stim |
| Miltown (*see* meprobamate) | Trade | |
| Mirapex (*see* pramipexole) | Trade | |
| mirtazapine | Generic | AD |
| mixed amphetamine salts | Generic | Stim |
| Moban (*see* molindone) | Trade | |
| modafinil | Generic | Stim |
| molindone | Generic | Antipsych |
| naltrexone | Generic | Opiate addiction, alcohol abuse |
| Nardil (*see* phenelzine) | Trade | |
| Navane (*see* thiothixene) | Trade | |
| nefazodone | Generic | Novel AD |
| Neurotin (*see* gabapentin) | Trade | |
| Noctec (*see* chloral hydrate) | Trade | |
| Nolvadex (*see* tamoxifen) | Trade | |
| Norpramin (*see* desipramine) | Trade | |
| nimodipine | Generic | Acute mania, mood stabilizer |
| Nimotop (*see* nimodipine) | Trade | |

| Medication name | Trade/generic | Medication class |
|---|---|---|
| nortriptyline | Generic | Cyclic AD |
| Nuvigil (*see* armodafinil) | Trade | |
| olanzapine | Generic | Acute mania, maintenance treatment |
| olanzapine/fluoxetine | Generic | Bipolar depression |
| Orap (*see* pimozide) | Trade | |
| oxazepam | Generic | BZP antianx/hyp |
| oxcarbazepine | Generic | Anticonvulsant mood stabilizer |
| paliperidone | Generic | Acute mania |
| Pamelor (*see* nortriptyline) | Trade | |
| Parnate (*see* tranylcypromine) | Trade | |
| paroxetine | Generic | SSRI AD |
| Paxil (*see* paroxetine) | Trade | |
| Paxipam (*see* halazepam) | Trade | |
| pemoline | Generic | Stim |
| perphenazine | Generic | Antipsyc |
| Pertofrane (*see* desipramine) | Trade | |
| phenelzine | Generic | MAO inhibitor AD |
| phentermine | Generic | Stim |
| pimozide | Generic | TS |
| pramipexole | Generic | Bipolar depression |
| Pristiq (*see* desmethylvenlafaxine) | Trade | |
| Prolixin (*see* fluphenazine) | Trade | |
| propranolol | Generic | Antianx, anti-SE |
| Prosom (*see* estazolam) | Trade | |
| protriptyline | Generic | Cyclic AD |

| Medication name | Trade/generic | Medication class |
|---|---|---|
| Proviqil (*see* modafinil) | Trade | |
| Prozac (*see* fluoxetine) | Trade | |
| quazepam | Generic | BZD hyp |
| quetiapine | Generic | Acute mania, maintenance treatment, bipolar depression |
| Remeron (*see* mirtazapine) | Trade | |
| Restoril (*see* temazepam) | Trade | |
| ReVia (*see* naltrexone) | Trade | |
| Risperdal (*see* risperidone) | Trade | |
| risperidone | Generic | Antipsych, acute mania, maintenance treatment |
| Ritalin (*see* methylphenidate) | Trade | |
| Saphris (*see* asenapine) | Trade | |
| S-citalopram | Generic | AD |
| selegiline | Generic | MAO inhibitor AD |
| Serax (*see* oxazepam) | Trade | |
| Serentil (*see* mesoridazine) | Trade | |
| Seroque (*see* quetapine) | Trade | |
| sertraline | Generic | SSRI AD |
| Serzone (*see* nefazodone) | Trade | |
| Sinequan (*see* doxepin) | Trade | |
| Stelazine (*see* trifluoperazine) | Trade | |
| Surmontil (*see* trimipramine) | Trade | |
| Suboxone (*see* buprenorphine) | Trade | |
| Subutex (*see* buprenorphine) | Trade | |
| Symbyax (*see* olanzapine/ fluoxetine) | Trade | |

| Medication name | Trade/generic | Medication class |
|---|---|---|
| Symmetrel (*see* amantadine) | Trade | |
| tamoxifen | Generic | Acute mania |
| Tegretol (*see* carbamazepine) | Trade | |
| temazepam | Generic | BZP antianx/hyp |
| Tenex (*see* guanfacine) | Trade | |
| Tenuate (*see* diethylproprion) | Trade | |
| Tenormin (*see* atenolol) | Trade | |
| thioridazine | Generic | Antipsych |
| thiothixene | Generic | Antipsych |
| Thorazine (*see* chlorpromazine) | Trade | |
| Tofranil (*see* imipramine) | Trade | |
| Topamax (*see* topiramate) | | |
| topiramate | Generic | Anticonvulsant, weight loss agent |
| Tranxene (*see* clorazepate) | Trade | |
| tranylcypromine | Generic | MAO inhibitor AD |
| trazodone | Generic | Cyclic AD |
| Triavil (*see* amitriptyline and pherphenazine [combination]) | Trade | |
| triazolam | Generic | BZP hyp |
| trifluoperazine | Generic | Antipsych |
| trifluopromazine | Generic | Antipsych |
| trihexyphenidyl | Generic | Antipark |
| Trilafon (*see* perphenazine) | Trade | |
| Trileptal (*see* oxcarbazepine) | Trade | |
| trimipramine | Generic | Cyclic AD |
| Valium (*see* diazepam) | Trade | |

| Medication name | Trade/generic | Medication class |
| --- | --- | --- |
| valproate | Generic | Mood stabilizer |
| venlafaxine | Generic | Novel AD |
| verapamil | Generic | Mood stabilizer |
| Vesprin (*see* trifluopromazine) | Trade | |
| Viibryd (*see* vilazodone) | Trade | |
| vilazodone | Generic | AD |
| Vistaril (*see* hydroxyzine) | Trade | |
| Vivactil (*see* protriptyline) | Trade | |
| vortioxetine | Generic | AD |
| Vyvanse (*see* lisdexamfetamine) | Trade | |
| Wellbutrin (*see* bupropion) | Trade | |
| Xanax (*see* alprazolam) | Trade | |
| ziprasidone | Generic | Acute mania, maintenance treatment |
| Zoloft (*see* sertraline) | Trade | |
| zolpidem | Generic | Hyp |
| Zyprexa (*see* olanzapine) | Trade | |

# References

## CHAPTER 1

1. Lish JD, Dime-Meenan S, Whybrow PC, et al. The National Depressive and Manic-Depressive Association (NDMDA) survey of bipolar members. *Journal of Affective Disorders.* 1994;31:281–294.
2. Geddes JR, Miklowitz DJ. Treatment of bipolar disorder. *Lancet.* 2013;381(9878):1672–1682.
3. Gitlin MJ, Mintz J, Sokolski K, et al. Subsyndromal depressive symptoms after symptomatic recovery from mania are associated with delayed functional recovery. *Journal of Clinical Psychiatry.* 2011;72(5):692–697.

## CHAPTER 2

1. American Psychiatric Association. *Diagnostic and Statistical Manual of Mental Disorders.* 5th ed. Arlington, VA: Author; 2013.
2. Angst J, Preisig M. Course of a clinical cohort of unipolar, bipolar and schizoaffective patients. Results of a prospective study from 1959 to 1985. *Schweizer Archiv für Neurologie und Psychiatrie.* 1995;146(1):5–16.
3. Goodwin FK, Jamison KR. *Manic–Depressive Illness.* 2nd ed. New York: Oxford University Press; 2007.
4. Cavanagh JT, Carson AJ, Sharpe M, et al. Psychological autopsy studies of suicide: a systematic review. *Psychological Medicine.* 2003;33(3):395–405.
5. Harris EC, Barraclough B. Suicide as an outcome for mental disorders: a meta-analysis. *British Journal of Psychiatry.* 1997;170:205–208.
6. Casper RC, Redmond DE Jr., Katz MM, et al. Somatic symptoms in primary affective disorder: presence and relationship to the classification of depression. *Archives of General Psychiatry.* 1985;42(11):1098–1104.
7. Coryell W, Keller M, Endicott J, et al. Bipolar II illness: course and outcome over a five-year period. *Psychological Medicine.* 1989;19(1):129–141.
8. Kupka RW, Luckenbaugh DA, Post RM, et al. Rapid and non-rapid cycling bipolar disorder: a meta-analysis of clinical studies. *Journal of Clinical Psychiatry.* 2003;64(12):1483–1494.

9.  Coryell CW, Endicott J, Keller M. Rapidly cycling affective disorder: demographics, diagnosis, family history, and course. *Archives of General Psychiatry.* 1992;49:126–131.

10. Ghaemi SN, Ko JY, Goodwin FK. The bipolar spectrum and the antidepressant view of the world. *Journal of Psychiatric Practice.* 2001;7(5):287–297.

11. Swann AC, Lafer B, Perugi G, et al. Bipolar mixed states: an international society for bipolar disorders task force report of symptom structure, course of illness, and diagnosis. *American Journal of Psychiatry.* 2013;170:31–42.

12. Baldessarini RJ, Leahy L, Arcona S, et al. Patterns of psychotropic drug prescription for U.S. patients with diagnoses of bipolar disorders. *Psychiatric Services.* 2007;58(1):85–91.

13. Pagel T, Baldessarini RJ, Franklin J, et al. Characteristics of patients diagnosed with schizoaffective disorder compared with schizophrenia and bipolar disorder. *Bipolar Disorders.* 2013;15:229–239.

14. Tsuang D, Coryell W. An 8-year follow-up of patients with DSM-III-R psychotic depression, schizoaffective disorder, and schizophrenia. *American Journal of Psychiatry.* 1993;150(8):1182–1188.

15. Schwartz JE, Fennig S, Tanenberg-Karant M, et al. Congruence of diagnoses 2 years after a first-admission diagnosis of psychosis. *Archives of General Psychiatry.* 2000;57(6):593–600.

16. White CN, Gunderson JG, Zanarini MC, et al. Family studies of borderline personality disorder: A review. *Harvard Review of Psychiatry.* 2003;11:8–19.

17. Bourne C, Aydemir O, Balanzi-Martinez V, et al. Neuropsychological testing of cognitive impairment in euthymic bipolar disorder: an individual patient data meta-analysis. *Acta Psychiatrica Scandinavica.* 2013;128:149–162.

18. Rice J, Reich T, Andreasen NC, et al. The familial transmission of bipolar illness. *Archives of General Psychiatry.* 1987;44:441–447.

19. Bertelsen A, Harvald B, Hauge M. A Danish twin study of manic–depressive disorders. *British Journal of Psychiatry.* 1977;130:330–351.

20. McGuffin P, Rijsdijk F, Andrew M, et al. The heritability of bipolar affective disorder and the genetic relationship to unipolar depression. *Archives of General Psychiatry.* 2003;60:497–502.

21. Mendlewicz J, Rainer JD. Adoption study supporting genetic transmission in manic–depressive illness. *Nature.* 1977;268:327–329.

22. Merikangas KR, Cui L, Kattan G, et al. Mania with and without depression in a community sample of US adolescents. *Archives of General Psychiatry.* 2012; 69(9):943–951.

23. Shulman KI, Schaffer A, Levitt A, et al. Effects of gender and age on phenomenology and management of bipolar disorder: a review. In: Maj M, Akiskal HS, Lopez-Ibor JJ Jr., et al. eds. *Bipolar Disorder.* New York: Wiley; 2002:359–440.

24. Tohen M, Shulman KI, Satlin A. First-episode mania in late life. *American Journal of Psychiatry.* 1994;151:130–132.

25. Post RM. Transduction of psychosocial stress into the neurobiology of recurrent affective disorder. *American Journal of Psychiatry.* 1992;149:999–1010.

26. Roy-Byrne P, Post RM, Uhde TW, et al. The longitudinal course of recurrent affective illness: life chart data from research patients at the NIMH. *Acta Psychiatrica Scandinavica Supplementum.* 1985;317:1–34.

27. Hammen C, Gitlin MJ. Stress reactivity in bipolar patients and its relation to prior history of the disorder. *American Journal of Psychiatry.* 1997;154:856–857.
28. Coryell W, Solomon D, Turvey C, et al. The long-term course of rapid-cycling bipolar disorder. *Archives of General Psychiatry.* 2003;60:914–920.
29. Baldessarini RJ, Salvatore P, Khalsa HM, et al. Morbidity in 303 first-episode bipolar I disorder patients. *Bipolar Disorders.* 2010;12(1):264–270.
30. Judd LL, Akiskal HS, Schettler PJ, et al. The long-term natural history of the weekly symptomatic status of bipolar I disorder. *Archives of General Psychiatry.* 2002;59:530–537.
31. Judd LL, Akiskal HS, Schettler PJ, et al. A prospective investigation of the natural history of the long-term weekly symptomatic status of bipolar II disorder. *Archives of General Psychiatry.* 2003;60:261–269.
32. Johnson SL, Cuellar A, Ruggero C, et al. Life events as predictors of mania and depression in bipolar I disorder. *Journal of Abnormal Psychology.* 2008;117:268–277.
33. Hosang GM, Korszun A, Jones L, et al. Life-event specificity: bipolar disorder compared with unipolar depression. *British Journal of Psychiatry.* 2012;201(6):458–465.
34. Hammen C, Brennan PA. Interpersonal dysfunction in depressed women: impairments independent of depressive symptoms. *Journal of Affective Disorders.* 2002;72(2):145–156.
35. Barbini B, Bertelli S, Colombo C, et al. Sleep loss, a possible factor in augmenting manic episode. *Psychiatry Research.* 1996;65(2):121–125.
36. Miklowitz DJ, Goldstein MJ, Nuechterlein KH, et al. Family factors and the course of bipolar affective disorder. *Archives of General Psychiatry.* 1988;45:225–231.
37. Yan LJ, Hammen C, Cohen AN, et al. Expressed emotion versus relationship quality variables in the prediction of recurrence in bipolar patients. *Journal of Affective Disorders.* 2004;83:199–206.
38. Miklowitz DJ, Johnson SL. Social and familial risk factors in bipolar disorder: basic processes and relevant interventions. *Clinical Psychology: Science and Practice.* 2009;16(2):281–296.
39. Judd LL, Schettler PJ, Solomon DA, et al. Psychosocial disability and work role function compared across the long-term course of bipolar I, bipolar II and unipolar major depressive disorders. *Journal of Affective Disorders.* 2008;108(1-2):49–58.
40. Tohen M, Hennen J, Zarate CM Jr., et al. Two-year syndromal and functional recovery in 219 cases of first-episode major affective disorder with psychotic features. *American Journal of Psychiatry.* 2000;157:220–228.
41. Strakowski SM, Keck PE, McElroy SL, et al. Twelve-month outcome after a first hospitalization for affective psychosis. *Archives of General Psychiatry.* 1998;55:49–55.
42. Schoeyen HK, Birkenaes AB, Vaaler AE, et al. Bipolar disorder patients have similar levels of education but lower socio-economic status than the general population. *Journal of Affective Disorders.* 2011;129(1-3):68–74.
43. Coryell W, Scheftner W, Keller M, et al. The enduring psychosocial consequences of mania and depression. *American Journal of Psychiatry.* 1993;150:720–727.

44. Whisman MA. Marital distress and DSM-IV psychiatric disorders in a population-based national survey. *Journal of Abnormal Psychology.* 2007;116:638–643.

45. Perlick DA, Miklowitz DJ, Link BG, et al. Perceived stigma and depression among caregivers of patients with bipolar disorder. *British Journal of Psychiatry.* 2007;190:535–536.

46. Gitlin MJ, Swendsen J, Heller TL, et al. Relapse and impairment in bipolar disorder. *American Journal of Psychiatry.* 1995;152(11):1635–1640.

47. Altshuler LL, Post RM, Black DO, et al. Subsyndromal depressive symptoms are associated with functional impairment in patients with bipolar disorder: results of a large, multisite study. *Journal of Clinical Psychiatry.* 2006;67(10):1551–1560.

48. Wingo AP, Wingo TS, Harvey PD, et al. Effects of lithium on cognitive performance: a meta-analysis. *Journal of Clinical Psychiatry.* 2009;70(11):1588–1597.

49. van Gorp WG, Altshuler L, Theberge DC, et al. Cognitive impairment in euthymic bipolar patients with and without prior alcohol dependence: a preliminary study. *Archives of General Psychiatry.* 1998;55:41–46.

## CHAPTER 3

1. First MB, Spitzer RL, Gibbon M, et al. *Structured Clinical Interview for DSM-IV Axis I Disorders.* New York: Biometrics Research Department, New York State Psychiatric Institute; 1995.

2. Duffy A, Alda M, Crawford L, et al. The early manifestations of bipolar disorder: a longitudinal prospective study of the offspring of bipolar parents. *Bipolar Disorders.* 2007;9:828–838.

3. Luby JL, Navsaria N. Pediatric bipolar disorder: evidence for prodromal states and early markers. *Journal of Child Psychology and Psychiatry.* 2010;51(4):459–471.

4. Malhi GS, Adams D, Berk M. Medicating mood with maintenance in mind: bipolar depression pharmacotherapy. *Bipolar Disorders.* 2009;11(suppl 2):55–76.

5. Marangell LB, Bauer M, Dennehy EB, et al. Prospective predictors of suicide and suicide attempts in 2000 patients with bipolar disorders followed for 2 years. *Bipolar Disorders.* 2006;8(5 pt 2):566–575.

6. Suppes T, Mintz J, McElroy SL, et al. Mixed hypomania in 908 patients with bipolar disorder evaluated prospectively in the Stanley Foundation Bipolar Treatment Network: a sex-specific phenomenon. *Archives of General Psychiatry.* 2005;62(10):1089–1096.

7. Birmaher B, Axelson D, Goldstein B, et al. Four-year longitudinal course of children and adolescents with bipolar spectrum disorders: the Course and Outcome of Bipolar Youth (COBY) study. *American Journal of Psychiatry.* 2009;166(7):795–804.

8. Brotman MA, Schmajuk M, Rich BA, et al. Prevalence, clinical correlates, and longitudinal course of severe mood dysregulation in children. *Biological Psychiatry.* 2006;60(9):991–997.

9. Miklowitz DJ, First MB. Specifiers as aids to treatment selection and clinical management in the ICD classification of mood disorders. *World Psychiatry.* 2012;11(suppl 1):11–16.

10. Linehan MM. *Cognitive-Behavioral Treatment of Borderline Personality Disorder.* New York: Guilford Press; 1993.

11. Geller B, Warner K, Williams M, Zimerman B. Prepubertal and young adolescent bipolarity versus ADHD: assessment and validity using the WASH-U-KSADS, CBCL and TRF. *Journal of Affective Disorders.* 1998;51:93–100.

12. Geller B, Zimerman B, Williams M, et al. DSM-IV mania symptoms in a prepubertal and early adolescent bipolar disorder phenotype compared to attention deficit hyperactive and normal controls. *Journal of the American Academy of Child and Adolescent Psychiatry.* 2002;12:11–25.

13. Hinshaw SP, Owens EB, Zalecki C, et al. Prospective follow-up of girls with attention-deficit/hyperactivity disorder into early adulthood: continuing impairment includes elevated risk for suicide attempts and self-injury. *Journal of Consulting and Clinical Psychology.* 2012;80(6):1041–1051.

14. Miklowitz DJ, Johnson SL. Social and familial risk factors in bipolar disorder: basic processes and relevant interventions. *Clinical Psychology: Science and Practice.* 2009;16(2):281–296.

15. Johnson SL, Cuellar A, Ruggero C, et al. Life events as predictors of mania and depression in bipolar I disorder. *Journal of Abnormal Psychology.* 2008;117:268–277.

16. Miklowitz DJ. The role of family systems in severe and recurrent psychiatric disorders: a developmental psychopathology view. *Development and Psychopathology.* 2004;16:667–688.

17. Miklowitz DJ. *Bipolar Disorder: A Family-Focused Treatment Approach.* 2nd ed. New York: Guilford Press; 2010.

18. Newman C, Leahy RL, Beck AT, et al. *Bipolar Disorder: A Cognitive Therapy Approach.* Washington, DC: American Psychological Association Press; 2001.

19. Frank E. *Treating Bipolar Disorder: A Clinician's Guide to Interpersonal and Social Rhythm Therapy.* New York: Guilford Press; 2005.

20. Hirschfeld RM, Williams JB, Spitzer RL, et al. Development and validation of a screening instrument for bipolar spectrum disorder: the Mood Disorder Questionnaire. *American Journal of Psychiatry.* 2000;157:1873–1875.

21. Zimmerman M, Galione JN, Ruggero CJ, et al. Screening for bipolar disorder and finding borderline personality disorder. *Journal of Clinical Psychiatry.* 2010;71(9):1212–1217.

22. Goldberg JF, Garakani A, Ackerman SH. Clinician-rated versus self-rated screening for bipolar disorder among inpatients with mood symptoms and substance misuse. *Journal of Clinical Psychiatry.* 2012;73(12):1525–1530.

23. Beck AT, Steer RA, Brown GK. *Beck Depression Inventory–II.* San Antonio, TX: Psychological Corporation; 1996.

24. Rush AJ, Trivedi MH, Ibrahim HM, et al. The 16-item Quick Inventory of Depressive Symptomatology (QIDS), clinician rating (QIDS-C), and self-report (QIDS-SR): a psychometric evaluation in patients with chronic major depression. *Biological Psychiatry.* 2003;54(5):573–583.

25. Beck AT, Steer RA, Beck JS, et al. Hopelessness, depression, suicidal ideation,

and clinical diagnosis of depression. *Suicide and Life Threatening Behavior.* 1993;23(2):139–145.

26. Altman EG, Hedeker D, Peterson JL, et al. The Altman Self-Rating Mania Scale. *Biological Psychiatry.* 1997;42:948–955.

27. Altshuler L, Mintz J, Leight K. The Life Functioning Questionnaire (LFQ): a brief, gender-neutral scale assessing functional outcome. *Psychiatry Research.* 2002;112:161–182.

28. Altshuler LL, Post RM, Black DO, et al. Subsyndromal depressive symptoms are associated with functional impairment in patients with bipolar disorder: results of a large, multisite study. *Journal of Clinical Psychiatry.* 2006;67(10):1551–1560.

29. Gitlin MJ, Mintz J, Sokolski K, et al. Subsyndromal depressive symptoms after symptomatic recovery from mania are associated with delayed functional recovery. *Journal of Clinical Psychiatry.* 2011;72(5):692–697.

## CHAPTER 4

1. Malkoff-Schwartz S, Frank E, Anderson B, et al. Stressful life events and social rhythm disruption in the onset of manic and depressive bipolar episodes: a preliminary investigation. *Archives of General Psychiatry.* 1998;55:702–707.

2. Young RC, Biggs JT, Ziegler VE, et al. A rating scale for mania: reliability, validity, and sensitivity. *British Journal of Psychiatry.* 1978;133:429–435.

3. Chengappa KNR, Baker RW, Shao L, et al. Rates of response, euthymia and remission in two placebo-controlled olanzapine trials for bipolar mania. *Bipolar Disorders.* 2003;5(1):1–5.

4. Swann AC, Bowden CL, Morris D, et al. Depression during mania: treatment response to lithium or divalproex. *Archives of General Psychiatry.* 1997;54:37–42.

5. Grof P, Duffy A, Cavazzoni P, et al. Is response to prophylactic lithium a familial trait? *Journal of Clinical Psychiatry.* 2002;63:942–947.

6. Cade JFJ. Lithium salts in the treatment of psychotic excitement. *Medical Journal of Australia.* 1949;36:349–352.

7. Bowden CL, Brugger AM, Swann AC, et al. Efficacy of divalproex vs lithium and placebo in the treatment of mania. *Journal of the American Medical Association.* 1994;271(12):918–924.

8. Cipriani A, Barbui C, Salanti G, et al. Comparative efficacy and acceptability of antimanic drugs in acute mania: a multiple-treatments meta-analysis. *Lancet.* 2011;378(9799):1306–1315.

9. Yildiz A, Vieta, E, Leucht S, et al. Efficacy of antimanic treatments: meta-analysis of randomized, controlled trials. *Neuropsychopharmacology.* 2011;36:375–389.

10. Perlis RH, Welge JA, Vornik LA, et al. Atypical antipsychotics in the treatment of mania: a meta-analysis of randomized, placebo-controlled trials. *Journal of Clinical Psychiatry.* 2006;67:509–516.

11. Scherk H, Pajonk FG, Leucht S. Second-generation antipsychotic agents in the treatment of acute mania: a systematic review and meta-analysis of randomized controlled trials. *Archives of General Psychiatry.* 2007;64(4):442–455.

12. Gitlin M. Lithium and the kidney. *Drug Safety.* 1999;20(3):231–243.

13. Gitlin MJ, Cochran SD, Jamison KR. Maintenance lithium treatment: side effects and compliance. *Journal of Clinical Psychiatry.* 1989;50(4):127–131.

14. Allen MH, Hirschfeld RM, Wozniak PJ, et al. Linear relationship of valproate serum concentration to response and optimal serum levels for acute mania. *American Journal of Psychiatry.* 2006;163:272–275.

15. Vieta E, Nuamah IF, Lim P, et al. A randomized, placebo- and active-controlled study of paliperidone extended release for the treatment of acute manic and mixed episodes of bipolar I disorder. *Bipolar Disorders.* 2010;12(3):230–243.

16. Hirschfeld RM, Keck PE Jr, Kramer M, et al. Rapid antimanic effect of risperidone monotherapy: a 3-week multicenter, double-blind, placebo-controlled trial. *American Journal of Psychiatry.* 2004;161:1057–1065.

17. Khanna S, Vieta E, Lyons B, Eerdekens M, Kramer M. Risperidone in the treatment of acute mania: double-blind, placebo-controlled study. *British Journal of Psychiatry.* 2005;187:229–234.

18. Tohen M, Sanger TM, McElroy SL, et al. Olanzapine versus placebo in the treatment of acute mania. *American Journal of Psychiatry.* 1999;156:702–709.

19. Tohen M, Jacobs TG, Grundy SL, et al. Efficacy of olanzapine in acute bipolar mania: a double-blind, placebo-controlled study. The Olanzapine HGGW Study Group. *Archives of General Psychiatry.* 2000;57(9):841–849.

20. Bowden CL, Grunze H, Mullen J, et al. A randomized, double-blind, placebo-controlled efficacy and safety study of quetiapine or lithium as monotherapy for mania in bipolar disorder. *Journal of Clinical Psychiatry.* 2005;66:111–121.

21. McIntyre RS, Brecher M, Paulsson B, et al. Quetiapine or haloperidol as monotherapy for bipolar mania—a 12-week, double-blind, randomised, parallel-group, placebo-controlled trial. *European Neuropsychopharmacology.* 2005;15(5):573–585.

22. Keck PE Jr, Versiani M, Potkin S, et al. Ziprasidone in the treatment of acute bipolar mania: a three-week, placebo-controlled, double-blind, randomized trial. *American Journal of Psychiatry.* 2003;160:741–748.

23. Potkin SG, Keck PE Jr, Segal S, et al. Ziprasidone in acute bipolar mania: a 21-day randomized, double-blind, placebo-controlled replication trial. *Journal of Clinical Psychopharmacology.* 2005;25(4):301–310.

24. Camm J, Karayal ON, Meltzer H, et al. Ziprasidone and the corrected QT interval. *CNS Drugs.* 2012;26(4):351–365.

25. Suppes T, Eudicone J, McQuade R, et al. Efficacy and safety of aripiprazole in subpopulations with acute manic or mixed episodes of bipolar I disorder. *Journal of Affective Disorders.* 2008;107(1):145–154.

26. Vita A, De Peri L, Siracusano A, et al. Efficacy and tolerability of asenapine for acute mania in bipolar I disorder: Meta-analyses of randomized-controlled trials. *International Clinical Psychopharmacology* 2013;28(5):219–227.

27. Weisler RH, Hirschfeld R, Cutler AJ, et al. Extended-release carbamazepine capsules as monotherapy in bipolar disorder: pooled results from two randomised, double-blind, placebo-controlled trials. *CNS Drugs.* 2006;20(3):219–231.

28. Vasudev K, Goswami U, Kohli K. Carbamazepine and valproate

monotherapy: feasibility, relative safety and efficacy, and therapeutic drug monitoring in manic disorder. *Psychopharmacology (Berlin)*. 2000;150(1):15–23.

29. Ketter TA, Post RM, Worthington K. Principles of clinically important drug interactions with carbamazepine. Part I. *Journal of Clinical Psychopharmacology*. 1991;11(3):198–203.

30. Ketter TA, Post RM, Worthington K. Principles of clinically important drug interactions with carbamazepine: Part II. *Journal of Clinical Psychopharmacology*. 1991;11(5):306–313.

31. Goldsmith DR, Wagstaff AJ, Ibbotson T, et al. Lamotrigine: a review of its use in bipolar disorder. *Drugs*. 2003;63(19):2029–2050.

32. Kushner SF, Khan A, Lane R, et al. Topiramate monotherapy in the management of acute mania: results of four double-blind placebo-controlled trials. *Bipolar Disorders*. 2006;8(1):15–27.

33. Kakkar AK, Rehan HS, Unni KES, et al. Comparative efficacy and safety of oxcarbazepine versus divalproex sodium in the treatment of acute mania: a pilot study. *European Psychiatry*. 2009;24(3):178–182.

34. Yildiz A, Guleryuz S, Ankerst DP, et al. Protein kinase c inhibition in the treatment of mania. *Archives of General Psychiatry*. 2008;65(3):255–263.

35. Armollahi X, Rezaei F, Salehi B, et al. Double-blind, randomized, placebo-controlled 6-week study on the efficacy and safety of the tamoxifen adjunctive to lithium in acute bipolar mania. *Journal of Affective Disorders*. 2011;129:327–331.

36. Nielsen J, Kane JM, Correll CU. Real-world effectiveness of clozapine in patients with bipolar disorder: results from a 2-year mirror-image study. *Bipolar Disorders*. 2012;14:863–869.

37. Mukherjee S, Sackeim HA, Schnur DB. Electroconvulsive therapy of acute manic episodes: a review of 50 years' experience. *American Journal of Psychiatry*. 1994;151:169–176.

38. Suppes T, Baldessarini RJ, Faedda GL, et al. Discontinuation of maintenance treatment in bipolar disorder: risks and implications. *Harvard Review of Psychiatry*. 1993;1(3):131–144.

## CHAPTER 5

1. Bauer M, Ritter P, Grunze H, et al. Treatment options for acute depression in bipolar disorder. *Bipolar Disorders*. 2012;14(suppl 2):37–50.

2. Sanford M, Keating GM. Quetiapine: a review of its use in the management of bipolar depression. *CNS Drugs*. 2012;26(5):435–460.

3. Loebel A, Cucchiaro J, Silva R, et al. Lurasidone monotherapy in the treatment of bipolar I depression: a randomized, double-blind, placebo-controlled study. *American Journal of Psychiatry*. 2014;171(2):160–168.

4. Calabrese JR, Huffman RF, White RL, et al. Lamotrigine in the acute treatment of bipolar depression: results of five double-blind, placebo-controlled clinical trials. *Bipolar Disorders*. 2008;10(2):323–333.

5. Geddes JR, Calabrese JR, Goodwin GM. Lamotrigine for treatment of bipolar depression: independent meta-analysis and meta-regression of

individual patient data from five randomised trials. *British Journal of Psychiatry.* 2009;194(1):4–9.

6. Licht RW. Lithium: still a major option in the management of bipolar disorder. *CNS Neuroscience and Therapeutics.* 2012;18:219–226.

7. Young AH, McElroy SL, Bauer M, et al. A double-blind, placebo-controlled study of quetiapine and lithium monotherapy in adults in the acute phase of bipolar depression (EMBOLDEN I). *Journal of Clinical Psychiatry.* 2010;71(2):150–162.

8. Bond DJ, Lam RW, Yatham LN. Divalproex sodium versus placebo in the treatment of acute bipolar depression: a systematic review and meta-analysis. *Journal of Affective Disorders.* 2010;124(3):228–234.

9. Geddes JR, Miklowitz DJ. Treatment of bipolar disorder. *Lancet.* 2013;381(9878):1672–1682.

10. Tohen M, Vieta E, Calabrese J, et al. Efficacy of olanzapine and olanzapine-fluoxetine combination in the treatment of bipolar I depression. *Archives of General Psychiatry.* 2003;60:1079–1088.

11. Thase ME, Jonas A, Khan A, et al. Aripiprazole monotherapy in nonpsychotic bipolar I depression: results of 2 randomized, placebo-controlled studies. *Journal of Clinical Psychopharmacology.* 2008;28(1):13–20.

12. Lombardo I, Sachs G, Kolluri S, et al. Two 6-week, randomized, double-blind, placebo-controlled studies of ziprasidone in outpatients with bipolar I depression: Did baseline characteristics impact trial outcome? *Journal of Clinical Psychopharmacology.* 2012;32(4):470–478.

13. van der Loos ML, Mulder PG, Hartong EG, et al. Efficacy and safety of lamotrigine as add-on treatment to lithium in bipolar depression: a multicenter, double-blind, placebo-controlled trial. *Journal of Clinical Psychiatry.* 2009;70(2):223–231.

14. Loebel A, Cucchiaro J, Silva R, et al. Lurasidone as adjunctive therapy with lithium or valproate for the treatment of bipolar I depression: a randomized, double-blind, placebo-controlled study. *American Journal of Psychiatry.* 2014;171(2):169–177.

15. Baldessarini RJ, Leahy L, Arcona S, et al. Patterns of psychotropic drug prescription for U.S. patients with diagnoses of bipolar disorders. *Psychiatric Services.* 2007;58(1):85–91.

16. Bottlender R, Rudolf DA, Möller H. Mood-stabilisers reduce the risk of developing antidepressant-induced maniform states in acute treatment of bipolar I depressed patients. *Journal of Affective Disorders.* 2001;63(1–3):79–83.

17. Sidor MM, MacQueen GM. An update on antidepressant use in bipolar depression. *Current Psychiatry Reports.* 2012;14:696–704.

18. Sachs GS, Nierenberg AA, Calabrese JR, et al. Effectiveness of adjunctive antidepressant treatment for bipolar depression. *New England Journal of Medicine.* 2007;356(17):1711–1722.

19. Post RM, Altshuler LL, Leverich GS, et al. Mood switch in bipolar depression: comparison of adjunctive venlafaxine, bupropion and sertraline. *British Journal of Psychiatry.* 2006;189:124–131.

20. Vieta E, Martinez-Aran A, Goikolea JM, et al. A randomized trial comparing paroxetine and venlafaxine in the treatment of bipolar depressed patients taking mood stabilizers. *Journal of Clinical Psychiatry.* 2002;63:508–512.

21. Altshuler LL, Post RM, Leverich GS, et al. Antidepressant-induced mania and cycle acceleration: a controversy revisited. *American Journal of Psychiatry.* 1995;152:1130–1138.

22. Bond DJ, Noronha MM, Kauer-Sant'Anna M, et al. Antidepressant-associated mood elevations in bipolar II disorder compared with bipolar I disorder and major depressive disorder: a systematic review and meta-analysis. *Journal of Clinical Psychiatry.* 2008;69:1589–1601.

23. Parker G. Clinical models for managing bipolar II disorder: Model I. In: Parker G, ed. *Bipolar II Disorder.* 2nd ed. New York: Cambridge University Press; 2012:182–191.

24. GlaxoSmithKline. A multicenter, double-blind, placebo-controlled, fixed-dose, eight week evaluation of the efficacy and safety of lamotrigine in the treatment of bipolar II depression. Brentwood, UK: Author; 2006.

25. Amsterdam JD, Brunswick DJ. Antidepressant monotherapy for bipolar type II major depression. *Bipolar Disorders.* 2003;5(6):388–395.

26. Himmelhoch JM, Thase ME, Mallinger AG, et al. Tranylcypromine versus imipramine in anergic bipolar depression. *American Journal of Psychiatry.* 1991;148(7):910–916.

27. Gijsman HJ, Geddes JR, Rendell JM, et al. Antidepressants for bipolar depression: a systematic review of randomized, controlled trials. *American Journal of Psychiatry.* 2004;161:1537–1547.

28. Aronson R, Offman HJ, Joffe RT, et al. Triiodothyronine augmentation in the treatment of refractory depression: a meta-analysis. *Archives of General Psychiatry.* 1996;53(9):842–848.

29. Calabrese JR, Ketter TA, Youakim JM, et al. Adjunctive armodafinil for major depressive episodes associated with bipolar I disorder: a randomized, multicenter, double-blind, placebo-controlled, proof-of-concept study. *Journal of Clinical Psychiatry.* 2010;71:1363–1370.

30. Frye MA, Grunze H, Suppes T, et al. A placebo-controlled evaluation of adjunctive modafinil in the treatment of bipolar depression. *American Journal of Psychiatry.* 2007;164(8):1242–1249.

31. Dell'Osso B, Ketter TA. Use of adjunctive stimulants in adult bipolar depression. *International Journal of Neuropsychopharmacology.* 2013;16(1):55–68.

32. Daly JJ, Prudic J, Devanand DP, et al. ECT in bipolar and unipolar depression: differences in speed of response. *Bipolar Disorders.* 2001;3(2):95–104.

33. Sarris J, Mischoulon D, Schweitzer I. Omega-3 for bipolar disorder: meta-analyses of use in mania and bipolar depression. *Journal of Clinical Psychiatry.* 2012;73(1):81–86.

34. Goldberg JF, Burdick KE, Endick CJ. Preliminary randomized, double-blind, placebo-controlled trial of pramipexole added to mood stabilizers for treatment-resistant bipolar depression. *American Journal of Psychiatry.* 2004;161(3):564–566.

35. Zarate CA Jr, Payne JL, Singh J, et al. Pramipexole for bipolar II depression: a placebo-controlled proof of concept study. *Biological Psychiatry.* 2004;56(1):54–60.

36. Katalanic N, Lai R, Somogyi A, et al. Ketamine as new treatment for depression: a review of its efficacy and adverse effects. *Australian and New Zealand Journal of Psychiatry.* 2013;(8):710–727.

## CHAPTER 6

1. Goodwin GM, Malhi GS. What is a mood stabilizer? *Psychological Medicine.* 2007;37(5):609–614.
2. Gitlin M, Frye MA. Maintenance therapies in bipolar disorders. *Bipolar Disorders.* 2012;14(suppl 2):51–65.
3. Gitlin MJ, Swendsen J, Heller TL, et al. Relapse and impairment in bipolar disorder. *American Journal of Psychiatry.* 1995;152:1635–1640.
4. Keller MB, Lavori PW, Coryell W, et al. Bipolar I: a five-year prospective follow-up. *Journal of Nervous and Mental Disease.* 1993;181:238–245.
5. Perlis RH, Ostacher MJ, Patel J, et al. Predictors of recurrence in bipolar disorder: primary outcomes from the Systematic Treatment Enhancement Program for Bipolar Disorder (STEP-BD). *American Journal of Psychiatry.* 2006;163(2):217–224.
6. Gitlin MJ, Mintz J, Sokolski K, et al. Subsyndromal depressive symptoms after symptomatic recovery from mania are associated with delayed functional recovery. *Journal of Clinical Psychiatry.* 2011;72(5):692–697.
7. Popovic D, Reinares M, Goikolea JM, et al. Polarity index of pharmacological agents used for maintenance treatment of bipolar disorder. *European Neuropsychopharmacology.* 2012;22(5):339–346.
8. Malhi GS, Adams D, Berk M. Is lithium in a class of its own?: a brief profile of its clinical use. *Australian and New Zealand Journal of Psychiatry.* 2009;43:1096–1104.
9. Geddes JR, Burgess S, Hawton K, et al. Long-term lithium therapy for bipolar disorder: systematic review and meta-analysis of randomized controlled trials. *American Journal of Psychiatry.* 2004;161(2):217–222.
10. Kleindienst N, Engel RR, Greil W. Which clinical factors predict response to prophylactic lithium?: a systematic review for bipolar disorders. *Bipolar Disorders.* 2005;7:404–417.
11. Gelenberg AJ, Kane JN, Keller MB, et al. Comparison of standard and low serum levels of lithium for maintenance treatment of bipolar disorders. *New England Journal of Medicine.* 1989;321:1489–1493.
12. Gitlin MJ, Cochran SD, Jamison KR. Maintenance lithium treatment: side effects and compliance. *Journal of Clinical Psychiatry.* 1989;50(4):127–131.
13. Shaw ED, Mann JJ, Stokes PE, et al. Effects of lithium carbonate on associational productivity and idiosyncrasy in bipolar outpatients. *American Journal of Psychiatry.* 1986;143:1166–1169.
14. Vestergaard P, Amdisen A, Schou M. Clinically significant side effects of lithium treatment: a survey of 237 patients in long-term treatment. *Acta Psychiatrica Scandinavica Supplementum.* 1980;62:193–200.
15. Antel J, Hebebrand J. Weight-reducing side effects of the antiepileptic agents topiramate and zonisamide. *Handbook of Experimental Pharmacology.* 2012;209:433–466.
16. Kleiner J, Altshuler L, Hendrick V, et al. Lithium-induced subclinical hypothyroidism: review of the literature and guidelines for treatment. *Journal of Clinical Psychiatry.* 1999;60:249–255.
17. Gitlin M. Lithium and the kidney. *Drug Safety.* 1999;20(3):231–243.

18. Jefferson JW. Lithium: a therapeutic magic wand. *Journal of Clinical Psychiatry.* 1989;50:81–86.
19. Bendz H, Schön S, Attman PO, et al. Renal failure occurs in chronic lithium treatment but is uncommon. *Kidney International.* 2010;77:219–224.
20. Singh LK, Nizamie SH, Akhtar S, et al. Improving tolerability of lithium with a once-daily dosing schedule. *American Journal of Therapeutics.* 2011;18(4):288–291.
21. Hansen HE, Amdisen A. Lithium intoxication (report of 23 cases and review of 100 cases from the literature). *Quarterly Journal of Medicine.* 1978;47(186):123–144.
22. Goodwin GM, Bowden CL, Calabrese JR, et al. A pooled analysis of 2 placebo-controlled 18-month trials of lamotrigine and lithium maintenance in bipolar I disorder. *Journal of Clinical Psychiatry.* 2004;65(3):432–441.
23. Calabrese JR, Suppes T, Bowden CL, et al. A double-blind, placebo-controlled, prophylaxis study of lamotrigine in rapid-cycling bipolar disorder. Lamictal 614 Study Group. *Journal of Clinical Psychiatry.* 2000;61:841–850.
24. Bowden CL, Calabrese JR, McElroy SL, et al. A randomized, placebo-controlled 12-month trial of divalproex and lithium in treatment of outpatients with bipolar I disorder. Divalproex Maintenance Study Group. *Archives of General Psychiatry.* 2000;57:481–489.
25. Geddes JR, Goodwin GM, Rendell J, et al. Lithum plus valproate combination therapy versus montherapy for relapse prevention in bipolar I disorder (BALANCE): a randomised open-label trial. *Lancet.* 2010;375(9712):385–395.
26. Dreifuss FE, Langer DH. Side effects of valproate. *American Journal of Medicine.* 1988;84:34–41.
27. Joffe H, Cohen LS, Suppes T, et al. Valproate is associated with new-onset oligoamenorrhea with hyperandrogenism in women with bipolar disorder. *Biological Psychiatry.* 2006;59(11):1078–1086.
28. Correll CU, Leucht S, Kane JM. Lower risk for tardive dyskinesia associated with second-generation antipsychotics: a systematic review of 1-year studies. *American Journal of Psychiatry.* 2004;161:414–425.
29. Tohen M, Calabrese JR, Sachs GS, et al. Randomized, placebo-controlled trial of olanzapine as maintenance therapy in patients with bipolar I disorder responding to acute treatment with olanzapine. *American Journal of Psychiatry.* 2006;163:247–256.
30. Tohen M, Greil W, Calabrese JR, et al. Olanzapine versus lithium in the maintenance treatment of bipolar disorder: a 12-month, randomized, double-blind, controlled clinical trial. *American Journal of Psychiatry.* 2005;162:1281–1290.
31. American Diabetes Association, American Psychiatric Association, American Association of Clinical Endocrinologists, et al. Consensus development conference on antipsychotic drugs and obesity and diabetes. *Diabetes Care.* 2004;27(2):596–601.
32. Keck P, Calabrese JR, McQuade RD, et al. A randomized, double-blind, placebo-controlled 26-week trial of aripiprazole in recently manic patients with bipolar I disorder. *Journal of Clinical Psychiatry.* 2006;64:626–637.

33. Marcus R, Khan A, Rollin L, et al. Efficacy of aripiprazole adjunctive to lithium or valproate in the long-term treatment of patients with bipolar I disorder with an inadequate response to lithium or valproate monotherapy: a multicenter, double-blind, randomized study. *Bipolar Disorders.* 2011;13:133–144.

34. Weisler RH, Nolen WA, Neijber A, et al. Continuation of quetiapine versus switching to placebo or lithium for maintenance treatment of bipolar I disorder (Trial 144: a randomized controlled study). *Journal of Clinical Psychiatry.* 2011;72(11):1452–1464.

35. Vieta E, Suppes T, Eggens I, et al. Efficacy and safety of quetiapine in combination with lithium or divalproex for maintenance of patients with bipolar I disorder [International trial 126]. *Journal of Affective Disorders.* 2008;109:251–263.

36. Suppes T, Vieta E, Liu S, et al. Maintenance treatment for patients with bipolar I disorder: results from a North American study of quetiapine in combination with lithium or divalproex. *American Journal of Psychiatry.* 2009;166:476–488.

37. Brecher M, Leong RW, Stening G, et al. Quetiapine and long-term weight change: a comprehensive data review of patients with schizophrenia. *Journal of Clinical Psychiatry.* 2007;68:597–603.

38. Bowden CL, Vieta E, Ice KS, et al. Ziprasidone plus a mood stablilizer in subjects with bipolar I disorder: a 6-month, randomized, placebo-controlled, double-blind trial. *Journal of Clinical Psychiatry.* 2010;71:130–137.

39. Camm J, Karayal ON, Meltzer H, et al. Ziprasidone and the corrected QT interval. *CNS Drugs.* 2012;26(4):351–365.

40. Macfadden W, Alphs L, Haskins JT, et al. A randomized, double-blind, placebo-controlled study of maintenance treatment with adjunctive risperidone long-acting therapy in patients with bipolar I disorder who relapse frequently. *Bipolar Disorders.* 2009;11:827–839.

41. Quiroz JA, Yatham LN, Palumbo JM, et al. Risperidone long-acting injectable monotherapy in the maintenance treatment of bipolar I disorder. *Biological Psychiatry.* 2010;68:156–162.

42. Greil W, Ludwig-Mayerhofer W, Erazo N, et al. Lithium versus carbamazepine in the maintenance treatment of bipolar disorders—a randomized study. *Journal of Affective Disorders.* 1997;43:151–161.

43. Hartong EG, Moleman P, Hoogduin CA, et al. Prophylactic efficacy of lithium versus carbamazepine in treatment-naive bipolar patients. *Journal of Clinical Psychiatry.* 2003;64:144–151.

44. Kleindienst N, Greil W. Differential efficacy of lithium and carbamazepine in the prophylaxis of bipolar disorder: results of the MAP study [Supplement 1]. *Neuropsychobiology.* 2000;42:2–10.

45. Vieta E, Cruz N, Garcia-Campayo J, et al. A double-blind, randomized, placebo-controlled prophylaxis trial of oxcarbazepine as adjunctive treatment to lithium in the long-term treatment of bipolar I and II disorder. *International Journal of Neuropsychopharmacology.* 2008;11:445–452.

46. Ketter TA, Post RM, Worthington K. Principles of clinically important drug interactions with carbamazepine. Part I. *Journal of Clinical Psychopharmacology.* 1991;11(3):198–203.

47. Ketter TA, Post RM, Worthington K. Principles of clinically important drug interactions with carbamazepine: Part II. *Journal of Clinical Psychopharmacology.* 1991;11(5):306–313.

48. Mazza M, Di Nicola M, Martinotti G, et al. Oxcarbazepine in bipolar disorder: a critical review of the literature. *Expert Opinion on Pharmacotherapy.* 2007;8:649–656.

49. Altshuler L, Kiriakos L, Calcagno J, et al. The impact of antidepressant discontinuation versus antidepressant continuation on 1-year risk for relapse of bipolar depression: a retrospective chart review. *Journal of Clinical Psychiatry.* 2001;62(8):612–616.

50. Altshuler L, Suppes T, Black D, et al. Impact of antidepressant discontinuation after acute bipolar depression remission on rates of depressive relapse at 1-year follow-up. *American Journal of Psychiatry.* 2003;160:1252–1262.

51. Amsterdam JD, Shults J. Efficacy and safety of long-term fluoxetine versus lithium monotherapy of bipolar II disorder: a randomized, double-blind, placebo-substitution study. *American Journal of Psychiatry.* 2010;167(7):792–800.

52. Post RM, Altshuler LL, Frye MA, et al. Complexity of pharmacologic treatment required for sustained improvement in outpatients with bipolar disorder. *Journal of Clinical Psychiatry.* 2010;71:1176–1186.

53. Goldberg JF, Brooks JO, Kurita K, et al. Depressive illness burden associated with complex polypharmacy in patients with bipolar disorder: findings from the STEP-BD. *Journal of Clinical Psychiatry.* 2009;70(2):155–162.

54. Denicoff KD, Smith-Jackson EE, Disney ER, et al. Comparative prophylactic efficacy of lithium, carbamazepine, and the combination in bipolar disorder. *Journal of Clinical Psychiatry.* 1997;58:470–478.

55. Suppes T, Webb A, Paul B, et al. Clinical outcome in a randomized 1-year trial of clozapine versus treatment as usual for patients with treatment-resistant illness and a history of mania. *American Journal of Psychiatry.* 1999;156:1164–1169.

56. Nielsen J, Kane JM, Correll CU. Real-world effectiveness of clozapine in patients with bipolar disorder: results from a 2-year mirror-image study. *Bipolar Disorders.* 2012;14:863–869.

57. Schulte PFJ. What is an adequate trial with clozapine? *Clinical Pharmacokinetics.* 2003;42(7):607–618.

58. Lahdelma L, Appelberg B. Clozapine-induced agranulocytosis in Finland, 1982–2007: long-term monitoring of patients is still warranted. *Journal of Clinical Psychiatry.* 2012;73(6):837–842.

59. Nielsen J, Correll CU, Manu P, et al. Termination of clozapine treatment due to medical reasons: when is it warranted and how can it be avoided. *Journal of Clinical Psychiatry.* 2013;64(6):603–613.

60. Bauer MS, Whybrow PC. Rapid cycling bipolar affective disorder II: treatment of refractory rapid cycling with high-dose levothyroxine: a preliminary study. *Archives of General Psychiatry.* 1990;47:435–440.

61. Bauer M, Berghöfer A, Bschor T, et al. Supraphysiological doses of L-thyroxine in the maintenance treatment of prophylaxis-resistant affective disorders. *Neuropsychopharmacology.* 2002;27:620–628.

62. Levy NA, Janicak PG. Calcium channel antagonists for the treatment of bipolar disorder. *Bipolar Disorders.* 2000;2(2):108–119.
63. Keck PE Jr, Mintz J, McElroy SL, et al. Double-blind, randomized, placebo-controlled trials of ethyl-eicosapentanoate in the treatment of bipolar depression and rapid cycling bipolar disorder. *Biological Psychiatry.* 2006;60(9):1020–1022.
64. Vaidya NA, Mahableshwarkar AR, Shahid R. Continuation and maintenance ECT in treatment-resistant bipolar disorder. *Journal of ECT.* 2003;19(1):10–16.

## CHAPTER 7

1. Goodwin FK, Jamison KR. *Manic–Depressive Illness.* 2nd ed. New York: Oxford University Press; 2007.
2. Miklowitz DJ, Otto MW, Frank E, et al. Psychosocial treatments for bipolar depression: a 1-year randomized trial from the Systematic Treatment Enhancement Program. *Archives of General Psychiatry.* 2007;64:419–427.
3. Sachs GS, Nierenberg AA, Calabrese JR, et al. Effectiveness of adjunctive antidepressant treatment for bipolar depression. *New England Journal of Medicine.* 2007;356(17):1711–1722.
4. Geddes JR, Miklowitz DJ. Treatment of bipolar disorder. *Lancet.* 2013;381(9878):1672–1682.
5. Miklowitz DJ, Scott J. Psychosocial treatments for bipolar disorder: Cost-effectiveness, mediating mechanisms, and future directions. *Bipolar Disorders.* 2009;11:110–122.
6. Kaplan KA, Harvey AG. Behavioral treatment of insomnia in bipolar disorder. *American Journal of Psychiatry.* 2013;170(7):716–720.
7. Frank E. *Treating Bipolar Disorder: A Clinician's Guide to Interpersonal and Social Rhythm Therapy.* New York: Guilford Press; 2005.
8. Frank E, Soreca I, Swartz HA, et al. The role of interpersonal and social rhythm therapy in improving occupational functioning in patients with bipolar I disorder. *American Journal of Psychiatry.* 2008;165(12):1559–1565.
9. Monk TH, Flaherty JF, Frank E, et al. The social rhythm metric: an instrument to quantify daily rhythms of life. *Journal of Nervous and Mental Disease.* 1990;178:120–126.
10. Dimidjian S, Hollon SD, Dobson KS, et al. Randomized trial of behavioral activation, cognitive therapy, and antidepressant medication in the acute treatment of adults with major depression. *Journal of Consulting and Clinical Psychology.* 2006;74(4):658–670.
11. Simoneau TL, Miklowitz DJ, Richards JA, et al. Bipolar disorder and family communication: effects of a psychoeducational treatment program. *Journal of Abnormal Psychology.* 1999;108:588–597.
12. Simon GE, Ludman EJ, Bauer MS, et al. Long-term effectiveness and cost of a systematic care program for bipolar disorder. *Archives of General Psychiatry.* 2006;63(5):500–508.
13. Bauer MS, McBride L, Williford WO, et al. Collaborative care for bipolar

disorder: Part II. Impact on clinical outcome, function, and costs. *Psychiatric Services.* 2006;57:937–945.

14. Colom F, Vieta E, Martinez-Aran A, et al. A randomized trial on the efficacy of group psychoeducation in the prophylaxis of bipolar disorder: a five year follow-up. *British Journal of Psychiatry.* 2009;194(3):260–265.

15. Scott J, Colom F, Popova E, et al. Long-term mental health resource utilization and cost of care following group psychoeducation or unstructured group support for bipolar disorders: a cost–benefit analysis. *Journal of Clinical Psychiatry.* 2009;70(3):378–386.

## CHAPTER 8

1. Foster A, Sheehan L, Johns L. Promoting treatment adherence in patients with bipolar disorder. *Current Psychiatry.* 2011;10(7):45–53.

2. Tondo L, Baldessarini RJ. Reducing suicide risk during lithium maintenance treatment. *Journal of Clinical Psychiatry.* 2000;61(suppl 9):97–104.

3. Suppes T, Dennehy EB, Gibbons EW. The longitudinal course of bipolar disorder. *Journal of Clinical Psychiatry.* 2000;61:23–30.

4. Cade JF. Lithium salts in the treatment of psychotic excitement. *Medical Journal of Australia.* 1949;36:349–352.

5. Colom F, Vieta E, Martinez-Aran A, et al. Clinical factors associated with treatment noncompliance in euthymic bipolar patients. *Journal of Clinical Psychiatry.* 2000;61:549–555.

6. Strakowski SM, Keck PE, McElroy SL, et al. Twelve-month outcome after a first hospitalization for affective psychosis. *Archives of General Psychiatry.* 1998;55:49–55.

7. Weiss RD, Greenfield SF, Najavits LM, et al. Medication compliance among patients with bipolar disorder and substance use disorder. *Journal of Clinical Psychiatry.* 1998;59:172–174.

8. Perlis RH, Ostacher MJ, Miklowitz DJ, et al. Clinical features associated with poor pharmacologic adherence in bipolar disorder: results from the STEP-BD study. *Journal of Clinical Psychiatry.* 2010;71(3):296–303.

9. Millett K. *The Loony-Bin Trip.* New York: Simon & Schuster; 1990.

10. Miklowitz DJ, Goldstein MJ, Nuechterlein KH, et al. Family factors and the course of bipolar affective disorder. *Archives of General Psychiatry.* 1988;45:225–231.

11. Thompson K, Kulkarni J, Sergejew AA. Reliability and validity of a new Medication Adherence Rating Scale (MARS) for the psychoses. *Schizophrenia Research.* 2000;42(3):241–247.

12. Byerly MJ, Nakonezny PA, Rush AJ. The Brief Adherence Rating Scale (BARS) validated against electronic monitoring in assessing the antipsychotic medication adherence of outpatients with schizophrenia and schizoaffective disorder. *Schizophrenia Research.* 2008;100(1–3):60–69.

13. Tondo L, Baldessarini RJ, Floris G. Long-term clinical effectiveness of lithium maintenance treatment in types I and II bipolar disorders. *British Journal of Psychiatry.* 2001;41(suppl):s184–s190.

14. Baldessarini RJ, Tondo L, Hennen J. Effects of lithium treatment and its

discontinuation on suicidal behavior in bipolar manic–depressive disorders. *Journal of Clinical Psychiatry.* 1999;60(suppl 2):77–84.

15. Bartzokis G, Lu PH, Amar CP, et al. Long acting injection versus oral risperidone in first-episode schizophrenia: differential impact on white matter myelination trajectory. *Schizophrenia Research.* 2011;132(1):35–41.

16. Miklowitz DJ. *Bipolar Disorder: A Family-Focused Treatment Approach.* 2nd ed. New York: Guilford Press; 2008.

17. Koukopoulos A, Reginaldi D, Tondo L, et al. Course sequences in bipolar disorder: Depressions preceding or following manias or hypomanias. *Journal of Affective Disorders.* 2013;151(1):105–110.

18. Miklowitz DJ. *The Bipolar Disorder Survival Guide: What You and Your Family Need to Know.* 2nd ed. New York: Guilford Press; 2011.

19. Jamison KR. *Touched with Fire: Manic–Depressive Illness and the Artistic Temperament.* New York: Maxwell Macmillan; 1993.

20. Johnson SL, Murray G, Fredrickson B, et al. Creativity and bipolar disorder: touched by fire or burning with questions? *Clinical Psychology Review.* 2012;32(1):1–12.

21. Thase ME. Pharmacotherapy for adults with bipolar depression. In: Miklowitz DJ, Cicchetti D, eds. *Understanding Bipolar Disorder: A Developmental Psychopathology Perspective.* New York: Guilford Press; 2010:445–465.

22. Frank E. *Treating Bipolar Disorder: A Clinician's Guide to Interpersonal and Social Rhythm Therapy.* New York: Guilford Press; 2005.

23. Miller WR, Rollnick S. *Motivational Interviewing: Preparing People for Change.* 2nd ed. New York: Guilford Press; 2002.

## CHAPTER 9

1. Di Florio A, Jones I. Is sex important? Gender differences in bipolar disorder. *International Review of Psychiatry.* 2010;22(5):437–452.

2. Schneck CD, Miklowitz DJ, Calabrese JR, et al. Phenomenology of rapid cycling bipolar disorder: data from the first 500 participants in the Systematic Treatment Enhancement Program for Bipolar Disorder. *American Journal of Psychiatry.* 2004;161:1902–1908.

3. Kenna HA, Jiang B, Rasgon NL. Reproductive and metabolic abnormalities associated with bipolar disorder and its treatment. *Harvard Review of Psychiatry.* 2009;17:138–146.

4. Cohen LS, Altshuler LL, Harlow BL, et al. Relapse of major depression during pregnancy in women who maintain or discontinue antidepressant treatment. *Journal of the American Medical Association.* 2006;295(5):499–507.

5. Viguera AC, Tondo L, Koukopoulos AE, et al. Episodes of mood disorders in 2,252 pregnancies and postpartum periods. *American Journal of Psychiatry.* 2011;168(11):1179–1185.

6. Viguera AC, Whitfield T, Baldessarini RJ, et al. Risk of recurrence in women with bipolar disorder during pregnancy: prospective study of mood stabilizer discontinuation. *American Journal of Psychiatry.* 2007;164(12):1817–1824.

7. Chaudron LH. Complex challenges in treating depression during pregnancy. *American Journal of Psychiatry.* 2013;170(1):12–20.

8. Di Florio AD, Forty L, Gordon-Smith K, et al. Perinatal episodes across the mood disorder spectrum. *Archives of General Psychiatry.* 2013;70(2):168–175.

9. Bergink V, Bouvy PF, Vervoort JSP, et al. Prevention of postpartum psychosis and mania in women at high risk. *American Journal of Psychiatry.* 2012;169:609–615.

10. Viguera AC, Nonacs R, Cohen LS, et al. Risk of recurrence of bipolar disorder in pregnant and nonpregnant women after discontinuing lithium maintenance. *American Journal of Psychiatry.* 2000;157(2):179–184.

11. Steiner M. Postpartum psychiatric disorders. *Canadian Journal of Psychiatry.* 1990;35(1):89–95.

12. Harlow BL, Vitonis AF, Sparen P, et al. Incidence of hospitalization for postpartum psychotic and bipolar episodes in women with and without prior prepregnancy or prenatal psychiatric hospitalizations. *Archives of General Psychiatry.* 2007;64(1):42–48.

13. Munk-Olsen T, Laursen TM, Meltzer-Brody S, et al. Psychiatric disorders with postpartum onset: possible early manifestations of bipolar affective disorders. *Archives of General Psychiatry.* 2012;69(4):428–434.

14. Segal ZV, Williams JMG, Teasdale JD. *Mindfulness-Based Cognitive Therapy for Depression: A New Approach to Preventing Relapse.* New York: Guilford Press; 2002.

15. Teasdale JD, Segal ZV, Williams JM, et al. Prevention of relapse/recurrence in major depression by mindfulness-based cognitive therapy. *Journal of Consulting and Clinical Psychology.* 2000;68(4):615–623.

16. Segal ZV, Bieling P, Young T, et al. Antidepressant monotherapy v. sequential pharmacotherapy and mindfulness-based cognitive therapy, or placebo, for relapse prophylaxis in recurrent depression. *Archives of General Psychiatry.* 2010;67(12):1256–1264.

17. Miklowitz DJ, Alatiq Y, Goodwin GM, et al. A pilot study of mindfulness-based cognitive therapy for bipolar disorder. *International Journal of Cognitive Therapy.* 2009;2(4):373–382.

18. Stewart DE. Depression during pregnancy. *New England Journal of Medicine.* 2011;365:1605–1611.

19. Yonkers KA, Wisner KL, Stowe Z, et al. Management of bipolar disorder during pregnancy and the postpartum period. *American Journal of Psychiatry.* 2004;161(4):608–620.

20. Holmes LB, Harvey EA, Coull BA, et al. The teratogenicity of anticonvulsant drugs. *New England Journal of Medicine.* 2001;344(15):1132–1138.

21. Holmes LB, Baldwin EJ, Smith CR, et al. Increased frequency of isolated cleft palate in infants exposed to lamotrigine during pregnancy. *Neurology.* 2008;70(22, pt 2):2152–2158.

22. Jones KL, Lacro RV, Johnson KA, et al. Pattern of malformations in the children of women treated with carbamazepine during pregnancy. *New England Journal of Medicine.* 1989;320:1661–1666.

23. Habermann D, Fritzsche J, Fuhlbruck F, et al. Atypical antipsychotic drugs and pregnancy outcome: a prospective, cohort study. *Journal of Clinical Psychopharmacology.* 2013; 33:453–462.

24. Einarson A, Boskovic R. Use and safety of antipsychotic drugs during pregnancy. *Journal of Psychiatric Practice.* 2009;15(3):183–192.

25. Newport DJ, Calamaras MR, DeVane CL, et al. Atypical antipsychotic administration during late pregnancy: placental passage and obstetrical outcomes. *American Journal of Psychiatry.* 2007;164:1214–1220.
26. Altshuler LL, Cohen L, Szuba MP, et al. Pharmacologic management of psychiatric illness during pregnancy: dilemmas and guidelines. *American Journal of Psychiatry.* 1996;153(5):592–606.
27. Byatt N, Derligiannidis KM, Freeman MP. Antidepressant use in pregnancy: a critical review focused on risks and controversies. *Acta Psychiatrica Scandinavica.* 2013;127:94–114.
28. Hemels EH, Einarson A, Koren G, et al. Antidepressant use during pregnancy and the rates of sponaneous abortions: a meta-analysis. *Annals of Pharmacotherapy.* 2005;39:803–809.
29. Grote NK, Bridge JA, Melville JL, et al. A meta-analysis of depression during pregnancy and the risk of preterm birth, low birth weight, and intrauterine growth restriction. *Archives of General Psychiatry.* 2010;67(10):1012–1024.
30. Gentile S, Galbally M. Prenatal exposure to antidepressant medications and neurodevelopmental outcomes: a systematic review. *Journal of Affective Disorders.* 2011;128(1–2):1–9.
31. American College of Obstetricians and Gynecologists. Use of psychiatric medications during pregnancy and lactation. *Obstetrics and Gynecology.* 2008;111(4):1011–1020.
32. Bar-Oz B, Einarson T, Einarson A, et al. Paroxetine and congenital malformations: meta-analysis and consideration of potential confounding factors. *Clinical Therapeutics.* 2007;29(5):918–926.
33. Occhiogrosso M, Omran SS, Altemus M. Persistent pulmonary hypertension of the newborn and selective serotonin reuptake inhibitors: lessons from clinical and translational studies. *American Journal of Psychiatry.* 2012;169:134–140.
34. Moses-Kolko EL, Bogen D, Perel J, et al. Neonatal signs after late in utero exposure to serotonin reuptake inhibitors: literature review and implications for clinical applications. *Journal of the American Medical Association.* 2005;293(19):2372–2383.
35. Anderson EL, Reti IM. ECT in pregnancy: a review of the literature from 1941 to 2007. *Psychosomatic Medicine.* 2009;71(2):235–242.
36. Hale TW. *Medications and mothers' milk.* 10th ed. Amarillo, TX: Pharmasoft; 2002.
37. Doucet S, Jones I, Letourneau N, et al. Interventions for the prevention and treatment of postpartum psychosis: a systematic review. *Archives of Women's Mental Health.* 2011;14(2):89–98.
38. American Academy of Pediatrics Committee on Drugs. The transfer of drugs and other chemicals into human milk. *Pediatrics.* 2001;108(3):776–789.
39. Gentile S. Infant safety with antipsychotic therapy in breast-feeding: a systematic review. *Journal of Clinical Psychiatry.* 2008;69(4):666–673.
40. Kelly LE, Poon S, Madadi P, et al. Neonatal benzodiazepines exposure during breastfeeding. *Journal of Pediatrics.* 2012;161(3):448–451.
41. Davanzo R, Copertino M, De Cunto A, et al. Antidepressant drugs and breastfeeding: a review of the literature. *Breastfeeding Medicine.* 2011;6(2):89–98.

42. Kim DR, Epperson N, Paré E, et al. An open label pilot study of transcranial magnetic stimulation for pregnant women with major depressive disorder. *Journal of Women's Health.* 2011;20(2):255–261.
43. Miklowitz DJ. *The Bipolar Disorder Survival Guide: What You and Your Family Need to Know.* 2nd ed. New York: Guilford Press; 2011.

## CHAPTER 10

1. Allen MH, Chessick CA, Miklowitz DJ, et al. Contributors to suicidal ideation among bipolar patients with and without a history of suicide attempts. *Suicide and Life-Threatening Behavior.* 2005;35(6):671–680.
2. World Health Organization. World report on violence and health. 2002; *http://whqlibdoc.who.int/publications/2002/9241545615_eng.pdf.*
3. Hawton K, van Heeringen K. Suicide. *Lancet.* 2009;373(9672):1372–1381.
4. Goodwin FK, Jamison KR. *Manic–Depressive Illness.* 2nd ed. New York: Oxford University Press; 2007.
5. Roy A. Genetic and biologic risk factors for suicide in depressive disorders. *Psychiatric Quarterly.* 1993;64(4):345–358.
6. Brent DA, Mann JJ. Family genetic studies, suicide, and suicidal behavior. *American Journal of Medical Genetics C: Seminars in Medical Genetics.* 2005;133(1):13–24.
7. Cavanagh JT, Carson AJ, Sharpe M, et al. Psychological autopsy studies of suicide: a systematic review. *Psychological Medicine.* 2003;33(3):395–405.
8. Yang GH, Phillips MR, Zhou MG, et al. Understanding the unique characteristics of suicide in China: national psychological autopsy study. *Biomedical and Environmental Sciences.* 2005;18:379–389.
9. McGirr A, Alda M, Séguin M, et al. Familial aggregation of suicide explained by cluster B traits: A three-group family study of suicide controlling for major depressive disorder. *American Journal of Psychiatry.* 2009;166:1124–1134.
10. Gunnell D, Hawton K, Ho D, et al. Hospital admissions for self harm after discharge from psychiatric inpatient care: cohort study. *British Medical Journal.* 2008;337:a2278. [Published online]
11. Jamison KR. Suicide and bipolar disorder. *Journal of Clinical Psychiatry.* 2000;61(suppl 9):47–56.
12. Nock MK, Borges G, Bromet EJ, et al. Suicide and suicidal behavior. *Epidemiological Reviews.* 2008;30:133–154.
13. Wilcox HC, Kuramoto SJ, Brent D, et al. The interaction of parental history of suicidal behavior and exposure to adoptive parents' psychiatric disorders on adoptee suicide attempt hospitalizations. *American Journal of Psychiatry.* 2012;169:309–315.
14. Bridge JA, Goldstein TR, Brent DA. Adolescent suicide and suicidal behavior. *Journal of Child Psychology and Psychiatry.* 2006;47(3/4):372–394.
15. Palmer BA, Pankratz VS, Bostwick JM. The lifetime risk of suicide in schizophrenia: a reexamination. *Archives of General Psychiatry.* 2005;62(3):247–253.
16. Bostwick JM, Pankratz VS. Affective disorders and suicide risk: a reexamination. *American Journal of Psychiatry.* 2000;157(12):1925–1932.
17. Angst J, Angst F, Gerber-Werder R, et al. Suicide in 406 mood-disordered

patients with and without long-term medication: a 40 to 44 years' follow-up. *Archives of Suicide Research.* 2005;9(3):279–300.

18. Novick DM, Swartz HA, Frank E. Suicide attempts in bipolar I and bipolar II disorder: a review and meta-analysis of the evidence. *Bipolar Disorders.* 2010;12(1):1–9.

19. Ösby U, Brandt L, Correia N, et al. Excess mortality in bipolar and unipolar disorder in Sweden. *Archives of General Psychiatry.* 2001;58(9):844–850.

20. Isometsa ET, Henriksson MM, Hillevi MA, et al. Suicide in bipolar disorder in Finland. *American Journal of Psychiatry.* 1994;151:1020–1024.

21. Pokorny AD. Prediction of suicide in psychiatric patients: report of a prospective study. *Archives of General Psychiatry.* 1983;40(3):249–257.

22. Beck AT, Steer RA, Beck JS, et al. Hopelessness, depression, suicidal ideation, and clinical diagnosis of depression. *Suicide and Life-Threatening Behavior.* 1993;23(2):139–145.

23. Reynolds WM. *Suicidal Ideation Questionnaire: Professional Manual.* Odessa, FL: Psychological Assessment Resources; 1998.

24. Linehan MM. *Cognitive-Behavioral Treatment of Borderline Personality Disorder.* New York: Guilford Press; 1993.

25. Linehan MM, Comtois KA, Ward-Ciesielski EF. Assessing and managing risk with suicidal individuals. *Cognitive and Behavioral Practice.* 2012;19:218–232.

26. Xiong GL, Barnhorst A, Hilty D. Inpatient psychiatric treatment. In: Simon RI, Hales RE, eds. *The American Psychiatric Publishing Textbook of Suicide Assessment and Management.* Arlington, VA: American Psychiatric Publishing; 2012:315–330.

27. Baldessarini RJ, Tondo L, Davis P, et al. Decreased risk of suicides and attempts during long-term lithium treatment: a meta-analytic review. *Bipolar Disorders.* 2006;8(5 pt 2):625–639.

28. Cipriani A, Pretty H, Hawton K, et al. Lithium in the prevention of suicidal behavior and all-cause mortality in patients with mood disorders: a systematic review of randomized trials. *American Journal of Psychiatry.* 2005;162:1805–1819.

29. Cipriani A, Hawton K, Stockton S, et al. Lithium in the prevention of suicide in mood disorders: updated systematic review and meta-analysis. *British Medical Journal.* 2013 Jun 27;346:f3646.[Published online]

30. Lauterbach E, Felber W, Müller-Oerlinghausen B, et al. Adjunctive lithium treatment in the prevention of suicidal behaviour in depressive disorders: a randomised, placebo-controlled, 1-year trial. *Acta Psychiatrica Scandinavica.* 2008;118:469–479.

31. Müller-Oerlinghausen B, Lewitzka U. Lithium reduces pathological aggression and suicidality: a mini-review. *Neuropsychobiology.* 2010;62:43–49.

32. Goodwin FK, Fireman B, Simon GE, et al. Suicide risk in bipolar disorder during treatment with lithium and divalproex. *Journal of the American Medical Association.* 2003;290:1467–1473.

33. Oquendo MA, Galfalvy HC, Currier D, et al. Treatment of suicide attempters with bipolar disorder: A randomized clinical trial comparing lithium and valproate in the prevention of suicidal behavior. *American Journal of Psychiatry.* 2011;168:1050–1056.

34. Fountoulakis KN, Gonda X, Samara M, et al. Antiepileptic drugs and suicidality. *Journal of Psychopharmacology.* 2012;26(11):1401–1407.

35. Meltzer HY, Alphs L, Green AI, et al. Clozapine treatment for suicidality in schizophrenia: International Suicide Prevention Trial (InterSePT). *Archives of General Psychiatry.* 2003;60(1):82–91.

36. Nielsen J, Kane JM, Correll CU. Real-world effectiveness of clozapine in patients with bipolar disorder: results from a 2-year mirror-image study. *Bipolar Disorders.* 2012;14:863–869.

37. Angst F, Stassen HH, Clayton PJ, et al. Mortality of patients with mood disorders: follow-up over 34–38 years. *Journal of Affective Disorders.* 2002;68:167–181.

38. Teicher MH, Glod C, Cole JO. Emergence of intense suicidal preoccupation during fluoxetine treatment. *American Journal of Psychiatry.* 1990;147:207–210.

39. Hammad TA, Laughren T, Racoosin J. Suicidality in pediatric patients treated with antidepressant drugs. *Archives of General Psychiatry.* 2006;63(3):332–339.

40. Leon AC. The revised warning for antidepressants and suicidality: unveiling the black box of statistical analyses. *American Journal of Psychiatry.* 2007;164:1786–1789.

41. Mann JJ, Kapur S. The emergence of suicidal ideation and behavior during antidepressant pharmacotherapy. *Archives of General Psychiatry.* 1991;48(11):1027–1033.

42. Martin A, Young C, Leckman JF, et al. Age effects on antidepressant-induced manic conversion. *Archives of Pediatrics and Adolescent Medicine.* 2004;158(8):773–780.

43. Gray D, Achilles J, Keller T, et al. Utah youth suicide study, phase I: government agency contact before death. *Journal of the American Academy of Child and Adolescent Psychiatry.* 2002;41(4):427–434.

44. Isacsson G, Holmgren P, Ahlner J. Selective serotonin reuptake inhibitor antidepressants and the risk of suicide: a controlled forensic database study of 14,857 suicides. *Acta Psychiatrica Scandinavica.* 2005;111(4):286–290.

45. Leon AC, Marzuk PM, Tardiff K, et al. Paroxetine, other antidepressants, and youth suicide in New York City: 1993–1998. *Journal of Clinical Psychiatry.* 2004;65:915–918.

46. Søndergård L, Kvist K, Andersen PK, et al. Do antidepressants precipitate youth suicide?: A nationwide pharmacoepidemiological study. *European Child and Adolescent Psychiatry.* 2006;15(4):232–240.

47. Edwards SJ, Sachmann MD. No-suicide contracts, no-suicide agreements, and no-suicide assurances: a study of their nature, utilization, perceived effectiveness, and potential to cause harm. *Crisis.* 2010;31(6):290–302.

48. McMyler C, Pryjmachuk S. Do "no-suicide" contracts work? *Journal of Psychiatric and Mental Health Nursing.* 2008;15(6):512–522.

49. Linehan MM. The reasons for living inventory. In: Keller PA, Ri LG, eds. *Innovations in Clinical Practice: A Source Book.* Miami, FL: Professional Resource Exchange; 1985:321–330.

50. Linehan MM, Goodstein JL, Nielsen SL, et al. Reasons for staying alive when you are thinking of killing yourself: The Reasons for Living Inventory. *Journal of Consulting and Clinical Psychology.* 1983;51:276–286.

51. Mann JJ, Oquendo M, Underwood MD, et al. The neurobiology of suicide risk: a review for the clinician. *Journal of Clinical Psychiatry.* 1999;60(suppl 2):7–11.

## CHAPTER 11

1. Merikangas KR, Jin R, He JP, et al. Prevalence and correlates of bipolar spectrum disorder in the world mental health survey initiative. *Archives of General Psychiatry.* 2011;68(3):241–251.
2. Faraone SV, Biederman J, Wozniak J. Examining the comorbidity between attention deficit hyperactivity disorder and bipolar I disorder: a meta-analysis of family genetic studies. *American Journal of Psychiatry.* 2012;169(12):1256–1266.
3. Kowatch RA, Fristad M, Birmaher B, et al. Treatment guidelines for children and adolescents with bipolar disorder. *Journal of the American Academy of Child and Adolescent Psychiatry.* 2005;44(3):213–235.
4. Nierenberg AA, Miyahara S, Spencer T, et al. Clinical and diagnostic implications of lifetime attention-deficit/hyperactivity disorder comorbidity in adults with bipolar disorder: data from the first 1000 STEP-BD participants. *Biological Psychiatry.* 2005;57(11):1467–1473.
5. Bond DJ, Hadjipavlou G, Lam RW, et al. The Canadian Network for Mood and Anxiety Treatments (CANMAT) task force recommendations for the management of patients with mood disorders and comorbid attention-deficit/hyperactivity disorder. *Annals of Clinical Psychiatry.* 2012;24(1):23–37.
6. Scheffer RE, Kowatch RA, Carmody T, et al. Randomized, placebo-controlled trial of mixed amphetamine salts for symptoms of comorbid ADHD in pediatric bipolar disorder after mood stabilization with divalproex sodium. *American Journal of Psychiatry.* 2005;162(1):58–64.
7. Pettinati HM, O'Brien CP, Dundon WD. Current status of co-occurring mood and substance use disorders: a new therapeutic target. *American Journal of Psychiatry.* 2013;170:23–30.
8. Frye MA, Altshuler LL, McElroy SL, et al. Gender differences in prevalence, risk, and clinical correlates of alcoholism comorbidity in bipolar disorder. *American Journal of Psychiatry.* 2003;160:883–889.
9. Farren CK, Hill KP, Weiss RD. Bipolar disorder and alcohol use disorder: a review. *Current Psychiatry Reports.* 2012;14(6):659–666.
10. Strakowski SM, DelBello MP, Fleck DE, et al. The impact of substance abuse on the course of bipolar disorder. *Biological Psychiatry.* 2000;48:477–485.
11. Weiss RD, Mirin SM. Subtypes of cocaine abusers. *Psychiatric Clinics of North America.* 1986;9:491–501.
12. Dickerson F, Stallings CR, Origoni AE, et al. Cigarette smoking among persons with schizophrenia or bipolar disorder in routine clinical settings, 1999–2011. *Psychiatric Services.* 2013;64(1):44–50.
13. Baek JH, Eisner LR, Nierenberg AA. Smoking and suicidality in subjects with bipolar disorder: results from the National Epidemiological Survey on Alcohol and Related Conditions (NESARC). *Depression and Anxiety.* 2013;30(10):982–990.

14. George TP, Wu BS, Weinberger AH. A review of smoking cessation in bipolar disorder: implications for future research. *Journal of Dual Diagnosis.* 2012;8(2):126–130.

15. Weiss RD, Griffin ML, Kolodziej ME, et al. A randomized trial of integrated group therapy versus group drug counseling for patients with bipolar disorder and substance dependence. *American Journal of Psychiatry.* 2007;164(1):100–107.

16. Goldstein B, Goldstein TR, Collinger-Larson K, et al. Treatment development and feasibility study of family-focused treatment for adolescents with bipolar disorder and comorbid substance use disorders. *Journal of Psychiatric Practice.* in press.

17. O'Sullivan K, Rynne C, Miller J, et al. A follow-up study on alcoholics with and without co-existing affective disorder. *British Journal of Psychiatry.* 1988;152:813–819.

18. Hester RK, Lenberg KL, Campbell W, et al. Overcoming addictions, a Web-based application, and SMART Recovery, an online and in-person mutual help group for problem drinkers, part 1: three-month outcomes of a randomized controlled trial. *Journal of Medical Internet Resources.* 2013;157(7):e134.

19. Jones SH, Barrowclough C, Allott R, et al. Integrated motivational interviewing and cognitive-behavioural therapy for bipolar disorder with comorbid substance use. *Clinical Psychology and Psychotherapy.* 2011;18(5):426–437.

20. Fan AH, Hassell J. Bipolar disorder and comorbid personality psychopathology: a review of the literature. *Journal of Clinical Psychiatry.* 2008;69:1794–1803.

21. Brieger P, Ehrt U, Marneros A. Frequency of comorbid personality disorders in bipolar and unipolar affective disorders. *Comprehensive Psychiatry.* 2003;44(1):28–34.

22. Goldstein TR, Axelson DA, Birmaher B, et al. Dialectical behavior therapy for adolescents with bipolar disorder: a 1-year open trial. *Journal of the American Academy of Child and Adolescent Psychiatry.* 2007;46(7):820–830.

23. Swartz HA, Pilkonis PA, Frank E, et al. Acute treatment outcomes in patients with bipolar I disorder and co-morbid borderline personality disorder receiving medication and psychotherapy. *Bipolar Disorders.* 2005;7(2):192–197.

24. Bateman A, Fonagy P. *Psychotherapy for Borderline Personality Disorder: Mentalization-Based Treatment.* Oxford, UK: Oxford University Press; 2004.

25. Bateman A, Fonagy P. Mentalization based treatment for borderline personality disorder. *World Psychiatry.* 2010;9:11–15.

26. Rossouw TI, Fonagy P. Mentalization-based treatment for self-harming adolescents: a randomised controlled trial. *Journal of the American Academy of Child and Adolescent Psychiatry.* 2012;51(12):1304–1313.

27. Ingenhoven T, Lafay P, Rinne T, et al. Effectiveness of pharmacotherapy for severe personality disorders: meta-analyses of randomized controlled trials. *Journal of Clinical Psychiatry.* 2010;71(1):14–25.

28. Lieb K, Völlm B, Rücker G, et al. Pharmacotherapy for borderline personality disorder: Cochrane systematic review of randomised trials. *British Journal of Psychiatry.* 2010;196(1):4–12.

29. Colom F, Vieta E, Martinez-Aran A, et al. Clinical factors associated with

treatment noncompliance in euthymic bipolar patients. *Journal of Clinical Psychiatry.* 2000;61:549–555.

30. Sala R, Goldstein BI, Morcillo C, et al. Course of comorbid anxiety disorders among adults with bipolar disorder in the U.S. population. *Journal of Psychiatric Research.* 2012;46(7):865–872.

31. Judd LL, Akiskal HS. The prevalence and disability of bipolar spectrum disorders in the US population: re-analysis of the ECA database taking into account subthreshold cases. *Journal of Affective Disorders.* 2003;73(1–2):123–131.

32. Fagiolini A, Frank E, Rucci P, et al. Mood and anxiety spectrum as a means to identify clinically relevant subtypes of bipolar I disorder. *Bipolar Disorders.* 2007;9(5):462–467.

33. Otto MW, Simon NM, Wisniewski SR, et al. Prospective 12-month course of bipolar disorder in outpatients with and without comorbid anxiety disorders. *British Journal of Psychiatry.* 2006;189:20–25.

34. Craske MG, Barlow DH. Panic disorder and agoraphobia. In: Barlow DH, ed. *Clinical Handbook of Psychological Disorders.* 2nd ed. New York: Guilford Press; 1993:1–47.

35. Segal ZV, Williams JMG, Teasdale JD. *Mindfulness-Based Cognitive Therapy for Depression: A New Approach to Preventing Relapse.* New York: Guilford Press; 2002.

36. Miklowitz DJ, George EL. *The Bipolar Teen: What You Can Do to Help Your Child and Your Family.* New York: Guilford Press; 2008.

37. Williams JMG, Teasdale JD, Segal ZV, et al. *The Mindful Way through Depression: Freeing Yourself from Chronic Unhappiness.* New York: Guilford Press; 2007.

38. Magalhães PV, Kapczinski F, Nierenberg AA, et al. Illness burden and medical comorbidity in the Systematic Treatment Enhancement Program for Bipolar Disorder. *Acta Psychiatrica Scandinavica.* 2012;125(4):303–308.

39. Thompson WK, Kupfer DJ, Fagiolini A, et al. Prevalence and clinical correlates of medical comorbidities in patients with bipolar I disorder: analysis of acute-phase data from a randomized controlled trial. *Journal of Clinical Psychiatry.* 2006;67(5):783–788.

40. Gildengers AG, Whyte EM, Drayer RA, et al. Medical burden in late-life bipolar and major depressive disorders. *American Journal of Geriatric Psychiatry.* 2008;16(3):194–200.

41. Guloksuz S, Cetin EA, Cetin T, et al. Cytokine levels in euthymic bipolar patients. *Journal of Affective Disorders.* 2010;126:458–462.

42. Geddes JR, Miklowitz DJ. Treatment of bipolar disorder. *Lancet.* 2013;381(9878):1672–1682.

43. Gitlin M. *The Psychotherapist's Guide to Psychopharmacology.* 2nd ed. New York: Free Press; 1996.

44. Miklowitz DJ, Price J, Holmes EA, et al. Facilitated integrated mood management (FIMM) for adults with bipolar disorder. *Bipolar Disorders.* 2012;14(2):185–197.

# Index